THE ULTIMATE Calorie, Carb, and Fat Gram COUNTER

2ND EDITION

QUICK, EASY
MEAL PLANNING USING
COUNTS FOR YOUR
FAVORITE FOODS

Lea Ann Holzmeister, RD, CDE

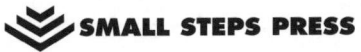 SMALL STEPS PRESS

Director, Book Publishing, Robert Anthony; *Managing Editor,* Abe Ogden; *Acquisitions Editor,* Victor Van Beuren; *Editor,* Rebekah Renshaw; *Production Manager,* Melissa Sprott; *Composition,* ADA; *Cover Design,* pixiedesign, llc; *Printer,* United Graphics, Inc.

Printed in the United States of America
3 5 7 9 10 8 6 4 2

Small Steps Press is an imprint of the American Diabetes Association. For information about Small Steps Press or the American Diabetes Association, in English or Spanish, call 1-800-342-2383. To order other Small Steps Press books, call 1-800-232-6733.

Consult a health care professional before trying any of the suggestions in this publication. Small Steps Press and ADA assume no responsibility or liability for personal or other injury, loss, or damage that may result from the suggestions or information in this publication.

⊚ The paper in this publication meets the requirements of the ANSI Standard Z39.48-1992 (permanence of paper).

Small Steps Press titles may be purchased for business or promotional use or for special sales. To purchase more than 50 copies of this book at a discount, or for custom editions of this book with your logo, contact Small Steps Press at the address below, at booksales@diabetes.org, or by calling 703-299-2046.

Small Steps Press
1701 North Beauregard Street
Alexandria, Virginia 22311

DOI: 10.2337/9781580403412

Library of Congress Cataloging-in-Publication Data

Holzmeister, Lea Ann.
  The ultimate calorie, carb, and fat gram counter / Lea Ann Holzmeister. -- 2nd ed.
      p. cm.
  Includes bibliographical references and index.
  ISBN 978-1-58040-341-2 (alk. paper)
  1. Food--Composition--Tables. I. American Diabetes Association. II. Title.
  TX551.H686 2010
  613.2--dc22

                                        2010032759

Dedication

To my family, my "ultimate" supporters.

Table of Contents

Introduction

Over the past twenty-five years, a disturbing trend has surfaced in our country and around the world—weight gain. As could be expected, as waistlines grow and we as a society eat more and exercise less, a variety of health problems have emerged in near epidemic proportions. Diabetes, cardiovascular disease, hypertension, stroke, cancer; the soaring prevalence of these conditions can be traced back to poor diet and a sedentary lifestyle.

To counteract these disturbing trends, more and more people are turning to meal planning as a way to avoid serious health problems, look better, and feel better. Fortunately, there are a number of options available for those looking to gain better control over their eating and enjoy the benefits weight loss can provide.

Just as there is no one diet that is right for everyone, there is also no one meal planning approach that meets everyone's needs. However, all meal-planning systems require one thing—a thorough knowledge of the nutrients in the foods you eat. To help provide this knowledge, I have created the *Ultimate Calorie, Carb, and Fat Gram Counter.*

If you are at risk for developing any of the so-called lifestyle diseases mentioned above, it is important to know your own nutrition goals. A registered dietitian (RD) can help you determine your individual nutrition goals and develop a meal plan based on your food preferences, lifestyle, overall health, and abilities. If you're not currently seeing a dietitian, your doctor may be able to recommend one. Or visit the American Dietetic Association's web site at www.eatright.org.

Types of Meal-Planning Approaches

Four types of meal planning approaches are described in this book:

+ Carbohydrate counting
+ Fat gram counting
+ Food exchange system
+ Calorie counting

The advantages and disadvantages of each are discussed, and information about where to learn more is provided.

It is important to select a meal planning approach that you are comfortable using and that will work toward achieving your goals. You do not have to use the same approach your entire life. As your individual nutrition goals change, so may your meal planning approach. Before switching though, it is a good idea to consult with a dietitian.

Carbohydrate Counting

Carbohydrate counting has been used for many years in Europe and is popular in the United States, especially for people with diabetes who need to pay attention to their carbohydrate intake to control their blood glucose levels. The three main nutrients in the foods we eat are carbohydrate, protein, and fat. In carbohydrate counting, you count only carbohydrate.

To use carbohydrate counting, you must know your total carbohydrate allotment for the day. A dietitian can help you determine this. Together, you and your dietitian will make a carbohydrate counting meal plan based on your usual food intake, lifestyle, and physical activity. Once you have your carbohydrate counting meal plan, you'll need to become familiar with the carbohydrate content in foods. Carbohydrate is found in many foods, such as grains, vegetables, fruits, milk, and table sugar. It is important to count all carbohydrate regardless of its source.

Carbohydrate counting has its advantages and disadvantages. Some people feel that focusing on only one nutrient makes this system easier. However, when you focus only on carbohydrate, it is easy to lose sight of the overall nutritional quality of foods. For example, counting the carbohydrate in foods like bacon or sausage but ignoring their fat content may lead you to eat these fatty foods more often. Too much fat in the diet increases your risk of heart disease, cancer, and weight gain. If you pay no attention to the overall nutritional quality of foods, you may end up eating a diet that is too high in fat or protein.

To learn more about carbohydrate counting, contact your dietitian. The American Diabetes Association and The American Dietetic Association have jointly published two instructional booklets on carbohydrate counting: *Count Your Carbs* and *Advanced Carbohydrate Counting*. You can obtain these booklets from your dietitian or by ordering them online at http://store.diabetes.org.

Fat Gram Counting
Fat gram counting has been around since the 1980s, when it was introduced as a tool to teach low-fat eating to reduce the risk of cancer. Since that time, it has also been used for heart-healthy eating for heart disease and reduced-calorie eating for weight reduction. Fat provides two and a half times as many calories per gram as carbohydrate or protein.

The first step in using fat gram counting is to establish a daily calorie requirement based on your height, weight, activity level, and weight goal. Your dietitian can help you determine this. Then, based on your nutrition goals, a daily fat gram goal will be determined. In fat gram counting, you keep a record of the foods you eat and their fat content.

There are some advantages to fat gram counting. It is simple, and it allows a considerable amount of flexibility and control over your food choices. With fat gram counting, you will usually improve the overall quality of your food choices, because you will tend to select low-fat foods, such as fruits, vegetables, grains, and low-fat dairy products. Like carbohydrate counting, you are focusing on only one nutrient, so the same advantages and disadvantages apply. There are many high-calorie foods that contain no fat, such as sodas, candies, and fat-free snacks. Even though these foods are fat-free, they can be loaded with calories and can still cause you to gain weight. Also, this approach does not focus on reducing unhealthy sources of fat such as saturated and trans fat.

To learn more about fat gram counting, contact your dietitian. Your local American Heart Association may also have additional information on fat gram counting programs.

Food Exchange System

For many years, the food exchange system has been used as a meal-planning approach for people with diabetes, though it works well for anyone trying to lose weight. This system groups foods with similar nutritional value into lists, with the goal of helping people with diabetes eat consistent amounts of nutrients. Each food has approximately the same number of calories, carbohydrate, protein, and fat as the other foods on the same list. Any food on a list can be traded or "exchanged" for any other food on the same list.

To use the exchange system, you need an individualized meal plan that tells you how many exchanges from each list to select for meals and snacks. A dietitian can help you design your individualized meal plan and teach you how to use this. The American Diabetes Association and The American Dietetic Association's *Choose Your Foods: Exchange Lists for Meal Planning* booklet groups food into three broad groups: the carbohydrate group, the meat and meat substitutes group, and the fat group.

The carbohydrate group includes five lists: the starch list, the fruit list, the milk list, the sweet desserts and other carbohydrates list, and the nonstarchy vegetable list. The meat and meat substitutes group includes four lists: the lean list, the medium-fat list, the high-fat list, and the plant-based proteins. The fat group includes a monounsaturated fats list, a polyunsaturated fats list, and a saturated fats list. In addition to these lists, there is a free foods list, a combination foods list, a fast foods list, and an alcohol list.

One advantage of the food exchange system is its emphasis on more than one nutrient and the importance of the overall nutritional content of foods. This system also encourages consistency in the timing and amount of your meals and snacks. If you're new to meal planning, you might find this approach useful for learning the caloric and fat values of foods. Food exchanges can also be used as a reference for those using carbohydrate counting. Each serving of a food in the carbohydrate group counts as 15 grams of carbohydrate.

One disadvantage of this system is the level of understanding needed to grasp the concept of "exchanging" foods. It also requires learning where a food that is not listed fits. To learn more about the food exchange system for meal planning, contact a dietitian.

Calorie Counting
Calorie counting has been used for many years as a way to achieve weight loss, weight gain, or weight maintenance. This can be the easiest, most straightforward way to lose weight.

To use calorie counting, you establish a calorie goal that will help you achieve the weight loss you feel is appropriate. Your weight goal will be based on your current weight, height, and activity level. If you desire to lose weight, your calorie goal will be set lower than your usual intake of calories. If you wish to maintain your current weight, your calorie goal will be set at a calorie level similar to your current intake of calories.

You keep records of the foods you eat and their calorie

content. A periodic comparison of your food records and weekly weight can give you feedback on how you are progressing toward your weight goal. These records can also help you identify problem areas. For example, you might realize after reviewing your records that you tend to overeat when away from home. Knowing this information will help you develop strategies for changing this behavior.

The main advantage of calorie counting is the expanded choice of foods, which gives you more flexibility in what you eat. You decide whether and how a food might fit into your meal plan. For example, say your daily calorie goal is 1,500 calories, and a food you want to eat contains 600 calories. You can eat that food as long as you plan that the other foods you'll eat that day will add up to the remaining 900 calories. Your serving size, too, is based on how you want to "spend" your calories. You might decide you can work in only half a serving of pasta salad, or you might choose to have a double serving of pasta salad and make up the difference at a later meal.

One disadvantage of calorie counting might be the amount of time involved in keeping records and calculating the calorie content of foods. Also, because this approach does not guide you toward making nutritionally balanced choices, you may end up with a high-fat diet or one low in essential vitamins and minerals. Your dietitian can provide you with basic nutrition guidelines by which to select your foods to ensure that you meet your nutrition goals as well.

Estimating Serving Sizes

The success of any meal planning approach depends on how accurately you estimate your serving sizes. Therefore, it is essential to train your eyes to do this. Equip your kitchen with measuring spoons, measuring cups, and a food scale. Use these tools to measure and weigh foods consistently for two weeks or until you have trained your eyes to recognize what a cup of pasta looks like on your plate or how much one cup of milk fills your favorite glass.

Without some practice, it is surprisingly easy to mistakenly pour yourself one cup instead of a half cup of juice. A cup of juice has twice the carbohydrate and calories of a half of a cup of juice. This might tip you over your calorie or carbohydrate goal. If you did this with two to three foods each day, it could spoil your efforts at weight loss.

Of course, it is not practical to measure servings when you eat out in a restaurant, but training your eyes will help. Fortunately, the serving sizes of fast foods are fairly standardized among restaurants, i.e., a taco at any Taco Bell restaurant is likely to be the same size.

Using This Book of Food Counts

This book is intended to be a comprehensive listing of both generic and brand name foods that are available nationally. The nutrition information in this book comes from several sources, including:

- The U.S. Department of Agriculture
- The Agricultural Research Service
- The USDA National Nutrient Database for Standard Reference, Release 21
- The American Diabetes Association and The American Dietetic Association's *Choose Your Foods: Exchange Lists for Diabetes* nutrient database
- A variety of food-processing companies and fast-food franchises
- Nutrition Facts from food labels

Foods are listed alphabetically by food category and manufacturer. Nutrient information for foods from mixes (for example, puddings and cakes) reflect values after the food has been prepared according to package directions.

This book lists the calories, carbohydrate, fat, calories from fat, saturated fat, trans fat, cholesterol, sodium, fiber, and protein of many foods. The nutrient values you use will depend on your meal planning approach. You may need one, two, or even more of the values to figure out how a food fits in your plan.

Values have been rounded to the nearest calorie, gram (g), or milligram (mg) per serving (a gram is a unit of mass and weight in the metric system; an ounce is about 30 grams). The serving sizes listed in this book are those most commonly used. Similar foods will have the same serving sizes. The serving size may be very different from the amount you serve yourself or eat. If your serving size is different, be sure to recalculate the numbers.

The exchange values of foods have been calculated using the "rounding off method" (Wheeler ML, Franz M, Barrier PH, Holler H, Cronmiller N, Delahanty LM: Macronutrient and energy database for the 1995 Exchange Lists for Meal Planning: A rationale for clinical practice decisions. *J Am Diet Assoc* 96:1167–1170, 1996). Table 1 shows the amount of nutrients in one serving from each list.

Some of the foods in this book have a nutrient claim, such as "reduced-fat" or "low-calorie," as part of their name. These claims have standard meanings set by the Food and Drug Administration (FDA). Some of these terms and their meanings are listed in Table 2.

TABLE 1. Nutrient Content of Exchange Lists

Groups/List	Carb. (g)	Prot. (g)	Fat (g)	Cal.
Carbohydrates				
Starch List	15	0–3	0–1	80
Fruit List	15	0	0	60
Milk List				
Fat-free, Low-Fat, 1%	12	8	0–3	100
Reduced-Fat, 2%	12	8	5	120
Whole	12	8	8	160
Sweets, Desserts, and Other Carbohydrate	15	Varies	Varies	Varies
Nonstarchy Vegetable List	5	2	0	25
Meat and Meat Substitutes				
Lean	0	7	0-3	45
Medium-Fat	0	7	4-7	75
High-Fat	0	7	8+	100
Plant-Based Proteins	Varies	7	Varies	Varies
Fats				
Monounsaturated Fats	0	0	5	45
Polyunsaturated Fats	0	0	5	45
Saturated Fats	0	0	5	45
Free Foods	5 or less	Varies	Varies	Less than 20
Combination Foods	Varies	Varies	Varies	Varies
Fast Foods	Varies	Varies	Varies	Varies
Alcohol	Varies	0	0	~100

Adapted from the American Diabetes Association and the American Dietetic Association: *Choose Your Foods: Exchange Lists for Diabetes.* Alexandria, VA, 2008, p. 4.

TABLE 2. Nutrient Claims on Food Labels

Term	Meaning
Calorie-Free	Less than 5 calories per serving
Cholesterol-Free	Less than 2 mg of cholesterol per serving and 2 g or less of saturated fat per serving
Extra Lean	Less than 5 g of fat, 2 g of saturated fat, and 95 mg of cholesterol per serving
Fat-Free	Less than 0.5 g of fat per serving
Lean	Less than 10 g of fat, 4 g of saturated fat, and 95 mg of cholesterol per serving
Light or Lite	33.3% fewer calories or 50% less fat per serving than comparison food
Low-Calorie	40 calories or less per serving
Low-Cholesterol	20 mg or less of cholesterol per serving and 2 g or less of saturated fat per serving
Low-Fat	3 g or less of fat per serving
Low-Saturated Fat	1 g or less of saturated fat per serving and 15% or less of calories from saturated fat
Low-Sodium	140 mg or less of sodium per serving
Reduced	25% less per serving than comparison food
Saturated Fat-Free	Less than 0.5 g of saturated fat and 0.5 g of trans fatty acids per serving
Sodium-Free	Less than 5 mg of sodium per serving
Sugar-Free	Less than 0.5 g of sugar per serving

ALCOHOL, BEER, SPIRITS, WINE

BEER

	Serving	Calories	Fat (g)	Cal. from Fat	Sat. Fat (g)	Trans Fat (g)	Chol. (mg)	Sod. (mg)	Carb. (g)	Fiber (g)	Prot. (g)	Servings/Exchanges
Beer, Light	12 oz	103	0	0	0	0	0	14	6	0	<1	1 alcohol, 1/2 carb
Beer, Non-alcoholic	12 oz	70	0	0	0	0	0	8	13	0	1	1 alcohol
Beer, Regular	12 oz	153	0	0	0	0	0	14	13	0	1	1 alcohol, 1 carb
Brands												
Bud Light	12 oz	110	0	0	0	0	0	11	7	0	1	1 alcohol, 1/2 carb
Budweiser	12 oz	145	0	0	0	0	0	11	11	0	1	1 alcohol, 1/2 carb
Budweiser Select	12 oz	95	0	0	0	0	0	NA	3	0	<1	1 alcohol
Coors Light	12 oz	102	0	0	0	0	0	NA	5	0	0	1 alcohol
Michelob Amber	12 oz	114	0	0	0	0	0	NA	4	0	1	1 alcohol
Michelob Light	12 oz	123	0	0	0	0	0	NA	9	0	1	1 alcohol, 1/2 carb
Michelob Ultra	12 oz	95	0	0	0	0	0	9	3	0	<1	1 alcohol

ALCOHOL, BEER, SPIRITS, WINE

	Serving	Calories	Fat (g)	Cal. from Fat	Sat. Fat (g)	Trans Fat (g)	Chol. (mg)	Sod. (mg)	Carb. (g)	Fiber (g)	Prot. (g)	Servings/Exchanges
Miller Genuine Draft Light	12 oz	110	0	0	0	0	0	NA	7	0	0	1 alcohol, 1/2 carb
Miller Light	12 oz	95	0	0	0	0	0	NA	3	0	<1	1 alcohol
O'Doul's Brew	12 oz	65	0	0	0	0	0	NA	13	0	<1	1 carb
O'Doul's Amber	12 oz	90	0	0	0	0	0	NA	18	0	2	1 carb
COCKTAILS												
Daiquiri, Canned	4 oz	152	0	0	0	0	0	49	19	0	0	1 carb
Piña Colada, Canned	4 oz	309	10	90	9	0	0	93	36	0	<1	2 1/2 carb, 2 fat
Piña Colada, from Mix	4 oz	219	2	18	2	0	0	8	29	0	0	2 carb
Tequila Sunrise, Canned	4 oz	137	0	0	0	0	0	71	14	0	<1	1 carb
Whiskey Sour, Canned	4 oz	147	0	0	0	0	0	54	17	0	0	1 carb
LIQUEURS												
Coffee Liqueur, 53 Proof	1.5 oz	170	0	0	0	0	0	4	24	0	0	1 1/2 carb

Crème de Menthe	1.5 oz	186	0	0	0	0	0	2	21	0	0	1 1/2 carb

MIXERS (NON-ALCOHOLIC)

Finest Call

Margarita Mix	4 oz	160	0	0	0	0	0	0	40	0	0	2 1/2 carb
Sweet & Sour Mix	4 oz	110	0	0	0	0	0	80	24	0	0	2 carb

Jose Cuervo

Margarita Mix	4 oz	110	0	0	0	0	0	55	28	0	0	2 carb
Strawberry Margarita Mix	4 oz	100	0	0	0	0	0	80	24	0	0	1 1/2 carb

Master of Mixes

Margarita Mixer	4 oz	140	0	0	0	0	0	25	34	0	0	2 carb
Piña Colada Mixer	4 oz	230	1.5	14	0	0	0	45	53	0	0	3 1/2 carb
Strawberry Daiquiri	4 oz	140	0	0	0	0	0	25	34	0	0	2 carb
Sweet 'N Sour Mixer	4 oz	110	0	0	0	0	0	55	26	0	0	2 carb

On the House

Bloody Mary Mix	4 oz	25	0	0	0	0	0	630	6	0	0	1 vegetable

ALCOHOL, BEER, SPIRITS, WINE

	Serving	Calories	Fat (g)	Cal. from Fat	Sat. Fat (g)	Trans Fat (g)	Chol. (mg)	Sod. (mg)	Carb. (g)	Fiber (g)	Prot. (g)	Servings/Exchanges
Mai Tai Cocktail Mix	4 oz	150	0	0	0	0	0	75	38	0	0	2 1/2 carb
Margarita Mix	4 oz	100	0	0	0	0	0	75	25	0	0	1 1/2 carb
Piña Colada Mix	4 oz	160	0	0	0	0	0	100	38	0	0	2 1/2 carb
Strawberry Daiquiri Mix	4 oz	200	0	0	0	0	0	75	50	0	0	3 carb
Sweet & Sour Cocktail Mix	4 oz	110	0	0	0	0	0	75	26	0	0	2 carb
Tom Collins Mix	3 oz	160	0	0	0	0	0	90	39	0	0	2 1/2 carb
Rose's												
Grenadine	2 Tbsp	90	0	0	0	0	0	10	22	0	0	1 1/2 carb
Sweetened Lime Juice	1 tsp	10	0	0	0	0	0	0	2	0	0	free
Sauza												
Blue Raspberry Margarita Mix	3 oz	80	0	0	0	0	0	45	19	0	0	1 carb

Margarita Mix	3 oz	70	0	0	0	0	65	18	0	1 carb
Strawberry Margarita Mix	3 oz	80	0	0	0	0	45	19	0	1 carb
Stirrings										
Bloody Mary Mix	4 oz	40	0	0	0	0	750	10	0	1/2 carb
Cosmopolitan	3 oz	60	0	0	0	0	0	16	0	1 carb
Pomegranate Martini	3 oz	60	0	0	0	0	0	15	0	1 carb
SPIRITS (GIN, RUM, VODKA, WHISKEY)										
100 Proof	1.5 oz	124	0	0	0	0	0	0	0	1 alcohol
86 Proof	1.5 oz	105	0	0	0	0	0	0	0	1 alcohol
80 Proof	1.5 oz	97	0	0	0	0	0	0	0	1 alcohol
WINE										
Cooking Wine	5 oz	72	0	0	0	0	908	9	0	<1	1 alcohol, 1/2 carb
Dry Dessert Wine	5 oz	224	0	0	0	0	13	17	0	0	1 alcohol, 1 carb
Light Wine	5 oz	72	0	0	0	0	10	2	0	0	1 alcohol
Non-alcoholic	5 oz	9	0	0	0	0	10	2	0	<1	1 alcohol

ALCOHOL, BEER, SPIRITS, WINE

	Serving	Calories	Fat (g)	Cal. from Fat	Sat. Fat (g)	Trans Fat (g)	Chol. (mg)	Sod. (mg)	Carb. (g)	Fiber (g)	Prot. (g)	Servings/Exchanges
Sake	1 oz	39	0	0	0	0	0	1	1.5	0	0	1/2 alcohol
Sweet Dessert wine	5 oz	236	0	0	0	0	0	13	20	0	0	1 alcohol, 1 carb
Wine Cooler	12 oz	20	0	0	0	0	0	5	35	0	0	1 alcohol, 2 carb
Red Table Wine												
Barbera	5 oz	125	0	0	0	0	0	NA	4	0	0	1 alcohol
Burgundy	5 oz	127	0	0	0	0	0	NA	6	0	0	1 alcohol
Cabernet Franc	5 oz	122	0	0	0	0	0	NA	4	0	0	1 alcohol
Cabernet Sauvignon	5 oz	120	0	0	0	0	0	NA	4	0	0	1 alcohol
Carignane	5 oz	109	0	0	0	0	0	NA	4	0	0	1 alcohol
Claret	5 oz	122	0	0	0	0	0	NA	5	0	0	1 alcohol
Gamay	5 oz	115	0	0	0	0	0	NA	4	0	0	1 alcohol
Lemberger	5 oz	118	0	0	0	0	0	NA	4	0	0	1 alcohol
Merlot	5 oz	122	0	0	0	0	0	6	4	0	0	1 alcohol
Mouvedre	5 oz	129	0	0	0	0	0	NA	4	0	0	1 alcohol

Petite Sirah	5 oz	125	0	0	0	NA	4	0	1 alcohol
Pinot Noir	5 oz	121	0	0	0	NA	3	0	1 alcohol
Sangiovese	5 oz	126	0	0	0	NA	4	0	1 alcohol
Syrah	5 oz	122	0	0	0	NA	4	0	1 alcohol
Zinfandel	5 oz	129	0	0	0	NA	4	0	1 alcohol
White Table Wine									
Chenin Blanc	5 oz	118	0	0	0	NA	4	0	1 alcohol
Fune Blanc	5 oz	121	0	0	0	NA	3	0	1 alcohol
Gewurztraminer	5 oz	119	0	0	0	NA	4	0	1 alcohol
Muller Thurgau	5 oz	112	0	0	0	NA	5	0	1 alcohol
Muscat	5 oz	123	0	0	0	NA	8	0	1 alcohol
Pinot Blanc	5 oz	119	0	0	0	NA	3	0	1 alcohol
Pinot Gris (Grigio)	5 oz	122	0	0	0	NA	3	0	1 alcohol
Reisling	5 oz	118	0	0	0	NA	6	0	1 alcohol
Sauvignon Blanc	5 oz	119	0	0	0	NA	3	0	1 alcohol

BEANS, PEAS, LENTILS

	Serving	Calories	Fat (g)	Cal. from Fat	Sat. Fat (g)	Trans Fat (g)	Chol. (mg)	Sod. (mg)	Carb. (g)	Fiber (g)	Prot. (g)	Servings/Exchanges
Baked Beans with Beef, Canned	1/2 cup	161	5	45	2	0	29	632	23	7	9	1 1/2 starch, 1 med-fat meat
Baked Beans, No Pork	1/2 cup	78	<1	0	0	0	0	333	17	4	4	1 starch
Baked Beans, Vegetarian, Canned	1/2 cup	119	<1	0	<1	0	0	436	27	5	6	2 starch
Black Beans, Cooked	1/2 cup	114	0.5	5	0	0	0	1	21	8	8	1 1/2 starch, 1 lean meat
Black-Eyed Peas, Cooked	1/2 cup	100	0.5	5	0	0	0	3	18	6	7	1 starch, 1 lean meat
Black Turtle Soup Beans, Cooked	1/2 cup	120	<1	0	<1	0	0	3	23	5	8	1 1/2 starch, 1 lean meat
Fava/Broadbeans, Canned	1/2 cup	91	<1	0	<1	0	0	580	16	5	7	1 starch, 1 lean meat

Food	Serving										Exchanges
French Beans, Cooked	1/2 cup	114	<1	0	0	0	5	21	8	6	1 1/2 starch
Garbanzo Beans/Chickpeas, Cooked	1/2 cup	134	2	20	0	0	6	23	6	7	1 1/2 starch
Great Northern Beans, Cooked	1/2 cup	104	<1	0	<1	0	2	19	6	7	1 starch, 1 lean meat
Hummus	1/2 cup	210	11	100	2	0	300	25	6	6	1 1/2 starch, 2 fat
Kidney Beans, California Red, Cooked	1/2 cup	110	<1	0	<1	0	4	20	8	8	1 starch, 1 lean meat
Kidney Beans, Red, Cooked	1/2 cup	112	<1	0	0	0	2	20	6	8	1 starch, 1 lean meat
Kidney Beans, Royal Red, Cooked	1/2 cup	109	<1	0	<1	0	4	19	8	8	1 starch, 1 lean meat
Lentils, Cooked	1/2 cup	115	<1	0	<1	0	2	20	8	9	1 starch, 1 lean meat
Lima Beans, Canned	1/2 cup	99	<1	0	0	0	280	18	6	7	1 starch, 1 lean meat
Lima Beans, Frozen	1/2 cup	76	<1	0	0	0	40	14	4	5	1 starch, 1 lean meat
Navy Beans, Cooked	1/2 cup	129	0.5	5	0	0	1	24	6	8	1 1/2 starch, 1 lean meat
Pink Beans, Cooked	1/2 cup	126	<1	0	<1	0	2	24	5	8	1 1/2 starch, 1 lean meat

BEANS, PEAS, LENTILS

	Serving	Calories	Fat (g)	Cal. from Fat	Sat. Fat (g)	Trans Fat (g)	Chol. (mg)	Sod. (mg)	Carb. (g)	Fiber (g)	Prot. (g)	Servings/Exchanges
Pinto Beans, Cooked	1/2 cup	122	0.5	5	0	0	0	1	22	8	8	1 1/2 starch, 1 lean meat
Pork & Beans in Sweet Sauce, Canned	1/2 cup	142	2	20	<1	0	9	423	27	5	7	2 starch
Pork & Beans in Tomato Sauce	1/2 cup	116	1	10	0	0	9	538	23	5	6	1 1/2 starch
Refried Beans/Frijoles	1/2 cup	100	0.5	5	0	0	10	570	17	6	6	1 starch, 1 lean meat
Split Peas, Cooked	1/2 cup	116	<1	0	0	0	0	2	21	8	8	1 1/2 starch, 1 lean meat
White Beans, Cooked	1/2 cup	125	<1	0	0	0	0	5	23	6	9	1 1/2 starch, 1 lean meat
White Beans, Small, Cooked	1/2 cup	127	0	0	0	0	0	2	23	9	8	1 1/2 starch, 1 lean meat
Yellow Beans, Cooked	1/2 cup	127	<1	0	<1	0	0	4	22	9	8	1 1/2 starch, 1 lean meat
Brands (Canned Beans)												
Allens												

Food	Serving	Cal	Fat (g)	Cal from Fat	Sat Fat (g)	Trans Fat (g)	Chol (mg)	Sodium (mg)	Carb (g)	Fiber (g)	Protein (g)	Exchanges
Baby Butter Beans	1/2 cup	120	0.5	5	0		0	460	22	6	7	1 1/2 starch, 1 lean meat
Black Beans	1/2 cup	100	0.5	5	0		0	400	19	8	6	1 starch, 1 lean meat
Black-Eyed Peas	1/2 cup	120	1	10	0		0	420	20	5	7	1 starch, 1 lean meat
Dark Red Kidney Beans	1/2 cup	130	0.5	5	0		0	310	22	8	8	1 1/2 starch, 1 lean meat
Garbanzo Beans	1/2 cup	120	2.5	25	0		0	330	19	8	5	1 starch
Great Northern Beans	1/2 cup	100	0.5	5	0		0	310	19	7	6	1 starch, 1 lean meat
Lima Beans	1/2 cup	120	0	0	0		0	370	23	8	7	1 1/2 starch, 1 lean meat
Navy Beans	1/2 cup	110	1	10	0		0	380	19	6	6	1 starch, 1 lean meat
Pinto Beans	1/2 cup	110	1	10	0		0	290	20	7	5	1 starch
Red Beans	1/2 cup	100	0.5	5	0		0	310	19	9	6	1 starch, 1 lean meat
Refried Beans	1/2 cup	150	2.5	25	1		0	260	24	11	7	1 1/2 starch, 1 lean meat
Refried Black Beans, No Fat Added	1/2 cup	120	0	0	0		0	500	23	8	7	1 1/2 starch, 1 lean meat
B & M												
Baked Beans, Bacon, Onion & Brown Sugar	1/2 cup	190	2	20	0.5	0	<5	450	36	8	8	2 1/2 starch

BEANS, PEAS, LENTILS

	Serving	Calories	Fat (g)	Cal. from Fat	Sat. Fat (g)	Trans Fat (g)	Chol. (mg)	Sod. (mg)	Carb. (g)	Fiber (g)	Prot. (g)	Servings/Exchanges
Baked Beans, Barbeque	1/2 cup	190	0.5	5	0	0	0	570	39	9	8	2 1/2 starch
Baked Beans, Country Style	1/2 cup	170	1.5	15	0.5	0	<5	710	35	7	7	2 starch
Baked Beans, Maple Flavor	1/2 cup	180	1	10	0	0	0	340	31	8	7	2 starch
Baked Beans, Original	1/2 cup	170	2	20	0.5	0	<5	400	31	8	7	2 starch
Baked Beans, Red Kidney	1/2 cup	200	3	25	1	0	<5	460	36	6	8	2 1/2 starch
Baked Beans, Vegetarian	1/2 cup	160	1	10	0	0	0	380	28	8	7	2 starch
Bush's												
Baked Beans, Bold & Spicy	1/2 cup	110	1	10	0	0	0	560	24	5	6	1 1/2 starch

Baked Beans, Boston Style	1/2 cup	150	1	10	0	0	440	31	5	6	2 starch
Baked Beans, Country Style	1/2 cup	160	1	10	0	0	680	33	5	6	2 starch
Baked Beans	1/2 cup	140	1	10	0	0	550	29	5	6	2 starch
Baked Beans, Honey Baked	1/2 cup	160	1	10	0	0	540	32	6	6	2 starch
Baked Beans, Maple Cured Bacon	1/2 cup	140	1	10	0	0	620	28	5	6	2 starch
Baked Beans, Onion	1/2 cup	140	1	10	0	0	550	29	5	6	2 starch
Baked Beans, Original	1/2 cup	140	1	10	0	0	550	29	5	6	2 starch
Baked Beans, Vegetarian	1/2 cup	130	0	0	0	0	550	29	5	6	2 starch
Black Beans	1/2 cup	110	0.5	5	0	0	450	23	7	8	1 1/2 starch
Black Beans, Frijoles Negros Condimentados	1/2 cup	110	0.5	5	0	0	450	23	7	8	1 1/2 starch, 1 lean meat

BEANS, PEAS, LENTILS

	Serving	Calories	Fat (g)	Cal. from Fat	Sat. Fat (g)	Trans Fat (g)	Chol. (mg)	Sod. (mg)	Carb. (g)	Fiber (g)	Prot. (g)	Servings/Exchanges
Black-Eyed Peas	1/2 cup	100	0	0	0	0	0	480	15	3	5	1 starch
Black-Eyed Peas with Bacon	1/2 cup	95	1.5	15	0	0	0	370	17	3	6	1 starch, 1 lean meat
Black-Eyed Peas with Snaps	1/2 cup	110	0.5	5	0	0	0	550	17	5	7	1 starch, 1 lean meat
Butter Beans, Baby	1/2 cup	120	0.5	5	0	0	0	510	19	5	7	1 starch, 1 lean meat
Cannellini Beans	1/2 cup	110	0.5	0	0	0	0	300	18	6	7	1 starch, 1 lean meat
Chili Beans	1/2 cup	120	1	10	0.5	0	0	480	20	6	6	1 starch, 1 lean meat
Chili Beans, Red Beans in Chili Sauce	1/2 cup	100	0.5	5	0	0	0	480	22	7	6	1 1/2 starch
Crowder Peas	1/2 cup	110	1	10	0	0	0	500	18	5	7	1 starch, 1 lean meat
Field Peas with Snaps	1/2 cup	80	0	0	0	0	0	430	16	2	5	1 starch
Garbanzo Beans	1/2 cup	105	2	15	0	0	0	470	20	5	6	1 starch, 1 lean meat
Great Northern Beans	1/2 cup	80	0	0	0	0	0	460	17	6	6	1 starch, 1 lean meat

Grillin' Beans, Bourbon & Brown Sugar	1/2 cup	170	0.5	5	0	0	480	35	6	7	1 starch, 1 lean meat
Grillin' Beans, Smokehouse Tradition	1/2 cup	170	1	10	0	0	570	34	5	7	2 starch
Grillin' Beans, Southern Pit BBQ	1/2 cup	170	0.5	5	0	0	550	35	6	6	2 starch
Grillin' Beans, Steakhouse Recipe	1/2 cup	180	0.5	5	0	0	510	39	5	6	2 1/2 starch
Kidney Beans, Dark Red	1/2 cup	105	0	0	0	0	260	22	8	7	1 1/2 starch, 1 lean meat
Kidney Beans, Light Red	1/2 cup	100	0	0	0	0	260	22	7	7	1 1/2 starch, 1 lean meat
Mixed Beans	1/2 cup	110	0	0	0	0	500	19	6	7	1 starch, 1 lean meat
Navy Beans	1/2 cup	80	0	0	0	0	470	17	7	6	1 starch, 1 lean meat
Pinto Beans	1/2 cup	110	0	0	0	0	390	19	6	6	1 starch, 1 lean meat
Pinto Beans with Pork	1/2 cup	120	2.5	25	1	5	530	17	6	6	1 starch, 1 lean meat
Pinto Beans, Frijoles Pintos	1/2 cup	80	0	0	0	0	450	18	7	6	1 starch, 1 lean meat

BEANS, PEAS, LENTILS

	Serving	Calories	Fat (g)	Cal. from Fat	Sat. Fat (g)	Trans Fat (g)	Chol. (mg)	Sod. (mg)	Carb. (g)	Fiber (g)	Prot. (g)	Servings/Exchanges
Purple Hull Peas	1/2 cup	90	0	0	0	0	0	460	19	5	6	1 starch, 1 lean meat
Red Beans	1/2 cup	110	0.5	5	0	0	0	460	19	6	6	1 starch, 1 lean meat
Refried Beans, Fat Free	1/2 cup	130	0	0	0	0	0	490	24	7	9	1 1/2 starch, 1 lean meat
Refried Beans, Traditional	1/2 cup	150	3	25	1	0	0	490	24	7	9	1 1/2 starch, 1 lean meat
Eden Organic												
Aduki Beans	1/2 cup	110	0	0	0	0	0	10	19	5	7	1 starch, 1 lean meat
Baked Beans with Sorghum & Mustard	1/2 cup	150	0	0	0	0	0	130	27	7	8	2 starch
Black Beans	1/2 cup	110	1	10	0	0	0	15	18	6	7	1 starch, 1 lean meat
Black Soy Beans	1/2 cup	120	6	50	1	0	0	30	8	7	11	1/2 starch, 1 lean meat
Black-Eyed Peas	1/2 cup	90	1	10	0	0	0	25	16	4	6	1 starch, 1 lean meat
Butter Beans	1/2 cup	100	1	10	0	0	0	35	17	4	5	1 starch
Cannellini	1/2 cup	100	1	10	0	0	0	40	17	4	5	1 starch

Caribbean Black Beans	1/2 cup	90	0.5	0	0	0	135	20	7	7	1 starch, 1 lean meat
Garbanzo Beans	1/2 cup	130	1	10	0	0	30	23	5	7	1 1/2 starch, 1 lean meat
Lentils with Onions & Bay Leaf	1/2 cup	90	0	0	0	0	210	13	4	8	1 starch, 1 lean meat
Pinto Beans	1/2 cup	110	1	0	0	0	15	18	6	6	1 starch, 1 lean meat
Refried Beans	1/2 cup	110	1.5	15	0	0	180	18	7	6	1 starch, 1 lean meat
Gebhardt											
Fat Free Refried Beans	1/2 cup	80	0	0	0	0	500	17	5	6	1 starch, 1 lean meat
Jalapeño Refried Beans	1/2 cup	100	2	20	1	0	400	17	5	6	1 starch, 1 lean meat
Refried Beans	1/2 cup	90	2	20	0.5	0	490	16	4	6	1 starch, 1 lean meat
Old El Paso											
Refried Beans, Fat-Free	1/2 cup	100	0	0	0	0	580	18	6	6	1 starch, 1 lean meat
Refried Beans, Fat-Free, Spicy	1/2 cup	90	0	0	0	0	510	16	5	5	1 starch
Refried Beans, Traditional	1/2 cup	90	0.5	5	0	0	580	16	5	5	1 starch

BEANS, PEAS, LENTILS

	Serving	Calories	Fat (g)	Cal. from Fat	Sat. Fat (g)	Trans Fat (g)	Chol. (mg)	Sod. (mg)	Carb. (g)	Fiber (g)	Prot. (g)	Servings/Exchanges
Refried Beans, Vegetarian	1/2 cup	90	0.5	5	0	0	0	570	16	5	5	1 starch
Progresso												
Black Beans	1/2 cup	100	0.5	5	0	0	0	400	17	5	6	1 starch, 1 lean meat
Chick Peas	1/2 cup	120	2.5	25	0	0	0	280	20	5	5	1 starch
Dark Red Kidney Beans	1/2 cup	110	0	0	0	0	0	340	20	6	8	1 starch, 1 lean meat
Fava Beans	1/2 cup	110	0.5	5	0	0	0	250	20	5	6	1 starch, 1 lean meat
Ranch Style												
Beans, Original	1/2 cup	130	3	25	0	0	0	600	19	5	5	1 starch
Beans with Sweet Onions	1/2 cup	130	3	25	0	0	<5	590	19	6	5	1 starch
Black Beans	1/2 cup	100	0.5	5	0	0	0	420	19	5	6	1 starch, 1 lean meat
Pinto Beans	1/2 cup	100	0	0	0	0	0	580	20	6	6	1 starch, 1 lean meat

Beans with Jalapeño Peppers	1/2 cup	120	2.5	25	0.5	0	740	19	6	5	1 starch
Rosarita											
No Fat Refried Beans	1/2 cup	100	0	0	0	0	510	19	6	7	1 starch, 1 lean meat
No Fat Refried Beans with Green Chili	1/2 cup	100	0	0	0	0	310	18	7	7	1 starch, 1 lean meat
No Fat Refried Beans with Spicy Jalapeño	1/2 cup	120	2	15	0.5	0	320	19	7	7	1 starch, 1 lean meat
No Fat Refried Black Beans	1/2 cup	110	0	0	0	0	320	19	8	7	1 starch, 1 lean meat
Refried Beans, Traditional	1/2 cup	120	2	20	0	0	310	18	6	7	1 starch, 1 lean meat
Refried Beans, Vegetarian	1/2 cup	120	2	20	0	0	540	19	7	7	1 starch, 1 lean meat
S & W											
Baked Beans	1/2 cup	160	1	5	0	0	510	32	8	8	2 starch

BEANS, PEAS, LENTILS

	Serving	Calories	Fat (g)	Cal. from Fat	Sat. Fat (g)	Trans Fat (g)	Chol. (mg)	Sod. (mg)	Carb. (g)	Fiber (g)	Prot. (g)	Servings/Exchanges
Baked Beans, Maple	1/2 cup	140	0.5	5	0	0	5	440	28	4	6	2 starch
Black Beans	1/2 cup	100	1	10	0	0	0	380	17	6	6	1 starch, 1 lean meat
Black Beans, 50% Less Sodium	1/2 cup	120	0.5	5	0	0	0	180	22	5	8	1 1/2 starch, 1 lean meat
Chili Beans, Pinto Beans & Chipotle	1/2 cup	110	1	10	0	0	0	530	23	6	7	1 1/2 starch, 1 lean meat
Garbanzo Beans	1/2 cup	110	2.5	20	0	0	0	460	15	3	7	1 starch, 1 lean meat
Garbanzo Beans, 50% Less Sodium	1/2 cup	110	2.5	20	0	0	0	220	15	3	7	1 starch, 1 lean meat
Kidney Beans	1/2 cup	120	1	10	0	0	0	380	20	6	7	1 starch, 1 lean meat
Kidney Beans, 50% Less Sodium	1/2 cup	110	1	5	0	0	0	180	21	5	7	1 1/2 starch, 1 lean meat
Pinquitos	1/2 cup	110	0.5	5	0	0	0	490	20	6	6	1 starch, 1 lean meat
Pinto Beans	1/2 cup	120	1	10	0	0	0	530	22	7	6	1 1/2 starch

Red Beans, Louisiana Style	1/2 cup	110	0.5	5	0	0	340	20	5	6	1 starch, 1 lean meat
White Beans	1/2 cup	110	0.5	5	0	0	480	19	6	7	1 starch, 1 lean meat
Trader Joe's											
Black Beans	1/2 cup	110	0	0	0	0	430	19	6	6	1 starch, 1 lean meat
Cannellini White Kidney Beans	1/2 cup	120	0	0	0	0	200	21	10	8	1 1/2 starch, 1 lean meat
Cuban Style Black Beans	1/2 cup	100	0.5	5	0	0	370	19	6	6	1 starch, 1 lean meat
Garbanzo Beans	1/2 cup	120	1	10	0	0	380	22	6	6	1 1/2 starch, 1 lean meat
Low Fat Vegetarian Refried Pinto Beans	1/2 cup	110	0.5	5	0	0	410	20	6	6	1 starch, 1 lean meat
Marinated Bean Salad	1/2 cup	140	2	15	0	0	410	24	6	6	1 1/2 starch, 1 lean meat
Organic Baked Beans	1/2 cup	140	0	0	0	0	450	29	7	7	2 starch
Organic Black Beans	1/2 cup	110	0	0	0	0	440	20	6	6	1 starch, 1 lean meat
Organic Pinto Beans	1/2 cup	110	0	0	0	0	220	22	7	6	1 1/2 starch, 1 lean meat

BEANS, PEAS, LENTILS

	Serving	Calories	Fat (g)	Cal. from Fat	Sat. Fat (g)	Trans Fat (g)	Chol. (mg)	Sod. (mg)	Carb. (g)	Fiber (g)	Prot. (g)	Servings/Exchanges
Refried Black Beans with Jalapeño Peppers	1/2 cup	120	0.5	5	0	0	0	440	22	7	8	1 1/2 starch, 1 lean meat
Van Camp's												
Baked Beans, Homestyle	1/2 cup	170	1	5	0	0	0	680	33	6	7	2 starch
Baked Beans, Original	1/2 cup	140	1	10	0	0	0	540	30	6	7	2 starch
Kidney Beans, Dark Red	1/2 cup	90	0	0	0	0	0	730	19	6	7	1 starch, 1 lean meat
New Orleans Red Kidney Beans	1/2 cup	90	0	0	0	0	0	450	19	6	6	1 starch, 1 lean meat

BEVERAGES, SODA, SPORTS/ENERGY DRINKS, MEAL-REPLACEMENT DRINKS, COCOA, COFFEE/CREAMER, TEA

COCOA, HOT CHOCOLATE, CHOCOLATE MILK

	Serving	Calories	Fat (g)	Cal. from Fat	Sat. Fat (g)	Trans Fat (g)	Chol. (mg)	Sod. (mg)	Carb. (g)	Fiber (g)	Prot. (g)	Servings/Exchanges
Hot Chocolate (Cocoa)	1 envelope	80	3	30	2	0	0	170	15	<1	<1	1 carb, 1 fat
Hot Chocolate (Cocoa), Sugar Free	1 envelope	50	<1	0	0	0	1	180	10	<1	2	1/2 carb
Hot Cocoa Mix, Lite	1 envelope	80	1	0	0	0	0	0	17	1	2	1 carb
Carnation												
Malted Milk	3 Tbsp	90	2	20	1	0	10	100	15	0	2	1 carb
Hershey's												
Chocolate Goodnight	1 envelope	140	2.5	20	1.5	0	<5	190	27	1	3	2 carb, 1 fat
Kisses Hot Cocoa												

BEVERAGES, SODA, SPORTS/ENERGY DRINKS

	Serving	Calories	Fat (g)	Cal. from Fat	Sat. Fat (g)	Trans Fat (g)	Chol. (mg)	Sod. (mg)	Carb. (g)	Fiber (g)	Prot. (g)	Servings/Exchanges
Nestlé												
Chocolate Caramel Hot Cocoa	1 envelope	100	3	25	2	0	0	190	19	<1	1	1 carb, 1 fat
Fat Free Hot Cocoa	1 envelope	25	0	0	0	0	0	150	5	<1	1	free
Hot Cocoa with Mini Marshmallows	1 envelope	80	2.5	25	2	0	0	160	14	<1	1	1 carb, 1 fat
Nesquik Chocolate	2 Tbsp	60	0.5	5	0	0	0	30	14	<1	<1	1 carb
Nesquik No Sugar Added Chocolate	2 Tbsp	35	1	10	0.5	0	0	70	7	1	1	1/2 carb
No Sugar Added Hot Cocoa	1 envelope	50	0	0	0	0	0	180	10	<1	2	1/2 carb
Rich Milk Chocolate Hot Cocoa	1 envelope	80	3	25	2	0	0	180	14	<1	1	1 carb, 1 fat

Ovaltine

Malted Milk Drink, Chocolate Malt	4 Tbsp	80	0	0	0	0	115	18	<1	1	1 carb
Malted Milk Drink, Rich Chocolate	4 Tbsp	80	0	0	0	0	140	19	0	<1	1 carb

Swiss Miss

Dark Chocolate Hot Cocoa	1 envelope	150	3.5	30	0	0	170	28	1	1	2 carb, 1 fat
Milk Chocolate Hot Cocoa	1 envelope	120	2	20	2	0	160	23	<1	1	1 1/2 carb

COFFEE

Coffee, Brewed	8 oz	2	0	0	0	0	5	0	0	0	free
Coffee, Instant	8 oz	5	0	0	0	0	10	<1	0	0	free

General Foods

Chai Latte	1 1/3 Tbsp	70	2	20	2	0	60	12	0	0	1 carb

BEVERAGES, SODA, SPORTS/ENERGY DRINKS

	Serving	Calories	Fat (g)	Cal. from Fat	Sat. Fat (g)	Trans Fat (g)	Chol. (mg)	Sod. (mg)	Carb. (g)	Fiber (g)	Prot. (g)	Servings/Exchanges
International Coffees, All Varieties	1 1/3 Tbsp	50–70	1.5	15–	0.5–	0	0	30–	10–	0	0–1	1 carb
International Coffees, Sugar-Free, Mocha	1 1/3 Tbsp	30	–3	30	2.5	0	0	110	12	0	0	free
Hills Brothers												
Cappuccino, French Vanilla	3 Tbsp	120	4.5	40	3.5	0	0	105	19	0	2	1 carb, 1 fat
Starbucks												
Coffee Frappuccino Coffee Drink	9.5-oz bottle	200	3	30	2	0	15	100	37	0	6	2 1/2 carb, 1 fat
Doubleshot Coffee Drink	6.5-oz can	140	6	50	3.5	0	20	70	18	0	4	1 carb, 1 fat
Mocha Frappuccino Coffee Drink	9.5-oz bottle	180	3	30	2	0	15	95	33	0	7	2 carb, 1 fat

Mocha Lite Frappuccino Coffee Drink	9.5-oz bottle	100	3	30	2	0	15	95	12	0	1 carb, 1 fat
Vanilla Frappuccino Coffee Drink	9.5-oz bottle	200	3	30	2	0	15	100	37	0	2 1/2 carb, 1 fat

COFFEE CREAMER

Cremora

Lite & Creamy	1 tsp	10	0	0	0	0	5	5	1	0	free
Original	1 tsp	10	0.5	5	0.5	0	0	10	0	0	free

International Delight Coffee House

Caramel Macchiato	1 Tbsp	40	1.5	15	1	0	0	5	7	0	1/2 carb
Vanilla Latte	1 Tbsp	40	1.5	15	1	0	0	5	7	0	1/2 carb

Nestlé Coffee-Mate (Liquid)

Cinnamon Vanilla Crème, Fat Free	1 Tbsp	25	0	0	0	0	0	25	5	0	free
French Vanilla	1 Tbsp	35	1.5	15	0	0	0	30	5	0	1 fat
Hazelnut	1 Tbsp	35	1.5	15	0	0	0	30	2	0	free

BEVERAGES, SODA, SPORTS/ENERGY DRINKS

	Serving	Calories	Fat (g)	Cal. from Fat	Sat. Fat (g)	Trans Fat (g)	Chol. (mg)	Sod. (mg)	Carb. (g)	Fiber (g)	Prot. (g)	Servings/Exchanges
Original	1 Tbsp	15	1	10	0	0	0	0	2	0	0	free
Vanilla Caramel	1 Tbsp	35	1.5	15	0	0	0	30	5	0	0	1 fat
Nestlé Coffee-Mate (Powder)												
Fat Free	1 tsp	10	0	0	0	0	0	0	2	0	0	free
French Vanilla	4 tsp	60	2.5	25	2	0	0	15	9	0	0	1/2 carb, 1 fat
Hazelnut	4 tsp	60	3	25	2.5	0	0	15	9	0	0	1/2 carb, 1 fat
Original	1 tsp	10	0.5	5	0.5	0	0	0	1	0	0	free
Vanilla Caramel	4 tsp	60	3	25	2.5	0	0	15	9	0	0	1/2 carb, 1 fat
FRUIT PUNCH & LEMONADE												
Fruit Punch Mix	8 oz	97	0	0	0	0	0	8	25	0	0	1 1/2 carb
Lemonade, Prepared	8 oz	112	0	0	0	0	0	19	29	0	0	2 carb
Country Time												
Lemonade, Powder	8 oz	60	0	0	0	0	0	25	16	0	0	1 carb
Lite Lemonade	8 oz	35	0	0	0	0	0	10	8	0	0	1/2 carb

Pink Lemonade	8 oz	60	0	0	0	0	16	0	0	1 carb
Crystal Light										
Crystal Light Bottles	8 oz	5	0	0	0	0	0	0	0	free
Crystal Light Drinks, Lemonades, or Teas	8 oz	5	0	0	0	0–35	0	0	0	free
Kool-Aid										
Drink Mix from Powder, All Varieties	8 oz	60	0	0	0	0	16	0	0	1 carb
Tang										
Orange Drink Mix, Powder	8 oz	40	0	0	0	0	9	0	0	1/2 carb
Orange Drink Mix, Sugar-Free, Powder	8 oz	5	0	0	0	0	0	0	0	free
Tropicana										
Lemonade	12-oz can	150	0	0	0	0	90	40	0	2 1/2 carb

BEVERAGES, SODAS SPORTS/ENERGY DRINKS

SODA DRINKS

Average (All Brands)

	Serving	Calories	Fat (g)	Cal. from Fat	Sat. Fat (g)	Trans Fat (g)	Chol. (mg)	Sod. (mg)	Carb. (g)	Fiber (g)	Prot. (g)	Servings/Exchanges
Soda Drink, Small	16 oz	207	0	0	0	0	0	20	53	0	0	2 1/2 carb
Soda Drink, Medium	22 oz	284	0	0	0	0	0	27	73	0	0	5 carb
Soda Drink, Large	32 oz	413	0	0	0	0	0	39	106	0	0	7 carb
Club Soda	12 oz	0	0	0	0	0	0	75	0	0	0	free
Cream Soda	12 oz	189	0	0	0	0	0	45	49	0	0	3 carb
Diet Cola/Coke with Aspartame	12 oz	4	0	0	0	0	0	21	<1	0	0	free
Ginger Ale	12 oz	124	0	0	0	0	0	26	32	0	0	3 carb
Grape Soda	12 oz	160	0	0	0	0	0	56	42	0	0	3 carb
Lemon-Lime Soda	12 oz	147	0	0	0	0	0	40	38	0	0	2 1/2 carb
Orange Soda	12 oz	179	0	0	0	0	0	45	46	0	0	3 carb
Root Beer	12 oz	152	0	0	0	0	0	48	39	0	0	2 1/2 carb

Brands										
7-Up	12 oz	140	0	0	0	0	40	39	0	0	2 1/2 carb
7-Up, Cherry	12 oz	140	0	0	0	0	40	39	0	0	2 1/2 carb
7-Up, Diet	12 oz	170	0	0	0	0	45	46	0	0	3 carb
A&W Root Beer	12 oz	170	0	0	0	0	47	65	0	0	3 carb
A&W Cream Soda	12 oz	190	0	0	0	0	70	47	0	0	3 carb
Barq's Root Beer	12 oz	160	0	0	0	0	70	45	0	0	3 carb
Canada Dry Ginger Ale	12 oz	140	0	0	0	0	50	36	0	0	2 1/2 carb
Coca-Cola										
Coca-Cola Classic	12 oz	140	0	0	0	0	50	39	0	0	2 1/2 carb
Coca-Cola Zero	12 oz	0	0	0	0	0	40	0	0	0	free
Cherry Coke	12 oz	150	0	0	0	0	35	42	0	0	3 carb
Diet Coke	12 oz	0	0	0	0	0	40	0	0	0	free
Diet Coke with Lime	12 oz	0	0	0	0	0	40	0	0	0	free
Vanilla Coke	12 oz	150	0	0	0	0	35	42	0	0	3 carb
Diet Rite	12 oz	0	0	0	0	0	0	0	0	0	free

BEVERAGES, SODA, SPORTS/ENERGY DRINKS

	Serving	Calories	Fat (g)	Cal. from Fat	Sat. Fat (g)	Trans Fat (g)	Chol. (mg)	Sod. (mg)	Carb. (g)	Fiber (g)	Prot. (g)	Servings/Exchanges
Dr. Pepper	12 oz	150	0	0	0	0	0	55	40	0	0	2 1/2 carb
Fanta Orange	12 oz	160	0	0	0	0	0	55	44	0	0	3 carb
Fresca	12 oz	0	0	0	0	0	0	35	0	0	0	free
Hansen's Natural Cane Soda												
Club Soda	8 oz	0	0	0	0	0	0	0	0	0	0	free
Creamy Root Beer	12 oz	160	0	0	0	0	0	0	43	0	0	3 carb
Diet Black Cherry	12 oz	0	0	0	0	0	0	0	0	0	0	free
Diet Green Tea Soda, Tangerine	8 oz	0	0	0	0	0	0	0	0	0	0	free
Ginger Ale	8 oz	90	0	0	0	0	0	0	24	0	0	1 1/2 carb
Mango Orange	12 oz	170	0	0	0	0	0	0	44	0	0	3 carb
Natural Green Tea Soda, Pomegranate	8 oz	90	0	0	0	0	0	0	22	0	0	1 1/2 carb
Natural Soda Tonic	8 oz	90	0	0	0	0	0	0	24	0	0	1 1/2 carb

Raspberry	12 oz	140	0	0	0	0	0	0	0	37	0	0	2 1/2 carb
Mountain Dew	12 oz	170	0	0	0	0	0	0	65	46	0	0	3 carb
Mountain Dew Code Red	12 oz	170	0	0	0	0	0	0	105	46	0	0	3 carb
Mountain Dew–Diet	12 oz	0	0	0	0	0	0	0	50	0	0	0	free
MUG Root Beer	12 oz	160	0	0	0	0	0	0	65	43	0	0	3 carb

Pepsi

Diet Pepsi	12 oz	0	0	0	0	0	0	0	35	0	0	0	free
Pepsi	12 oz	150	0	0	0	0	0	0	30	41	0	0	3 carb
Pepsi Max	12 oz	0	0	0	0	0	0	0	35	0	0	0	2 carb
Pepsi Natural	12 oz	150	0	0	0	0	0	0	35	39	0	0	2 1/2 carb
Wild Cherry Pepsi	12 oz	160	0	0	0	0	0	0	30	42	0	0	3 carb
Sierra Mist	12 oz	140	0	0	0	0	0	0	35	39	0	0	2 1/2 carb
Slice Orange	12 oz	180	0	0	0	0	0	0	35	48	0	0	3 carb

Sprite

Sprite Zero	12 oz	0	0	0	0	0	0	0	35	0	0	0	free
Sprite	12 oz	140	0	0	0	0	0	0	65	38	0	0	2 1/2 carb

BEVERAGES, SODA, SPORTS/ENERGY DRINKS

	Serving	Calories	Fat (g)	Cal. from Fat	Sat. Fat (g)	Trans Fat (g)	Chol. (mg)	Sod. (mg)	Carb. (g)	Fiber (g)	Prot. (g)	Servings/Exchanges
Squirt	12 oz	140	0	0	0	0	0	50	39	0	0	2 1/2 carb
Sunkist Orange	12 oz	190	0	0	0	0	0	65	52	0	0	3 carb
TAB	12 oz	0	0	0	0	0	0	40	0	0	0	free
SPORTS/NUTRITION/ENERGY DRINKS												
Accelerade	1 scoop (12 oz)	120	1	10	0	0	0	190	21	0	5	1 1/2 carb
Accelerade, Citrus Grapefruit	8 oz	80	0	0	0	0	0	120	15	0	4	1 carb
All Sport Body Quencher	8 oz	60	0	0	0	0	0	55	16	0	0	1 carb
All Sport Naturally Zero	8 oz	0	0	0	0	0	0	55	0	0	0	free
AMP Energy Drink	8 oz	110	0	0	0	0	0	65	29	0	0	2 carb
AMP Energy Drink, Sugar Free	8 oz	5	0	0	0	0	0	75	<1	0	0	free
Boost	8 oz	240	4	35	0.5	0	5	130	41	0	10	3 carb

Boost Glucose Control	8 oz	190	7	60	1	0	10	180	16	3	16	1 carb, 2 lean meat
Boost High Protein	8 oz	240	6	50	0.5	0	10	170	33	0	15	2 carb, 1 med-fat meat
Boost Plus	8 oz	360	14	130	1.5	0	10	170	45	0	14	3 carb, 1 med-fat meat, 2 fat
Carnation Instant Breakfast Essentials, Powder Mix	1 packet	130	0–1	0–10	0–0.5	0	<5	80–160	26–27	0–1	5	2 carb
Carnation Instant Breakfast Essentials, Ready-to-Drink	10.8-oz bottle	250–260	5	50	1.5	0	10	180	34–41	0–1	14	2 carb, 1 med-fat meat
Carnation Instant Breakfast Essentials, Sugar-Free	1 packet	60–70	0–1	0–10	0	0	<5	60–70	12	3–4	5	1 carb
Carnation Instant Breakfast, Sugar-Free, Ready-to-Drink	10.8-oz bottle	150	5	50	1.5	0	10	240	16	2	13	1 carb, 1 med-fat meat

BEVERAGES, SODA, SPORTS/ENERGY DRINKS

	Serving	Calories	Fat (g)	Cal. from Fat	Sat. Fat (g)	Trans Fat (g)	Chol. (mg)	Sod. (mg)	Carb. (g)	Fiber (g)	Prot. (g)	Servings/Exchanges
Clif Quench Sport Drink, All Varieties	8 oz	45	0	0	0	0	0	130	11	0	0	1 carb
CytoSport Cytomax Performance Ready-to-Drink	8 oz	50	0	0	0	0	0	55	13	0	0	1 carb
CytoSport Cytomax Powder	1 scoop	90	0	0	0	0	0	120	22	0	0	1 1/2 carb
CytoSport Muscle Milk Light Ready-to-Drink	14 oz	160	4.5	40	1	0	10	340	10	5	20	1/2 carb, 3 lean meat
CytoSport Muscle Milk Powder	1 scoop	150	6	55	3	0	8	115	8	2.5	16	1/2 carb, 2 lean meat
CytoSport Muscle Milk Ready-to-Drink	14 oz	230	9	80	1.5	0	10	350	12	2	25	1 carb, 3 lean meat
Gatorade (All Varieties)	8 oz	50	0	0	0	0	0	110	14	0	0	1 carb

Gatorade G2	8 oz	25	0	0	0	0	110	7	0	0	1/2 carb
Glaceau Vitamin Water (All Varieties)	8 oz	50	0	0	0	0	0	13	0	0	1 carb
KMX Energy Drink (All Varieties)	8.4 oz	120	0	0	0	0	75	31	0	0	2 carb
Monster Energy Drink	8 oz	100	0	0	0	0	180	27	0	0	2 carb
Monster Energy Drink, Lo-Carb	8 oz	10	0	0	0	0	180	3	0	0	free
No Fear	8 oz	130	0	0	0	0	115	36	0	0	2 1/2 carb
No Fear Blood Shot	8 oz	100	0	0	0	0	160	24	0	0	1 1/2 carb
No Fear Motherload	8 oz	130	0	0	0	0	100	34	0	0	2 carb
No Fear Sugar Free	8 oz	10	0	0	0	0	100	1	0	0	free
Powerade (All Varieties)	8 oz	50	0	0	0	0	100	14	0	0	1 carb
Powerade Zero	8 oz	0	0	0	0	0	55	0	0	0	free
Propel Fitness Water	8 oz	10	0	0	0	0	75	2	0	0	free
Red Bull Energy Drink	8.4 oz	110	0	0	0	0	100	28	0	<1	2 carb

BEVERAGES, SODA, SPORTS/ENERGY DRINKS

	Serving	Calories	Fat (g)	Cal. from Fat	Sat. Fat (g)	Trans Fat (g)	Chol. (mg)	Sod. (mg)	Carb. (g)	Fiber (g)	Prot. (g)	Servings/Exchanges
Rockstar Energy Drink	8 oz	140	0	0	0	0	0	40	31	0	0	2 carb
R.W. Knudsen												
Recharge Sports	8 oz	70	0	0	0	0	0	25	18	0	0	1 carb
Simply Nutritious Mega Green	8 oz	130	0	0	0	0	0	35	31	0	1	2 carb
Simply Nutritious Plum Boost	8 oz	120	0	0	0	0	0	10	33	0	0	2 carb
Simply Nutritious VitaJuice	8 oz	120	0	0	0	0	0	40	31	0	0	2 carb
Sparkling Essence Organic Blueberry	8 oz	0	0	0	0	0	0	0	0	0	0	free
Ross Products												
Ensure	8 oz	250	6	55	1	0	5	190	41	0	9	2 1/2 carb, 1 fat
Ensure High Calcium	8 oz	220	6	50	1	0	<5	290	31	0	10	2 carb, 1 med-fat meat

Ensure High Protein	8 oz	230	6	50	1	0	<5	290	31	0	12	2 carb, 1 med-fat meat
Ensure Plus	8 oz	350	11	100	1.5	0	10	220	50	0	13	3 carb, 2 fat
Glucerna, Chocolate	8 oz	200	7	60	0.5	0	<5	210	27	5	10	2 carb, 2 fat

Slim-Fast

Easy to Digest	10.8-oz can	180	5	45	1	0	<5	240	26	3	10	1 med-fat meat, 1 1/2 carb
High Protein Extra Creamy Chocolate	10.8-oz can	190	5	45	2	0	10	220	24	5	15	1 1/2 carb, 2 lean meat
Lower Carb Creamy Chocolate	10.8-oz can	190	9	80	1.5	0	15	260	6	4	20	1/2 carb, 3 lean meat
Optima Creamy Milk Chocolate	10.8-oz can	190	6	25	2.5	0	5	200	25	5	10	1 1/2 carb, 1 med-fat meat
Original Creamy Milk Chocolate	10.8-oz can	220	3	25	1	0	5	220	40	5	10	2 1/2 carb, 1 lean meat

Snapple Elements

Diet Ice Drinks	8 oz	10	0	0	0	0	0	10	2	0	0	free

BEVERAGES, SODA, SPORTS/ENERGY DRINKS

	Serving	Calories	Fat (g)	Cal. from Fat	Sat. Fat (g)	Trans Fat (g)	Chol. (mg)	Sod. (mg)	Carb. (g)	Fiber (g)	Prot. (g)	Servings/Exchanges
Juice Drinks (Spark)	8 oz	110–130	0	0	0	0	0	10–35	28–29	0	0	2 carb
SoBe												
Adrenaline Rush Energy	8 oz	130	7	60	4.5	0	0	95	34	0	0	2 carb
Energy	8 oz	110	0	0	0	0	0	15	27	0	0	2 carb
Lean Diet Energy	8 oz	5	0	0	0	0	0	15	1	0	0	free
Lifewater	8 oz	40	0	0	0	0	0	20	17	0	0	1 carb
Nirvana	8 oz	120	0	0	0	0	0	15	29	0	0	2 carb
Power	8 oz	110	0	0	0	0	0	15	27	0	0	2 carb
Starbucks												
DoubleShot Coffee Drink	8 oz	170	7	60	4.5	0	25	85	22	0	5	1 low-fat milk, 1/2 carb
Frappuccino-Vanilla	8 oz	170	2.5	25	1.5	0	10	85	31	0	5	1 low-fat milk, 1 carb

BREAD, BAGELS, ROLLS, BISCUITS, TORTILLAS, PANCAKES, WAFFLES, STUFFING, CROUTONS

	Serving	Calories	Fat (g)	Cal. from Fat	Sat. Fat (g)	Trans Fat (g)	Chol. (mg)	Sod. (mg)	Carb. (g)	Fiber (g)	Prot. (g)	Servings/Exchanges
Bagel, Cinnamon Raisin	1, 2–3 inches	97	1	10	0	0	0	114	20	<1	4	1 starch
Bagel, Plain	1, 2–3 inches	95	<1	0	0	0	0	184	18	<1	4	1 starch
Biscuit	1, 2 1/2 inches	127	6	55	<1	0	0	368	17	<1	2	1 starch, 1 fat
Bread Sticks, Plain	2, 4-inch	42	1	10	0	0	0	66	7	0	1	1/2 starch
Bread, Butter Croissant	1, small	171	9	80	5	0	28	312	19	1	3	1 starch, 2 fat
Bread, Corn	1.5-oz piece	113	3	30	1	0	17	280	19	1	3	1 starch, 1 fat
Bread, Cracked Wheat	1 slice	65	1	10	0	0	0	134	12	1	2	1 starch

BREAD, BAGELS, ROLLS, BISCUITS, TORTILLAS

	Serving	Calories	Fat (g)	Cal. from Fat	Sat. Fat (g)	Trans Fat (g)	Chol. (mg)	Sod. (mg)	Carb. (g)	Fiber (g)	Prot. (g)	Servings/Exchanges
Bread, French, Vienna, or Sourdough	1 small slice	92	1	10	<1	0	0	208	18	<1	4	1 starch
Bread, Italian	1 slice	81	1	10	<1	0	0	175	15	<1	3	1 starch
Bread, Multi Grain	1 slice	69	1	10	0	0	0	109	11	2	3	1 starch
Bread, Oatmeal	1 slice	73	1	10	0	0	0	162	13	1	2	1 starch
Bread, Pita	1/2	82	<1	0	0	0	0	161	17	1	3	1 starch
Bread, Pita, Whole Wheat	1, large	170	2	20	0	0	0	340	35	5	6	2 starch
Bread, Pumpernickel	1 slice	80	1	10	0	0	0	215	15	2	3	1 starch
Bread, Raisin	1 slice	71	1	10	0	0	0	101	14	1	2	1 starch
Bread, Rye	1 slice	83	1	10	0	0	0	211	16	2	3	1 starch
Bread, Wheat Bran	1 slice	89	1	10	0	0	0	175	17	1	3	1 starch
Bread, Wheat, Reduced Calorie	2 slices	91	1	10	0	0	0	235	20	6	4	1 starch
Bread, White	1 slice	67	1	10	0	0	0	134	12	1	2	1 starch

	Serving											
Bread, White, Reduced Calorie	2 slices	95	1	10	0	0	0	208	20	5	4	1 starch
Bread, Whole Wheat	1 slice	69	1	10	0	0	0	148	13	2	3	1 starch
Bun, Hamburger	1/2	60	1	10	0	0	0	103	11	<1	2	1 starch
Bun, Hot Dog	1/2	61	1	10	0	0	0	120	11	<1	2	1 starch
Chapati	1, 6-inch	71	<1	0	0	0	0	131	15	2	3	1 starch
Croutons	1 cup	122	2	20	<1	0	0	209	22	2	4	1 1/2 starch
Egg Bread/Challah	1 slice	113	2	20	<1	0	20	197	19	<1	4	1 starch
English Muffin	1/2	67	0.5	5	0	0	0	132	13	1	2	1 starch
French Toast, Frozen	1 slice	126	4	35	1	0	48	292	19	<1	4	1 starch, 1 fat
French Toast, Homemade with 2% Milk	1 slice	149	7	65	2	0	75	311	16	NA	5	1 starch, 1 fat
Naan	1/4, large	75	2	20	0	0	9	90	13	<1	2	1 starch
Pancakes, Plain, Frozen	1, 4-inch	82	1	10	0	0	3	183	16	<1	2	1 starch
Roll, Plain	1	85	2	20	0.5	0	0	148	14	1	2	1 starch
Roll, Whole Wheat	1	74	1	10	0	0	0	134	14	2	2	1 starch

BREAD, BAGELS, ROLLS, BISCUITS, TORTILLAS

	Serving	Calories	Fat (g)	Cal. from Fat	Sat. Fat (g)	Trans Fat (g)	Chol. (mg)	Sod. (mg)	Carb. (g)	Fiber (g)	Prot. (g)	Servings/Exchanges
Taco Shells	2	124	6	55	1	0	0	98	17	2	2	1 starch, 1 fat
Tortilla, Corn	1, 6-inch	52	0.5	5	0	0	0	11	11	2	1	1 starch
Tortilla, Flour	1, 6-inch	112	3	30	<1	0	0	229	19	1	3	1 starch
Tortilla, Flour	1/3 of 10 1/2-inch	185	4	40	1	0	0	272	32	2	5	2 starch, 1 fat
Waffles, Toaster Style	1, 4-inch	96	3	30	<1	0	3	217	15	1	2	1 starch, 1 fat
Brands												
Aunt Hattie's												
All Natural 100% Whole Grain	1 slice	100	1.5	10	0	0	0	240	19	3	4	1 starch
All Natural Dark 12 Grain	1 slice	120	2	20	0	0	0	200	20	1	4	1 starch
All Natural Double Fiber	1 slice	100	1.5	10	0	0	0	190	22	6	4	1 1/2 starch
Homestyle Potato	1 slice	80	1	5	0	0	0	180	15	0	3	1 starch

Food	Serving										
Homestyle Wheat	1 slice	70	1	10	0	0	140	13	1	2	1 starch
Homestyle White	1 slice	70	1	10	0	0	160	13	0	2	1 starch
Light 9 Grain	2 slices	90	0.5	5	0	0	260	16	4	4	1 starch
Low Carb	1 slice	45	0.5	5	0	0	120	7	2	4	1/2 starch
Potato Hamburger Buns	1	140	2	20	0	0	220	25	1	4	1 1/2 starch
Potato Hot Dog Buns	1	140	2	20	0	0	250	25	1	5	1 1/2 starch
Soft Wheat with Buttermilk	1 slice	70	1	10	0	0	150	13	1	3	1 starch
Wheat Berry	1 slice	110	1.5	10	0	0	230	20	2	4	1 starch
Aunt Jemima											
Pancake/Waffle Mix, Buttermilk	1/3 cup	110	0.5	5	0	0	480	23	1	4	1 1/2 starch
Pancake/Waffle Mix, Original	1/3 cup	150	0	0	0	0	740	33	1	4	2 starch
Pancake/Waffle Mix, Whole Wheat	1/4 cup	120	0.5	5	0	0	620	26	3	4	2 starch

BREAD, BAGELS, ROLLS, BISCUITS, TORTILLAS

	Serving	Calories	Fat (g)	Cal. from Fat	Sat. Fat (g)	Trans Fat (g)	Chol. (mg)	Sod. (mg)	Carb. (g)	Fiber (g)	Prot. (g)	Servings/Exchanges
Betty Crocker												
Bisquick, Original	1/3 cup	160	5	45	1.5	1.5	0	490	26	1	3	2 starch, 1 fat
Heart Smart	1/3 cup	140	2.5	25	0	0	0	340	27	<1	3	2 starch, 1 fat
Food for Life												
Ezekial 4:9 100% Whole Wheat Sprouted	1 slice	80	0.5	5	0	0	0	75	15	3	4	1 starch
Ezekial 4:9 Low Sodium	1 slice	80	0.5	5	0	0	0	0	15	3	4	1 starch
Healthy Choice												
Hearty 100% Whole Grain	1 slice	80	1	10	0	0	0	170	18	3	3	1 starch
Hearty 7 Grain	1 slice	80	1	10	0	0	0	170	18	3	4	1 starch
Holsum												
Hamburger Buns	1	110	1.5	15	0	0	0	220	20	1	4	1 starch
Hot Dog Buns	1	110	1.5	15	0	0	0	220	20	1	4	1 starch

Thin White Sandwich	1 slice	70	1	10	0	0	0	160	14	0	2	1 starch
Home Pride												
Butter Top White	1 slice	70	1	10	0	0	0	140	14	0	2	1 starch
Jiffy												
Buttermilk Biscuit Mix	1/3 cup	160	5	45	2	0	<5	420	27	<1	5	2 starch, 1 fat
Corn Muffin Mix	1/4 cup	150	4.5	40	2	0	<5	340	27	<1	2	1 starch, 1 fat
Kellogg's Eggo												
French Toast Sticks	2 slices	220	6	60	1.5	0	25	540	35	<1	5	2 starch, 1 fat
Pancakes, Blueberry	3	260	8	70	1.5	0	15	500	42	1	6	3 starch, 2 fat
Pancakes, Buttermilk	3	280	9	80	1.5	0	15	580	44	1	6	2 starch, 2 fat
Waffles, Apple Cinnamon	2	190	6	60	1.5	0	15	370	29	1	4	2 starch, 1 fat
Waffles, Blueberry	2	190	6	60	1.5	0	15	370	29	<1	4	2 starch, 1 fat
Waffles, Buttermilk	2	180	6	60	2	0	15	420	26	1	5	2 starch, 1 fat
Waffles, Chocolate Chip	2	210	7	60	2.5	0	15	380	32	1	4	2 starch, 1 fat
Waffles, Cinnamon Toast	3	300	11	100	3	0	20	490	45	1	5	3 starch, 2 fat

BREAD, BAGELS, ROLLS, BISCUITS, TORTILLAS

	Serving	Calories	Fat (g)	Cal. from Fat	Sat. Fat (g)	Trans Fat (g)	Chol. (mg)	Sod. (mg)	Carb. (g)	Fiber (g)	Prot. (g)	Servings/Exchanges
Waffles, French Toast	1	140	6	50	2	0	10	240	19	<1	3	1 starch, 1 fat
Waffles, Homestyle	2	190	7	70	2	0	20	430	27	<1	4	2 starch, 1 fat
Waffles, Minis Homestyle	3	260	10	90	2.5	0	25	610	38	1	6	2 1/2 starch, 2 fat
Waffles, Nutri-Grain Whole Wheat	2	170	6	50	1.5	0	0	400	26	3	4	2 starch, 1 fat
Waffles, Special K	3	160	2.5	20	0.5	0	20	440	29	<1	5	2 starch, 1 fat
Waffles, Waf-Fulls, Strawberry	1	170	5	45	1.5	0	10	300	27	<1	3	2 starch, 1 fat
Krusteaz												
Buttermilk Pancakes	3	280	4	35	0.5	0	10	710	52	3	8	3 1/2 starch, 1 fat
Homestyle French Toast	2	230	5	50	1	0	95	540	36	2	9	2 1/2 starch, 1 fat
Mini Pancakes	12	220	2.5	20	0.5	0	0	580	43	2	6	3 starch, 1 fat
Marshall's												

Biscuits, Buttermilk	3	240	12	110	3	3.5	0	600	29	1	4	2 starch, 2 fat
Biscuits, Homestyle	1	120	6	50	3	1.5	0	330	15	0	2	1 starch, 1 fat
Milton's												
Gourmet White	1 slice	110	0.5	5	0	0	0	110	23	1	4	1 1/2 starch
Multi-Grain 100% Whole Wheat Bread	1 slice	110	0.5	5	0	0	0	220	22	5	5	1 1/2 starch
Whole Grain Plus	1 slice	90	0.5	5	0	0	0	125	16	5	4	1 starch
Mission												
96% Fat Free Flour Tortilla, Large Burrito Size	1	180	2.5	20	0.5	0	0	450	35	5	5	2 starch, 1 fat
96% Fat Free Flour Tortilla, Medium Soft Taco Size	1	130	1.5	15	0	0	0	330	26	3	4	2 starch
96% Fat Free Whole Wheat Flour Tortilla, Soft Taco Size	1	130	2	15	0	0	0	340	25	3	4	1 1/2 starch

BREAD, BAGELS, ROLLS, BISCUITS, TORTILLAS

	Serving	Calories	Carb. (g)	Fat (g)	Cal. from Fat	Sat. Fat (g)	Trans Fat (g)	Chol. (mg)	Sod. (mg)	Fiber (g)	Prot. (g)	Servings/Exchanges
Carb Balance Flour Tortilla, Fajita Size	1	80	2	15	0	0	0	220	12	7	3	1 starch
Carb Balance Flour Tortilla, Medium Soft Taco Size	1	120	3.5	25	1.5	0	0	330	18	11	5	1 starch, 1 fat
Carb Balance Whole Wheat Flour Tortilla, Small Fajita Size	1	80	2	10	0	0	0	220	12	8	3	1 starch
Life Balance Flour Tortilla, Medium Soft Taco Size	1	130	3	30	1.5	0	0	290	20	3	4	1 starch, 1 fat
Life Balance Whole Wheat Tortilla, Soft Taco Size	1	130	3	30	1.5	0	0	310	19	4	4	1 starch, 1 fat
Multi-Grain Flour Tortilla, Soft Taco Size	1	150	4.5	35	1.5	0	0	460	23	5	5	1 1/2 starch, 1 fat

Tortilla Wraps, Jalapeño Cheddar	1	210	4.5	40	2	0	850	35	1	5	2 starch, 1 fat
Tortilla Wraps, Multi-Grain	1	210	6	50	2.5	0	660	32	7	6	2 starch, 1 fat
Tortilla Wraps, Sun Dried Tomato Basil	1	210	4.5	40	2	0	570	35	2	6	2 starch, 1 fat
Tortilla, Large Burrito Size	1	210	5	45	2	0	630	36	1	6	2 1/2 starch, 1 fat
Tortilla, Medium Soft Taco	1	150	3.5	35	1.5	0	440	25	1	4	1 1/2 starch, 1 fat
Tortilla, Small Fajita	1	110	3	25	1	0	320	18	1	3	1 starch, 1 fat
White Corn Tortilla	2	90	1	10	0	0	10	17	3	2	1 starch
Yellow Corn Tortilla	2	110	1.5	15	0	0	10	22	3	2	1 1/2 starch
Mrs. Cubbinson's											
Caesar Salad	5	35	0	0	0	0	65	4	0	<1	1/2 starch
Fat Free Herb Seasoned	5	30	0	0	0	0	105	5	0	1	1/2 starch

BREAD, BAGELS, ROLLS, BISCUITS, TORTILLAS

	Serving	Calories	Fat (g)	Cal. from Fat	Sat. Fat (g)	Trans Fat (g)	Chol. (mg)	Sod. (mg)	Carb. (g)	Fiber (g)	Prot. (g)	Servings/Exchanges
Nature's Own												
100% Whole Wheat	1 slice	60	1	10	0	0	0	125	11	2	4	1 starch
Double Fiber Wheat	1 slice	50	0.5	5	0	0	0	135	13	5	3	1 starch
Honey Wheat	1 slice	70	0.5	5	0	0	0	120	14	<1	2	1 starch
White Wheat	2 slices	100	2	15	0	0	0	230	22	5	6	1 1/2 starch
Old El Paso												
Taco Shells, Corn	3	150	7	60	3	0	0	135	19	1	2	1 starch, 1 fat
Tostada Shells, Corn	3	150	7	60	3	0	0	135	19	1	2	1 starch, 1 fat
Oroweatx												
100% Whole Wheat English Muffin	1	130	1.5	15	0	0	0	240	25	4	5	1 1/2 starch
100% Whole Wheat Hamburger Buns	1	180	3	25	0.5	0	0	370	32	6	9	2 starch, 1 fat
Country Buttermilk	1 slice	100	1	10	0	0	0	180	19	<1	3	1 starch

Country Potato	1 slice	100	1	10	0	0	190	20	<1	3	1 starch
Country White	1 slice	110	1.5	15	0	0	240	20	<1	3	1 starch
Double Fiber	1 slice	70	1	10	0	0	160	16	6	3	1 starch
Health Nut	1 slice	100	2	20	0	0	190	18	2	4	1 starch
Jewish Rye	1 slice	80	1	10	0	0	170	15	1	3	1 starch
Oatnut	1 slice	100	1.5	15	0	0	190	19	1	4	1 starch
Russian Rye	1 slice	70	1	10	0	0	200	13	<1	2	1 starch
Seven Grain	1 slice	100	1	10	0	0	180	20	2	3	1 starch
Whole Grain & Flax Seed	1 slice	100	1.5	15	0	0	160	17	3	4	1 starch
Ortega											
Taco Shells, Corn	2	120	6	50	1	0	170	16	2	2	1 starch, 1 fat
Tostada Shells	2	120	6	50	1	0	170	19	2	2	1 starch, 1 fat
Pepperidge Farm											
9 Grain	1 slice	100	2	15	0	0	130	20	3	4	1 starch
German Dark Wheat	1 slice	100	1.5	15	0	0	150	20	3	4	1 starch

BREAD, BAGELS, ROLLS, BISCUITS, TORTILLAS

	Serving	Calories	Fat (g)	Cal. from Fat	Sat. Fat (g)	Trans Fat (g)	Chol. (mg)	Sod. (mg)	Carb. (g)	Fiber (g)	Prot. (g)	Servings/Exchanges
Honey Flax	1 slice	100	2	15	0	0	0	120	19	3	5	1 starch
Bagels and Rolls												
Bagel, Cinnamon and Raisin	1	270	1	10	0	0	0	450	57	3	8	4 starch
Bagel, Everything	1	260	1.5	15	0.5	0	0	480	53	2	9	3 1/2 starch
Bagel, Mini Plain	1	110	0.5	5	0	0	0	200	22	1	4	1 1/2 starch
Bagel, Plain	1	260	1	10	0	0	0	500	54	3	9	3 1/2 starch
Buns, Sandwich with Sesame Seeds	1	130	3	30	0.5	0	0	220	22	1	5	1 1/2 starch, 1 fat
Buns, Classic 100% Whole Wheat Hamburger	1	120	2	20	0	0	0	190	18	2	6	1 starch
English Muffin, 100% Whole Wheat	1	140	1.5	15	0.5	0	0	210	26	3	6	2 starch

English Muffin, Original	1	130	1.5	15	0.5	0	170	25	1	5	1 1/2 starch
Mini Bagel, Brown Sugar Cinnamon	1	120	0.5	5	0	0	150	24	2	4	1 1/2 starch
Rolls, Hamburger Classic	1	120	2	20	0.5	0	180	22	1	5	1 1/2 starch
Rolls, Soft Country Dinner	1	90	1.5	15	0	0	150	17	1	3	1 starch
Rolls, Soft Hoagie with Sesame Seeds	1	210	6	55	1.5	0	350	35	2	7	2 starch, 1 fat
Croutons											
Seasoned	6	30	1	10	0	0	75	5	0	<1	1/2 starch
Whole Grain	6	30	1	10	0	0	70	5	<1	1	1/2 starch
Farm House Hearty Sliced Bread											
12 Grain	1 slice	120	2	15	0	0	180	21	3	4	1 starch
7 Grain	1 slice	110	1.5	15	0.5	0	170	21	2	4	1 starch
Crunchy Oat	1 slice	120	1.5	15	0.5	0	160	21	2	5	1 starch
Hearty White	1 slice	120	1.5	15	0.5	0	250	22	1	4	1 starch

BREAD, BAGELS, ROLLS, BISCUITS, TORTILLAS

	Serving	Calories	Fat (g)	Cal. from Fat	Sat. Fat (g)	Trans Fat (g)	Chol. (mg)	Sod. (mg)	Carb. (g)	Fiber (g)	Prot. (g)	Servings/Exchanges
Soft 100% Whole Wheat	1 slice	110	2	15	0.5	0	0	150	19	3	5	1 starch
Soft Oatmeal	1 slice	120	1.5	15	0.5	0	0	200	21	1	4	1 starch
Sourdough	1 slice	120	1.5	15	0.5	0	0	220	22	1	4	1 starch
Sweet Buttermilk	1 slice	120	1.5	15	0.5	0	0	190	23	1	4	1 starch
Hot & Crusty Breads												
Twin French	4-inch slice	150	1.5	15	0	0	0	260	29	1	5	1 starch
Light Style Breads												
Extra Fiber	3 slices	120	1	10	0	0	0	250	26	6	6	1 1/2 starch
Oatmeal	3 slices	140	1	10	0	0	0	260	27	2	7	2 starch
Seven Grain	3 slices	130	1	10	0	0	0	270	26	4	7	
Soft Wheat	3 slices	130	1.5	15	0	0	0	270	25	4	8	1 1/2 starch
Party Breads												
Dark Pumpernickel	5 slices	130	1.5	15	0	0	0	320	23	3	5	1 1/2 starch

Jewish Rye	5 slices	130	2	18	0	0	460	25	2	4	1 1/2 starch
Rye & Pumpernickel											
Deli Swirl	1 slice	80	1	10	0	0	180	14	1	3	1 starch
Pumpernickel	1 slice	80	1	10	0	0	190	15	1	3	1 starch
Seedless Rye	1 slice	80	1	10	0	0	180	14	1	3	1 starch
Variety Breads											
100% Whole Wheat Thin Sliced	1 slice	70	1	10	0	0	65	12	2	2	1 starch
Oatmeal	1 slice	70	1	10	0	0	85	12	1	2	1 starch
Very Thin Breads											
100% Whole Wheat	3 slices	110	2	20	0.5	0	230	20	3	4	1 starch
White	3 slices	120	1	10	0	0	250	24	1	4	1 1/2 starch
White Breads											
Italian Bread	1 slice	90	1	10	0	0	190	17	<1	3	1 starch
Original Whole Grain White	2 slices	110	2	20	0.5	0	200	22	3	4	1 1/2 starch

BREAD, BAGELS, ROLLS, BISCUITS, TORTILLAS

	Serving	Calories	Fat (g)	Cal. from Fat	Sat. Fat (g)	Trans Fat (g)	Chol. (mg)	Sod. (mg)	Carb. (g)	Fiber (g)	Prot. (g)	Servings/Exchanges
Sandwich	2 slices	130	2.5	25	0.5	0	0	250	23	<1	4	1 1/2 starch, 1 fat
Pillsbury												
Bread, Crusty French	1/6 batch	120	1.5	15	0.5	0	0	300	24	<1	4	1 1/2 starch
Crescent Rolls, Original	1	110	6	60	2	1.5	0	220	11	0	2	1 starch, 1 fat
Crescent Rolls, Reduced Fat	1	90	4.5	35	0.5	0	0	220	12	0	2	1 starch, 1 fat
Crescent Rounds	1	110	6	60	2	1.5	0	220	11	0	2	1 starch, 1 fat
Pizza Crust, Thin	1/5 can	180	5	45	1	0	0	360	29	1	5	2 starch, 1 fat
Pillsbury Grands												
Big Biscuits, Butter Tastin	1	180	8	70	2	3.5	0	580	25	<1	3	1 1/2 starch, 2 fat
Big Biscuits, Buttermilk	1	180	8	70	2	2	0	540	25	<1	3	1 1/2 starch, 2 fat
Big Biscuits, Flaky Layers	1	180	8	70	2	2	0	540	25	<1	4	1 1/2 starch, 2 fat

Big Biscuits, Reduced Fat Flaky Layers	1	160	6	50	2	0	0	570	26	<1	4	2 starch, 1 fat
Biscuits, Buttermilk	1	100	4	40	1	1	0	360	14	<1	2	1 starch, 1 fat
Biscuits, Honey Butter	1	110	4	35	1	1	0	290	15	0	2	1 starch, 1 fat
Progresso												
Bread Crumbs, Italian Style	1/4 cup	110	1.5	15	0.5	0	0	470	20	1	4	1 starch
Bread Crumbs, Parmesan	1/4 cup	110	1.5	15	0.5	0	0	870	19	1	4	1 starch
Bread Crumbs, Plain	1/4 cup	110	1.5	15	0.5	0	0	220	19	1	4	1 starch
Roman Meal												
Sandwich Bread	1 slice	60	1	5	0	0	0	140	12	1	3	1 starch
Whole Grain Bread	2 slices	130	2	15	0	0	0	240	24	2	5	1 1/2 starch
Rudi's Organic												
100% Whole Wheat bread	1 slice	100	1	10	0	0	0	140	19	3	4	1 starch

BREAD, BAGELS, ROLLS, BISCUITS, TORTILLAS

	Serving	Calories	Fat (g)	Cal. from Fat	Sat. Fat (g)	Trans Fat (g)	Chol. (mg)	Sod. (mg)	Carb. (g)	Fiber (g)	Prot. (g)	Servings/Exchanges
7 Grain Flax	1 slice	100	1.5	15	0	0	0	150	18	4	4	1 starch
Honey Whole Wheat	1 slice	100	1	10	0	0	0	170	19	3	5	1 starch
Multigrain Oat	1 slice	110	1	10	0	0	0	180	21	2	4	1 starch
Spelt	1 slice	100	1	10	0	0	0	210	22	2	3	1 starch
Spelt Ancient Grain	1 slice	120	2.5	25	0	0	0	170	20	2	4	1 starch, 1 fat
Wheat & Oat	1 slice	90	1	10	0	0	0	190	18	4	3	1 starch
Sara Lee												
Classic White	2 slices	160	2	20	0.5	0	0	270	30	1	5	2 starch
Whole Grain White	2 slices	150	2	20	0.5	0	0	220	28	2	5	2 starch
Shake 'N Bake												
Coating Mix, Classic Italian	1/8 pkt	35	0.5	5	0	0	0	280	7	0	<1	1/2 starch
Coating Mix, Original Chicken	1/8 pkt	40	1	10	0	0	0	220	7	0	<1	1/2 starch

Coating Mix, Original Pork	1/8 pkt	40	0	0	0	0	240	8	0	1	1/2 starch
Coating Mix, Parmesan	1/8 pkt	35	0.5	5	0	0	290	7	0	1	1/2 starch
Stove Top											
Stuffing Mix for Pork	1/2 cup	160	7	60	1.5	0	510	21	1	3	1 starch, 2 fat
Stuffing Mix for Turkey	1/2 cup	160	7	60	1.5	0	520	21	1	3	1 starch, 2 fat
Stuffing Mix, Chicken Flavor	1/2 cup	150	7	60	1	0	520	20	<1	3	1 starch, 2 fat
Stuffing Mix, Corn Bread	1/2 cup	160	7	60	1.5	0	570	22	<1	3	1 1/2 starch, 2 fat
Stuffing Mix, Herbs	1/2 cup	160	7	60	1.5	0	530	21	1	3	1 starch, 2 fat
Trader Joe's											
100% Stone Ground Whole Grain	1 slice	100	0.5	5	0	0	200	22	3	4	1 1/2 starch
100% Whole Grain Fiber Bread	1 slice	90	1	10	0	0	160	20	5	4	1 starch

BREAD, BAGELS, ROLLS, BISCUITS, TORTILLAS

	Serving	Calories	Fat (g)	Cal. from Fat	Sat. Fat (g)	Trans Fat (g)	Chol. (mg)	Sod. (mg)	Carb. (g)	Fiber (g)	Prot. (g)	Servings/Exchanges
California Style Complete Protein	1 slice	90	0.5	5	0	0	0	160	15	2	5	1 starch
Gourmet White	1 slice	120	3.5	35	0	0	0	260	19	1	3	1 starch, 1 fat
Harvest Whole Wheat	1 slice	90	1	10	0	0	0	180	19	3	3	1 1/2 starch
Multi-Grain	1 slice	120	1	10	0	0	0	170	24	1	3	1 1/2 starch
Omega Seed Bread	1 slice	140	4	35	0.5	0	0	140	22	3	4	1 1/2 starch, 1 fat
Organic Flourless Sprouted 7 Grain	1 slice	80	0.5	5	0	0	0	65	16	3	4	1 starch
Potato	1 slice	110	1.5	10	0	0	0	180	20	1	4	1 starch
Seeded Harvest	2 oz	130	2	20	0	0	0	250	25	2	5	1 1/2 starch
Sprouted Multigrain	1 slice	90	0.5	5	0	0	0	170	15	2	5	1 starch
Sprouted Wheat Berry	1 slice	90	1	10	0	0	0	140	18	2	4	1 starch
Whole Grain	1 slice	90	0.5	5	0	0	0	200	19	3	3	1 starch
Whole Wheat	1 slice	100	1.5	15	0	0	0	190	20	3	5	1 starch

Wonder

Classic White	1 slice	70	1	10	0	0	0	150	14	0	2	1 starch
Made with Whole Grain White	2 slices	130	2	20	0.5	0	0	300	25	4	6	1 1/2 starch
Texas Toast	1 slice	100	1	10	0	0	0	200	19	<1	3	1 starch

BREAKFAST CEREAL, READY-TO-EAT CEREAL, HOT CEREAL

	Serving	Calories	Fat (g)	Cal. from Fat	Sat. Fat (g)	Trans Fat (g)	Chol. (mg)	Sod. (mg)	Carb. (g)	Fiber (g)	Prot. (g)	Servings/Exchanges
Bran, 100%, Wheat,	1/2 cup	63	1	10	0	0	0	1	19	12	5	1 starch
Bran, Oat, Uncooked	1/4 cup	58	2	20	0	0	0	1	16	4	4	1 starch
Bulgur, Cooked	1/2 cup	76	0	0	0	0	0	5	17	4	3	1 starch
Corn Grits, White or Yellow, Cooked	1/2 cup	71	0	0	0	0	0	2	16	<1	2	1 starch
Cream of Rice, Cooked	1/2 cup	63	0	0	0	0	0	1	14	<1	1	1 starch
Cream of Wheat, Cooked	1/2 cup	65	0	0	0	0	0	69	13	<1	2	1 starch
Farina, Cooked	1/2 cup	56	0	0	0	0	0	2	12	<1	2	1 starch
Granola, Homemade	1/2 cup	298	15	135	2.5	0	0	15	33	6	9	2 starch, 3 fat
Kasha or Buckwheat Groats, Cooked	1/2 cup	77	0.5	5	0	0	0	3	17	2	3	1 starch
Millet, Cooked	1/4 cup	52	0.5	5	0	0	0	1	10	<1	2	1/2 starch

Muesli	1/4 cup	74	1	10	0	0	0	64	15	2	2	1 starch
Oatmeal Cereal, Cooked	1/2 cup	73	1	10	<1	0	0	1	13	2	3	1 starch
Puffed Rice	1 1/2 cup	80	0	0	0	0	0	1	18	<1	2	1 starch
Puffed Wheat	1 1/2 cup	66	0.5	5	0	0	0	1	14	2	3	1 starch
Shredded Wheat, Plain	1/2 cup	83	0	0	0	0	0	2	20	3	3	1 starch
Wheatena, Cooked	1/2 cup	68	0.5	5	0	0	0	2	14	3	2	1 starch

Brands

Active Lifestyle

Original	1 cup	110	0	0	0	0	0	220	22	<1	7	1 1/2 starch
Strawberry	1 cup	110	0	0	0	0	0	220	25	1	3	1 1/2 starch

General Mills

Basic 4	1 cup	200	2	20	1	0	0	320	43	3	4	3 starch
Boo Berry	1 cup	130	1	10	0	0	0	190	28	1	1	2 starch
Cheerios	1 cup	100	2	15	0	0	0	190	20	3	3	1 starch
Cheerios Plus, Multi-Grain	1 cup	110	1	10	0	0	0	200	24	3	2	1 1/2 starch

BREAKFAST CEREAL, READY-TO-EAT CEREAL, HOT CEREAL

	Serving	Calories	Fat (g)	Cal. from Fat	Sat. Fat (g)	Trans Fat (g)	Chol. (mg)	Sod. (mg)	Carb. (g)	Fiber (g)	Prot. (g)	Servings/Exchanges
Cheerios, Apple Cinnamon	3/4 cup	120	1.5	15	0	0	0	120	25	1	2	1 1/2 starch
Cheerios, Banana Nut	3/4 cup	100	1	10	0	0	0	160	23	1	1	1 1/2 starch
Cheerios, Berry Burst Triple Berry	1 cup	100	1	10	0	0	0	170	22	2	2	1 1/2 starch
Cheerios, Frosted	3/4 cup	110	1	10	0	0	0	170	23	2	2	1 1/2 starch
Cheerios, Fruity	3/4 cup	100	1.5	15	0	0	0	135	23	2	1	1 1/2 starch
Cheerios, Honey Nut	3/4 cup	110	1.5	15	0	0	0	190	22	2	2	1 1/2 starch
Cheerios, Oat Cluster Crunch	3/4 cup	100	1	10	0	0	0	135	22	2	2	1 1/2 starch
Cheerios, Yogurt Burst Strawberries	3/4 cup	120	1.5	15	0.5	0	0	180	24	2	2	1 1/2 starch
Chex, Chocolate	3/4 cup	130	2.5	25	0.5	0	0	240	26	<1	2	2 starch, 1 fat
Chex, Cinnamon	3/4 cup	120	2	20	0	0	0	190	25	0	2	1 1/2 starch

Chex, Corn	1 cup	120	0.5	0	0	0	290	26	1	2	2 starch
Chex, Honey Nut	3/4 cup	120	0.5	5	0	0	230	28	1	2	2 starch
Chex, Multi-Bran	1 cup	160	1.5	10	0	0	310	39	6	3	2 1/2 starch
Chex, Rice	1 cup	100	0	0	0	0	250	23	0	2	1 1/2 starch
Chex, Strawberry	3/4 cup	130	2	15	0	0	200	26	<1	1	2 starch
Chex, Wheat	1 cup	160	1	10	0	0	340	38	5	5	2 1/2 starch
Cinnamon Toast Crunch	3/4 cup	130	3	30	0.5	0	220	25	1	1	1 1/2 starch, 1 fat
Cinnamon Toast Crunch, Reduced Sugar	3/4 cup	110	2.5	20	0	0	170	23	3	2	1 1/2 starch, 1 fat
Cocoa Puffs	1 cup	110	1.5	10	0	0	150	23	1	1	1 1/2 starch
Cookie Crisp	1 cup	100	1	10	0	0	150	22	1	1	1 1/2 starch
Cookie Crisp, Sprinkles	3/4 cup	100	1	10	0	0	150	23	1	1	1 1/2 starch
Count Chocula	3/4 cup	110	1	10	0	0	160	23	1	1	1 1/2 starch
Country Corn Flakes	1 cup	120	0.5	5	0	0	300	28	1	2	2 starch
Dora the Explorer	3/4 cup	100	1.5	15	0	0	180	23	3	1	1 1/2 starch
Fiber One	1/2 cup	60	1	10	0	0	105	25	14	2	1 1/2 starch

BREAKFAST CEREAL, READY-TO-EAT CEREAL, HOT CEREAL

	Serving	Calories	Fat (g)	Cal. from Fat	Sat. Fat (g)	Trans Fat (g)	Chol. (mg)	Sod. (mg)	Carb. (g)	Fiber (g)	Prot. (g)	Servings/Exchanges
Fiber One, Caramel Delight	1 cup	180	3	25	0	0	0	260	41	9	3	2 1/2 starch, 1 fat
Fiber One, Frosted Shredded Wheat	1 cup	200	1	10	0	0	0	0	50	9	5	3 starch
Fiber One, Honey Clusters	1 cup	160	1.5	15	0	0	0	290	42	13	5	3 starch
Fiber One, Raisin Bran Clusters	1 cup	170	1	10	0	0	0	260	45	11	4	3 starch
Frankenberry	1 cup	130	1.5	10	0	0	0	190	28	1	1	2 starch
Golden Grahams	3/4 cup	120	1	10	0	0	0	270	26	1	2	2 starch
Honey Kix	1 1/4 cup	120	1	10	0	0	0	230	28	3	2	2 starch
Honey Nut Clusters	1 cup	210	1	10	0	0	0	290	49	3	4	3 starch
Kaboom	1 1/4 cup	110	1	10	0	0	0	210	28	4	1	2 starch
Kix	1 1/4 cup	110	1	5	0	0	0	210	26	3	2	1 1/2 starch

Food	Serving										Exchanges
Kix, Berry Berry	3/4 cup	100	1	10	0	0	180	22	1	1	1 1/2 starch
Lucky Charms	1 cup	110	1	10	0	0	190	22	1	2	1 1/2 starch
Lucky Charms, Chocolate	1 cup	110	1	10	0	0	160	24	1	1	1 1/2 starch
Oatmeal Crisp, Almond	1 cup	240	5	45	0	0	250	47	4	5	3 starch, 1 fat
Oatmeal Crisp, HeartyRaisin	1 cup	230	2.5	20	0.5	0	135	51	4	5	3 1/2 starch, 1 fat
Para Su Familia Raisin Bran	1 1/4 cup	170	1	10	0	0	300	41	6	4	2 1/2 starch
Raisin Nut Bran	3/4 cup	180	3	30	0.5	0	230	38	5	4	2 1/2 starch, 1 fat
Reese's Puffs	3/4 cup	120	3	30	0.5	0	180	22	1	2	1 1/2 starch, 1 fat
Total Blueberry Pomegranate	1 cup	170	2	15	0	0	95	38	4	5	2 1/2 starch
Total Cinnamon Crunch	1 cup	190	2.5	25	0	0	200	40	4	4	2 1/2 starch, 1 fat
Total Cranberry Crunch	1 1/4 cup	190	1.5	15	0	0	230	44	4	4	3 starch
Total Raisin Bran	1 cup	160	1	5	0	0	230	40	5	3	2 1/2 starch

BREAKFAST CEREAL, READY-TO-EAT CEREAL, HOT CEREAL

	Serving	Calories	Fat (g)	Cal. from Fat	Sat. Fat (g)	Trans Fat (g)	Chol. (mg)	Sod. (mg)	Carb. (g)	Fiber (g)	Prot. (g)	Servings/Exchanges
Total Whole-Grain	3/4 cup	100	0.5	5	0	0	0	190	23	3	2	1 1/2 starch
Trix	1 cup	120	1	10	0	0	0	190	28	1	1	2 starch
Wheaties	3/4 cup	100	0.5	5	0	0	0	190	22	3	3	1 1/2 starch
Health Valley Organic												
Cranberry Crunch	3/4 cup	190	4	35	0	0	0	100	38	3	4	2 1/2 starch, 1 fat
Heart Wise	1 cup	200	3	25	0	0	0	140	37	5	11	2 1/2 starch, 1 fat
Low Fat Date Almond Flavor Granola	2/3 cup	180	1	10	0	0	0	90	43	6	5	3 starch
Low Fat Raisin Cinnamon Fruit Granola	2/3 cup	180	1	10	0	0	0	90	43	6	5	3 starch
Organic Amaranth Flakes	1 cup	100	1	10	0	0	0	90	23	3	3	1 1/2 starch
Organic Blue Corn Flakes	3/4 cup	100	0	0	0	0	0	10	24	3	3	1 1/2 starch

Organic Chocolate Blast-Ems	3/4 cup	120	1.5	15	0	0	0	90	25	3	3	1 1/2 starch
Organic Fiber 7	1 cup	160	1	10	0	0	0	100	37	7	6	2 1/2 starch
Organic Golden Flax Cereal	1 cup	180	3.5	30	0	0	0	65	37	6	6	2 1/2 starch, 1 fat
Organic Multi-Grain Apple Cinnamon Square-Ems	1 1/4 cup	210	3	30	0	0	0	125	44	8	5	3 starch, 1 fat
Organic Oat Bran Flakes	1 cup	190	1.5	15	0.5	0	0	190	39	4	5	2 1/2 starch
Kashi												
7 Grain Puffs	1 cup	70	0.5	5	0	0	0	0	15	1	2	1 starch
7 Whole Grain Flakes	1 cup	180	1	10	0	0	0	150	41	6	6	2 1/2 starch
Cinnamon Harvest	1 cup	190	1	10	0	0	0	0	44	5	4	3 starch
GoLean	1 cup	140	1	10	0	0	0	85	30	10	13	2 starch
GoLean Crunch	1 cup	190	3	25	0	0	0	100	37	8	9	2 1/2 starch, 1 fat
GoLean Crunch Honey Almond Flax	1 cup	200	4.5	40	0	0	0	140	36	8	9	2 1/2 starch, 1 fat

BREAKFAST CEREAL, READY-TO-EAT CEREAL, HOT CEREAL

	Serving	Calories	Fat (g)	Cal. from Fat	Sat. Fat (g)	Trans Fat (g)	Chol. (mg)	Sod. (mg)	Carb. (g)	Fiber (g)	Prot. (g)	Servings/Exchanges
Good Friends	1 cup	160	1.5	15	0	0	0	110	42	12	5	3 starch
Good Friends Cinna-Raisin Crunch	1 cup	170	1.5	15	0	0	0	105	41	8	4	3 starch
Heart to Heart Honey Toasted	3/4 cup	110	1.5	15	0	0	0	90	25	5	4	1 1/2 starch
Heart to Heart Oat Flakes & Wild Blueberry Clusters	1 cup	200	2	15	0	0	0	135	44	4	6	3 starch
Heart to Heart Warm Cinnamon	3/4 cup	110	1.5	15	0	0	0	80	24	5	4	1 1/2 starch
Honey Sunshine	3/4 cup	100	1.5	10	0	0	0	135	25	6	2	1 1/2 starch
Island Vanilla	27 biscuits	180	1	5	0	0	0	0	44	6	6	3 starch
Organic Promise Autumn Wheat	29 biscuits	180	1	10	0	0	0	0	43	6	6	3 starch

Organic Promise Strawberry Fields	1 cup	120	0	0	0	0	200	28	1	2	2 starch
Vive Toasted Graham & Vanilla	1 1/4 cup	170	2.5	25	1	0	100	43	12	4	3 starch, 2 fat
Kellogg's											
All-Bran	1/2 cup	80	1	10	0	0	80	23	10	4	1 1/2 starch
All-Bran Bran Buds	1/3 cup	70	1	10	0	0	200	24	13	2	1 1/2 starch
All-Bran Complete Wheat Flakes	3/4 cup	90	0.5	5	0	0	210	23	5	3	1 1/2 starch
All-Bran Yogurt Bites	1 1/4 cup	190	3	30	0	0	240	44	10	6	3 starch, 1 fat
Apple Jacks	1 cup	100	0.5	5	0	0	130	25	3	1	1 1/2 starch
Cocoa Krispies	3/4 cup	120	1	10	0.5	0	150	27	1	1	2 starch
Corn Flakes	1 cup	100	0	0	0	0	200	24	1	2	1 1/2 starch
Corn Flakes Touch of Honey	1 cup	120	0	0	0	0	220	27	<1	2	2 starch
Corn Pops	1 cup	110	0	0	0	0	110	26	0	1	2 starch

BREAKFAST CEREAL, READY-TO-EAT CEREAL, HOT CEREAL

	Serving	Calories	Fat (g)	Cal. from Fat	Sat. Fat (g)	Trans Fat (g)	Chol. (mg)	Sod. (mg)	Carb. (g)	Fiber (g)	Prot. (g)	Servings/Exchanges
Cracklin' Oat Bran	3/4 cup	200	7	60	3	0	0	150	35	6	4	2 starch, 1 fat
Crispix	1 cup	110	0	0	0	0	0	220	25	<1	2	2 starch
Eggo Cinnamon Toast	1 cup	130	3	30	0	0	0	130	26	2	2	2 starch, 1 fat
Froot Loops	1 cup	110	1	10	0.5	0	0	135	25	3	1	1 1/2 starch
Frosted Flakes	3/4 cup	110	0	0	0	0	0	140	27	1	1	2 starch
Frosted Flakes, 1/3 Less Sugar	1 cup	120	0	0	0	0	0	180	28	<1	1	2 starch
Frosted Mini-Wheats Little Bites Chocolate	52 biscuits	200	2	15	1	0	0	200	45	6	5	3 starch
Frosted Mini-Wheats Little Bites Honey Nut	46 biscuits	190	1	10	0	0	0	120	47	6	5	3 starch
Frosted Mini-Wheats Strawberry Delight	24 biscuits	180	1	10	0	0	0	0	43	5	4	3 starch
Honey Smacks	3/4 cup	100	0.5	5	0	0	0	50	24	1	2	1 1/2 starch

Keebler Cookie Crunch	1 cup	110	1	10	0	0	0	170	26	1	2	2 starch
Mini-Wheats, Big Bite	5 biscuits	180	1	10	0	0	0	5	41	5	5	3 starch
Mini-Wheats, Blueberry	24 biscuits	180	1	10	0	0	0	0	43	5	4	3 starch
Mini-Wheats, Frosted Bite Size	24 biscuits	200	1	10	0	0	0	5	48	6	6	3 starch
Mini-Wheats, Frosted Maple & Brown Sugar	24 biscuits	190	1	10	0	0	0	0	44	5	4	3 starch
Product 19	1 cup	100	0	0	0	0	0	210	25	1	2	1 1/2 starch
Raisin Bran	1 cup	190	1.5	15	0	0	0	350	45	7	5	3 starch
Raisin Bran Crunch	1 cup	190	1	9	0	0	0	210	45	4	3	3 starch
Raisin Bran Extra	1 cup	190	3	25	1.5	0	0	350	44	7	5	3 starch
Rice Krispies	1 1/4 cup	130	0	0	0	0	0	220	29	<1	2	2 starch
Smart Start Original	1 cup	190	0.5	5	0	0	0	280	43	3	3	3 starch
Smart Start Strong Heart Strawberry Bites	30 biscuits	200	2.5	20	0.5	0	0	130	43	6	6	3 starch, 1 fat

BREAKFAST CEREAL, READY-TO-EAT CEREAL, HOT CEREAL

	Serving	Calories	Fat (g)	Cal. from Fat	Sat. Fat (g)	Trans Fat (g)	Chol. (mg)	Sod. (mg)	Carb. (g)	Fiber (g)	Prot. (g)	Servings/Exchanges
Smart Start Toasted Oat	1 1/4 cup	220	2.5	20	0.5	0	0	140	48	5	6	3 starch, 1 fat
Special K	1 cup	120	0.5	5	0	0	0	220	23	1	6	1 1/2 starch
Special K Chocolatey Delight	3/4 cup	120	2	20	2	0	0	180	25	1	2	1 1/2 starch
Special K Fruit & Yogurt	3/4 cup	120	1	10	0.5	0	0	135	27	1	2	2 starch
Special K Red Berries	1 cup	120	0	0	0	0	0	220	25	1	3	1 1/2 starch
Special K Vanilla Almond	1 cup	110	1.5	15	0	0	0	160	25	1	2	1 1/2 starch
Malt-O-Meal												
Apple Zings	1 cup	130	1	5	0	0	0	150	30	1	1	2 starch
Berry Colossal Crunch	3/4 cup	120	1.5	15	0	0	0	230	26	0	1	2 starch
Blueberry Muffin Tops	3/4 cup	130	3.5	30	0.5	0	0	140	24	1	1	1 1/2 starch, 1 fat
Cinnamon Toasters	3/4 cup	130	3.5	30	0.5	0	0	140	24	1	1	1 1/2 starch, 1 fat
Cocoa Roos	3/4 cup	120	1.5	15	0	0	0	135	26	<1	1	2 starch

Creamy Hot Wheat	3 Tbsp	130	0	0	0	0	0	27	1	4	2 starch
Crispy Rice	1 1/4 cup	130	0	0	0	0	300	26	0	2	2 starch
Dyno Bites	3/4 cup	120	1	0	10	0	150	26	0	1	2 starch
Frosted Flakes	3/4 cup	120	0	0	0	0	180	28	1	1	2 starch
Frosted Mini Spooners	1 cup	190	1	0	10	0	10	45	6	5	3 starch
Golden Puffs	3/4 cup	110	0	0	0	0	65	24	0	2	2 starch
Honey & Oat Blenders	3/4 cup	120	1.5	0	15	0	150	25	1	2	1 1/2 starch
Honey Buzzers	1 1/3 cup	110	0.5	0	5	0	220	26	1	1	2 starch
Honey Graham Squares	3/4 cup	130	3	0.5	25	0	270	25	1	1	1 1/2 starch, 1 fat
Honey Nut Scooters	1 cup	110	1.5	0	10	0	210	24	2	2	1 1/2 starch
Hot Wheat Cereal, Chocolate	3 Tbsp dry	130	0	0	0	0	0	27	1	4	2 starch
Hot Wheat Cereal, Maple & Brown Sugar	1/4 cup dry	170	0	0	0	0	0	37	1	4	2 1/2 starch
Hot Wheat Cereal, Quick Original	3 Tbsp dry	130	0.5	0	5	0	0	27	1	5	2 starch

BREAKFAST CEREAL, READY-TO-EAT CEREAL, HOT CEREAL,

	Serving	Calories	Fat (g)	Cal. from Fat	Sat. Fat (g)	Trans Fat (g)	Chol. (mg)	Sod. (mg)	Carb. (g)	Fiber (g)	Prot. (g)	Servings/Exchanges
Marshmallow Mateys	1 cup	120	1	10	0	0	0	200	25	1	2	1 1/2 starch
Raisin Bran	1 cup	220	1.5	10	0	0	0	340	49	6	5	3 starch
Tootie Fruities	1 cup	130	1	10	0	0	0	150	28	1	2	2 starch
Nature's Path Organic												
Organic Flax Plus Multibran	3/4 cup	110	1.5	15	0	0	0	135	23	5	4	1 1/2 starch
Organic Flax Plus Raisin Bran	3/4 cup	190	2.5	20	0	0	0	190	41	8	6	2 1/2 starch, 1 fat
Organic Hemp Plus Granola	3/4 cup	260	10	90	1.5	0	0	35	36	5	6	2 1/2 starch, 2 fat
Organic Heritage Heirloom Whole Grains	3/4 cup	120	1	10	0	0	0	130	24	5	4	1 1/2 starch
Organic Optimum Blueberry Cinnamon	1 cup	200	3	25	0	0	0	230	38	7	9	2 1/2 starch, 1 fat

Organic Pumpkin Flax Plus Granola	3/4 cup	260	10	90	1.5	0	0	45	37	5	6	2 1/2 starch, 2 fat
Post												
Alpha-Bits	1 cup	110	1	10	0	0	0	160	23	2	2	1 1/2 starch
Banana Nut Crunch	1 cup	240	6	50	0.5	0	0	230	44	4	5	3 starch, 1 fat
Blueberry Morning	1 1/4 cup	220	3	30	0	0	0	280	45	2	3	3 starch, 1 fat
Bran Flakes	3/4 cup	100	0.5	5	0	0	0	220	24	5	3	1 1/2 starch
Cocoa Pebbles	3/4 cup	110	1.5	10	1	0	0	180	26	3	1	2 starch
Cranberry Almond Crunch	3/4 cup	200	2.5	35	0	0	0	115	39	3	4	2 1/2 starch, 1 fat
Fruity Pebbles	3/4 cup	110	1	10	1	0	0	180	26	3	1	2 starch
Golden Crisp	3/4 cup	110	0	0	0	0	0	25	24	<1	2	1 1/2 starch
Grape Nuts	1/2 cup	200	1	10	0	0	0	290	48	7	6	3 starch
Grape Nuts Flakes	3/4 cup	110	1	10	0	0	0	110	24	3	3	1 1/2 starch
Great Grains, Crunchy Pecan	1/2 cup	220	6	60	0.5	0	0	150	38	4	5	2 1/2 starch, 1 fat

BREAKFAST CEREAL, READY-TO-EAT CEREAL, HOT CEREAL

	Serving	Calories	Fat (g)	Cal. from Fat	Sat. Fat (g)	Trans Fat (g)	Chol. (mg)	Sod. (mg)	Carb. (g)	Fiber (g)	Prot. (g)	Servings/Exchanges
Great Grains, Raisin/Date/Pecan	1/2 cup	210	4.5	40	0	0	0	130	40	4	4	2 1/2 starch, 1 fat
Honey Bunches of Oats, Honey Roasted	3/4 cup	120	1.5	15	0	0	0	150	25	2	2	1 1/2 starch
Honeycombs	1 1/3 cup	120	1.5	10	0	0	0	180	27	2	2	2 starch
Raisin Bran	1 cup	190	1	10	0	0	0	300	46	8	4	3 starch
Shredded Wheat	2 biscuits	160	1	10	0	0	0	0	40	6	5	2 1/2 starch
Shredded Wheat 'n Bran	1 1/4 cup	200	1	10	0	0	0	0	49	8	6	3 starch
Shredded Wheat, Frosted	1 cup	180	1	10	0	0	0	0	43	5	4	3 starch
Shredded Wheat, Honey Nut	1 cup	190	1.5	15	0	0	0	70	44	5	4	3 starch
Quaker												
High Fiber Oatmeal Cinnamon Swirl	1 pkt	160	2	20	0.5	0	0	210	34	10	4	2 starch

Instant Hot Oatmeal	1 pkt	100	2	20	0	0	0	80	19	3	4	1 starch
Instant Hot Oatmeal Express, Baked Apple	1 cup	200	2.5	25	0.5	0	0	250	41	4	5	2 1/2 starch, 1 fat
Instant Hot Oatmeal Express, Cinnamon	1 cup	200	2.5	25	0.5	0	0	250	41	4	5	2 1/2 starch, 1 fat
Instant Hot Oatmeal, Apple & Cinnamon	1 pkt	130	1.5	15	0.5	0	0	170	27	3	3	2 starch
Instant Hot Oatmeal, Apple & Cinnamon, Lower Sugar	1 pkt	110	1.5	15	0.5	0	0	170	22	3	3	1 1/2 starch
Instant Hot Oatmeal, Cinnamon Roll	1 pkt	160	2	20	0.5	0	0	240	33	3	4	2 starch
Instant Hot Oatmeal, Cinnamon Spice	1 pkt	170	2	20	0.5	0	0	250	35	3	4	2 starch
Instant Hot Oatmeal, Maple & Brown Sugar	1 pkt	160	2	20	0	0	0	270	33	3	4	2 starch

BREAKFAST CEREAL, READY-TO-EAT CEREAL, HOT CEREAL

	Serving	Calories	Fat (g)	Cal. from Fat	Sat. Fat (g)	Trans Fat (g)	Chol. (mg)	Sod. (mg)	Carb. (g)	Fiber (g)	Prot. (g)	Servings/Exchanges
Instant Hot Oatmeal, Maple & Brown Sugar, Low Sugar	1 pkt	120	2	20	0	0	0	290	24	3	4	1 1/2 starch
Instant Hot Oatmeal, Peaches & Cream	1 pkt	130	2	20	0.5	0	0	190	27	2	3	2 starch
Instant Hot Oatmeal, Raisin & Spice	1 pkt	150	2	20	0	0	0	240	33	3	3	2 starch
Instant Hot Oatmeal, Raisin/Date/Walnut	1 pkt	140	2.5	25	0	0	0	240	27	3	3	2 starch, 1 fat
Instant Hot Oatmeal, Strawberries & Cream	1 pkt	130	2	20	0.5	0	0	180	27	2	3	2 starch
Life	3/4 cup	120	1.5	15	0	0	0	160	25	2	3	1 1/2 starch
Life, Cinnamon	3/4 cup	120	1.5	15	0	0	0	150	25	2	3	1 1/2 starch
Life, Maple & Brown Sugar	3/4 cup	120	1.5	15	0	0	0	150	25	2	3	1 1/2 starch

Natural Granola Oats, Honey & Raisins	1/2 cup	210	6	50	3.5	0	0	25	38	3	5	2 1/2 starch, 1 fat
Natural Granola, Lowfat	2/3 cup	210	3	25	1.5	0	0	135	45	3	4	3 starch, 1 fat
Oat Bran	1 1/4 cup	210	3	25	0.5	0	0	210	43	6	7	3 starch
Old-Fashioned Hot Oats	1/2 cup	150	3	25	0.5	0	0	0	27	4	5	2 starch, 1 fat
Quick Hot Oats	1/2 cup	150	3	25	0.5	0	0	0	27	4	5	2 starch
Simple Harvest Apples & Cinnamon (Hot Cereal)	1 pkt	150	1.5	15	0	0	0	90	33	4	4	2 starch
Simple Harvest Maple Brown Sugar with Pecans (Hot Cereal)	1 pkt	160	3.5	30	0	0	0	75	30	4	4	2 starch, 1 fat
Take Heart Instant Oatmeal Blueberry	1 pkt	160	2.5	25	0.5	0	0	105	33	6	4	2 starch, 1 fat
Take Heart Instant Golden Maple	1 pkt	160	2.5	25	0.5	0	0	110	33	5	4	2 starch, 1 fat

BREAKFAST CEREAL, READY-TO-EAT CEREAL, HOT CEREAL

	Serving	Calories	Fat (g)	Cal. from Fat	Sat. Fat (g)	Trans Fat (g)	Chol. (mg)	Sod. (mg)	Carb. (g)	Fiber (g)	Prot. (g)	Servings/Exchanges
Toasted Oatmeal Squares, Brown Sugar	1 cup	210	2.5	25	0.5	0	0	250	44	5	6	3 starch, 1 fat
Toasted Oatmeal Squares, Cinnamon	1 cup	230	2.5	25	0.5	0	0	260	47	5	6	3 starch, 1 fat
Weight Control Instant Oatmeal Banana Bread	1 pkt	160	3	25	0.5	0	0	260	29	6	7	2 starch, 1 fat
Weight Control Instant Oatmeal Maple & Brown Sugar	1 pkt	160	3	25	0.5	0	0	310	29	6	7	2 starch, 1 fat
Trader Joe's												
Apple & Cinnamon Instant Oatmeal	1 pouch	130	1.5	15	0	0	0	170	27	3	3	2 starch
Banana Nut Clusters	1 cup	240	8	70	0.5	0	0	140	40	2	4	2 1/2 starch, 2 fat

Gluten Free Granola Loaded Fruit & Nut	3/4 cup	270	13	120	2	0	0	45	34	3	4	2 starch, 3 fat
Gourmet Flakes & Chocolate	1 1/4 cup	230	4.5	40	2.5	0	0	290	43	3	4	3 starch, 1 fat
High Fiber Cereal	2/3 cup	80	0.5	5	0	0	0	70	23	9	3	1 1/2 starch
High Fiber Fruit & Nut Medley	2/3 cup	90	1.5	15	0	0	0	55	25	7	2	1 1/2 starch
Honey Almond & Flax 9 Grain Crunch	1 cup	190	5	45	0	0	0	125	33	8	10	2 starch, 1 fat
Honey Nut O's	3/4 cup	120	1.5	15	0	0	0	200	24	2	2	1 1/2 starch
Joe's O's	1 cup	110	1.5	15	0	0	0	280	22	3	3	1 1/2 starch
Just The Clusters Maple Pecan Granola	2/3 cup	250	10	90	1	0	0	70	38	3	5	2 1/2 starch, 2 fat
Lowfat Granola Mixed Berry	3/4 cup	210	2.5	20	0	0	0	75	45	5	4	3 starch, 1 fat
Lowfat Granola with Almonds	3/4 cup	210	3	25	0	0	0	75	44	5	4	3 starch, 1 fat

BREAKFAST CEREAL, READY-TO-EAT CEREAL, HOT CEREAL

	Serving	Calories	Fat (g)	Cal. from Fat	Sat. Fat (g)	Trans Fat (g)	Chol. (mg)	Sod. (mg)	Carb. (g)	Fiber (g)	Prot. (g)	Servings/Exchanges
Oat 'n Wheat Bran Swirls	1/2 cup	200	7	60	0	0	0	135	34	4	4	2 starch, 1 fat
Organic Cinnamon Spice Instant Oatmeal	1 pkt	150	1.5	15	0	0	0	90	30	2.5	4	2 starch
Organic Corn Flakes	1 cup	110	0	0	0	0	0	280	26	<1	2	2 starch
Organic Golden Flax	3/4 cup	200	3.5	30	0.5	0	0	65	37	6	6	2 1/2 starch, 1 fat
Organic Granny's Apple Granola	2/3 cup	210	7	60	0.5	0	0	45	31	4	5	2 starch, 1 fat
Organic High Fiber O's	1 1/4 cup	190	1	10	0	0	0	115	44	9	6	3 starch
Organic Honey Crunch 'n Oats	3/4 cup	120	1	10	0	0	0	135	25	2	2	1 1/2 starch
Organic Morning Lite	1 cup	170	2.5	25	0	0	0	70	40	10	3	2 1/2 starch, 1 fat
Organic Oats & Flax	1 pkt	150	2	25	0	0	0	130	29	3	4	2 starch
Organic Raisin Bran	1 cup	170	1	10	0	0	0	120	44	8	4	3 starch

Organic Raisin Bran Clusters	1 cup	190	3	25	0	0	0	150	40	7	6	2 1/2 starch, 1 fat
Pomegranate Blueberry Flakes & Clusters	1 cup	210	2	20	0	0	0	110	46	4	4	3 starch
Quick Cook Steel Cut Oats	1/4 cup dry	150	2.5	25	0.5	0	0	0	27	4	5	2 starch, 1 fat
Shredded Bite Size Wheats	1 cup	180	1	10	0	0	0	0	38	5	5	2 1/2 starch
Soy & Flax Clusters	1 cup	190	3	25	0	0	0	135	38	6	7	2 1/2 starch, 1 fat
Strawberry Yogurt O's	3/4 cup	110	2.5	25	0	0	0	60	22	3	2	1 1/2 starch 1 fat
Super Nutty Toffee Clusters	3/4 cup	250	9	80	1.5	0	0	105	38	3	5	2 1/2 starch, 2 fat
Toasted Oatmeal Flakes	3/4 cup	110	1	10	0	0	0	190	23	3	3	1 1/2 starch
Triple Berry-O's	3/4 cup	110	1	10	0	0	0	180	25	3	2	1 1/2 starch
Triple Nut Reduced Sugar & Flakes	1/2 cup	130	4	35	0	0	0	55	21	2	3	1 1/2 starch, 1 fat

BREAKFAST CEREAL, READY-TO-EAT CEREAL, HOT CEREAL

	Serving	Calories	Fat (g)	Cal. from Fat	Sat. Fat (g)	Trans Fat (g)	Chol. (mg)	Sod. (mg)	Carb. (g)	Fiber (g)	Prot. (g)	Servings/Exchanges
Twigs, Flakes & Clusters	1 cup	170	1.5	15	0	0	0	105	41	12	5	2 1/2 starch
Vanilla Almond Clusters	1 cup	220	6	60	0.5	0	0	150	38	2	5	2 1/2 starch, 1 fat
Vanilla Almond Granola	2/3 cup	250	9	80	1	0	0	70	39	3	5	2 1/2 starch, 2 fat
Very Berry Clusters	1 cup	230	5	50	0.5	0	0	120	42	3	5	3 starch, 1 fat

BUTTER, MARGARINE, SOUR CREAM

	Serving	Calories	Fat (g)	Cal. from Fat	Sat. Fat (g)	Trans Fat (g)	Chol. (mg)	Sod. (mg)	Carb. (g)	Fiber (g)	Prot. (g)	Servings/Exchanges
Butter, Light	1 Tbsp	50	6	55	3.5	0	15	100	0	0	0	1 fat
Butter, Stick	1 tsp	34	4	35	2	0	10	27	0	0	0	1 fat
Butter, Whipped	2 tsp	33	4	35	2	0	10	33	0	0	0	1 fat
Margarine, Fat-Free	1 Tbsp	6	0	0	0	0	0	85	<1	0	0	free
Margarine, Liquid	1 tsp	34	4	35	<1	NA	0	37	0	0	0	1 fat
Margarine, Stick	1 tsp	30	3	25	<1	NA	0	37	0	0	0	1 fat
Margarine, Tub	1 tsp	24	3	27	<1	NA	0	29	0	0	0	1 fat
Margarine-like Spread, Light or Lower Fat	1 Tbsp	46	5	45	1	NA	0	86	0	0	0	1 fat
Sour Cream, Fat-Free	1 Tbsp	30	0	0	0	0	5	20	3	0	1	free
Sour Cream, Reduced-Fat or Light	3 Tbsp	45	4	35	3	0	18	38	3	0	3	1 fat
Sour Cream, Regular	2 Tbsp	62	5	45	3	0	19	14	1	0	<1	1 fat

BUTTER, MARGARINE, SOUR CREAM

	Serving	Calories	Fat (g)	Cal. from Fat	Sat. Fat (g)	Trans Fat (g)	Chol. (mg)	Sod. (mg)	Carb. (g)	Fiber (g)	Prot. (g)	Servings/Exchanges
Brands												
Benecol Spread												
Light	1 Tbsp	50	5	50	0.5	0	0	110	0	0	0	1 fat
Regular	1 Tbsp	70	8	70	1	0	0	110	0	0	0	2 fat
Blue Bonnet Margarine												
Light Stick	1 Tbsp	50	5	50	1	1	0	80	<1	0	0	1 fat
Regular Stick	1 Tbsp	80	9	80	2	1.5	0	110	0	0	0	2 fat
Regular Tub	1 Tbsp	60	7	60	1.5	1	0	125	0	0	0	1 fat
Breakstone's/Knudsen												
Sour Cream	2 Tbsp	60	5	50	3.5	0	20	10	1	0	1	1 fat
Sour Cream, Fat Free	2 Tbsp	30	0	0	0	0	5	25	6	0	1	1/2 carb
Sour Cream, Reduced Fat	2 Tbsp	40	3	30	2	0	15	20	2	0	1	free
Brummel & Brown Margarine Spread with Yogurt												

Tub	1 Tbsp	45	5	45	1.5	0	0	90	0	0	0	1 fat
Butter Buds												
Butter Replacement, Dry	1 Tbsp	15	0	0	0	0	0	360	6	0	0	free
Canola Harvest Margarine												
Baking Margarine	2 tsp	70	8	70	1.5	2.5	0	70	0	0	0	2 fat
Flaxseed Blend	2 tsp	70	8	70	1	0	0	70	0	0	0	2 fat
Olive Oil Blend	2 tsp	70	8	70	1	0	0	70	0	0	0	2 fat
Original	2 tsp	70	8	70	1	0	0	70	0	0	0	2 fat
Regular Soft Tub	1 Tbsp	100	11	100	1.5	0	0	100	0	0	0	2 fat
Canola												
100% Canola Margarine	1 Tbsp	100	11	100	2	0	0	120	0	0	0	2 fat
Daisy												
Sour Cream	2 Tbsp	60	5	45	3.5	0	20	15	1	0	1	1 fat
Sour Cream, Light	2 Tbsp	60	2.5	25	2.5	0	10	25	2	0	2	1 fat
Fleischmann's Margarine												
Original Tub	1 Tbsp	60	7	60	1	0	0	35	0	0	0	1 fat

BUTTER, MARGARINE, SOUR CREAM

	Serving	Calories	Fat (g)	Cal. from Fat	Sat. Fat (g)	Trans Fat (g)	Chol. (mg)	Sod. (mg)	Carb. (g)	Fiber (g)	Prot. (g)	Servings/Exchanges
Original Tub with Olive Oil	1 Tbsp	60	6.5	60	1	0	0	45	0	0	0	1 fat
Gold n Soft												
Original Tub	1 Tbsp	100	10	90	2.5	0	0	90	0	0	0	2 fat
I Can't Believe It's Not Butter												
Light Spread	1 Tbsp	50	5	45	1	0	0	85	0	0	0	1 fat
Original Spread	1 Tbsp	70	8	70	2	0	0	90	0	0	0	2 fat
Regular Stick	1 Tbsp	100	11	90	3.5	0	0	95	0	0	0	2 fat
Spray Original	5 sprays	0	0	0	0	0	0	15	0	0	0	free
IMO												
Sour Cream Substitute	2 Tbsp	60	5	50	5	0	0	30	2	0	1	1 fat
Imperial												
Regular Stick	1 Tbsp	80	8	80	1.5	2	0	105	0	0	0	2 fat
Land O'Lakes												

Food	Serving											
Country Morning Blend Soft Spread	1 Tbsp	100	11	100	2.5	2	0	80	0	0	0	2 fat
Country Morning Blend Stick	1 Tbsp	100	11	100	2.5	2.5	0	90	0	0	0	2 fat
Fresh Buttery Taste Soft Spread	1 Tbsp	70	8	70	2	0	0	80	0	0	0	2 fat
Fresh Buttery Taste Stick Spread	1 Tbsp	90	10	90	2	2	0	95	0	0	0	2 fat
Garlic Butter Tub	1 Tbsp	90	10	90	5	0	20	110	0	0	0	2 fat
Honey Butter Tub	1 Tbsp	90	8	70	4	0.5	15	40	4	0	0	2 fat
Light Butter Stick	1 Tbsp	50	6	50	3.5	0	15	100	0	0	0	1 fat
Margarine Soft Tub	1 Tbsp	100	11	100	3	0	0	125	0	0	0	2 fat
Margarine Stick	1 Tbsp	100	11	100	2	2.5	0	105	0	0	0	2 fat
Salted Butter Stick	1 Tbsp	100	11	100	7	0	30	95	0	0	0	2 fat
Salted Whipped Light Butter	1 Tbsp	45	5	45	3	0	15	85	0	0	0	1 fat

BUTTER, MARGARINE, SOUR CREAM

	Serving	Calories	Fat (g)	Cal. from Fat	Sat. Fat (g)	Trans Fat (g)	Chol. (mg)	Sod. (mg)	Carb. (g)	Fiber (g)	Prot. (g)	Servings/Exchanges
Spreadable Butter with Canola Oil	1 Tbsp	100	11	100	4.5	0	20	90	0	0	0	2 fat
Spreadable Butter with Olive Oil	1 Tbsp	90	10	90	4	0	15	90	0	0	0	2 fat
Spreadable Light Butter with Canola Oil	1 Tbsp	50	5	50	2	0	5	90	0	0	0	1 fat
Unsalted Butter Stick	1 Tbsp	100	11	100	7	0	30	0	0	0	0	2 fat
Whipped Salted Butter	1 Tbsp	50	6	50	3.5	0	15	50	0	0	0	1 fat
Nucoa Margarine												
Regular Stick	1 Tbsp	100	11	100	2	1.5	0	160	0	0	0	2 fat
Parkay												
Squeeze	1 Tbsp	70	8	70	1.5	0	0	110	0	0	0	2 fat
Promise												
Activ	1 Tbsp	45	5	45	1	0	<5	85	0	0	0	1 fat

Fat Free Spread	1 Tbsp	5	0	0	5	0	90	0	0	free
Light Spread	1 Tbsp	45	5	1	45	0	85	0	0	1 fat
Regular Spread	1 Tbsp	80	8	1.5	80	0	85	0	0	2 fat

Shedd's Spread Country Crock

Calcium Plus Vitamin D Spread	1 Tbsp	50	5	1	45	0	95	0	0	1 fat
Churn Style Spread	1 Tbsp	80	8	1.5	80	0	95	0	0	2 fat
Honey Spread	1 Tbsp	50	5	1	45	0	95	0	0	1 fat
Light Spread	1 Tbsp	50	5	1.5	50	0	85	0	0	1 fat
Omega Plus Light Spread	1 Tbsp	50	5	1	45	0	80	0	0	1 fat
Omega Plus Spread	1 Tbsp	70	8	1.5	70	0	100	0	0	2 fat
Regular Tub	1 Tbsp	60	7	1.5	60	0	110	0	0	1 fat
Spreadable Butter	1 Tbsp	80	9	3.5	80	15	65	0	0	2 fat
Spreadable Sticks	1 Tbsp	80	8	1.5	80	0	90	0	0	2 fat
Whipped Easy Squeeze	1 Tbsp	60	7	1	60	0	85	0	0	1 fat

BUTTER, MARGARINE, SOUR CREAM

	Serving	Calories	Fat (g)	Cal. from Fat	Sat. Fat (g)	Trans Fat (g)	Chol. (mg)	Sod. (mg)	Carb. (g)	Fiber (g)	Prot. (g)	Servings/Exchanges
Smart Balance												
67% Buttery Spread	1 Tbsp	80	9	80	2.5	0	0	90	0	0	0	2 fat
Butter Blend Regular Stick	1 Tbsp	100	11	100	5	0	15	100	0	0	0	2 fat
Butter Blend Regular Stick with Omega-3	1 Tbsp	100	11	100	5	0	15	100	0	0	0	2 fat
Heart Right Buttery Spread	1 Tbsp	80	8	80	2.5	0	0	85	0	0	0	2 fat
Light 32% Buttery Spread	1 Tbsp	45	5	45	1.5	0	0	85	0	0	0	1 fat
Low Sodium Buttery Spread	1 Tbsp	65	7	65	2	0	0	30	0	0	0	1 fat
Omega Plus	1 Tbsp	80	9	80	2.5	0	0	90	0	0	0	2 fat
Omega-3 Buttery Spread	1 Tbsp	80	9	80	2.5	0	0	85	0	0	0	2 fat

Food	Serving											
Omega-3 Light Buttery Spread	1 Tbsp	50	5	50	1.5	0	0	80	0	0	0	1 fat
Omega-3 with Extra Virgin Olive Oil Buttery Spread	1 Tbsp	60	7	60	2	0	0	70	0	0	0	1 fat
Omega-3 with Extra Virgin Olive Oil Light Buttery Spread	1 Tbsp	50	5	50	1.5	0	0	70	0	0	0	1 fat
Organic Buttery Spread	1 Tbsp	80	9	80	2.5	0	0	100	0	0	0	2 fat
Regular Buttery Spread Light with Flax Oil	1 Tbsp	45	5	45	1.5	0	0	90	0	0	0	1 fat
Regular Buttery Spread with Flax Oil	1 Tbsp	80	9	80	2.5	0	0	85	0	0	0	2 fat
Smart Beat												
Smart Squeeze	1 Tbsp	5	0	0	0	0	0	100	0	0	0	free

CANDY, SWEETS

	Serving	Calories	Fat. (g)	Cal. from Fat	Sat. Fat (g)	Trans Fat (g)	Chol. (mg)	Sod. (mg)	Carb. (g)	Fiber (g)	Prot. (g)	Servings/Exchanges
Almond Roca	1 oz	124	5	45	3	0	3	51	19	<1	2	1 carb, 1 fat
Almonds, Chocolate Coated	1/4 cup	234	18	162	3	0	<1	24	16	4	5	1 carb, 4 fat
Almonds, Sugar Coated	7	116	4	35	<1	0	0	3	20	<1	2	1 carb, 1 fat
Butterscotch	5 pieces	119	1	10	<1	0	3	13	29	0	<1	2 carb
Candies, Chocolate Covered, Caramel with Nuts	3 pieces	197	9	80	2	0	0	10	26	2	4	2 carb, 2 fat
Candy Corn	26 pieces	140	0	0	0	0	0	80	36	0	0	2 1/2 carb
Caramels	3	116	3	30	2	0	2	74	23	<1	1	1 1/2 carb, 1 fat
Cherries, Chocolate Covered	2	110	4	35	3	0	0	15	18	2	<1	1 carb, 1 fat
Chewing Gum	1 piece	10	<1	0	0	0	0	<1	3	0	0	free

Food	Amount	Cal.	Fat (g)	% Cal. Fat	Sat. Fat (g)	Chol. (mg)	Sod. (mg)	Carb. (g)	Fiber (g)	Pro. (g)	Exchanges
Chewing Gum, Sugar Free	1 piece	11	<1	0	0	0	<1	4	0	<1	free
Divinity, Homemade	3 pieces	120	0	0	0	0	11	29	0	0	2 carb
Fruit Leather	1 oz	102	<1	0	0	0	114	24	0	0	1 1/2 carb
Fudge, Chocolate, Homemade	3 pieces	210	5	45	3	7	23	40	0	1	2 1/2 carb, 1 fat
Fudge, Vanilla, Homemade	1 oz	105	2	20	<1	5	19	23	0	<1	1 1/2 carb
Gumdrops, Sugar Free	10 small	81	0	0	0	0	16	44	0	0	3 carb
Gummy Bears	10 small	85	0	0	0	0	15	22	0	0	1 1/2 carb
Hard Candy, All Flavors	1 oz	106	0	0	0	0	11	28	0	0	2 carb
Jellybeans	10	40	<1	0	0	0	3	10	0	0	1/2 carb
Lollipops	1	22	0	0	0	0	2	6	0	0	1/2 carb
Peanut Brittle, Homemade	1 oz	122	5	45	1	3	111	18	<1	2	1 carb, 1 fat
Peanuts, Milk Chocolate Coated	1/4 cup	193	13	115	5	3	15	18	2	5	1 carb, 3 fat

CANDY, SWEETS

	Serving	Calories	Fat (g)	Cal. from Fat	Sat. Fat (g)	Trans Fat (g)	Chol. (mg)	Sod. (mg)	Carb. (g)	Fiber (g)	Prot. (g)	Servings/Exchanges
Peanuts, Yogurt Covered	1/4 cup	194	13	115	3	0	1	15	16	2	4	1 carb, 3 fat
Praline, Homemade	1 oz	129	7	65	<1	0	0	18	18	<1	<1	1 carb, 1 fat
Raisins, Milk Chocolate Covered	1/4 cup	185	7	65	4	0	1	17	33	2	2	2 carb, 1 fat
Raisins, Yogurt Covered	1/4 cup	176	7	65	5	0	1	16	31	1	2	2 carb, 1 fat
Taffy, Homemade	1 oz	11	<1	0	<1	0	3	15	26	0	0	2 carb
Toffee, Homemade	1 oz	157	9	80	6	0	29	38	18	0	0	1 carb, 2 fat
Truffles, Homemade	1 oz	143	10	90	5	0	15	19	13	<1	2	1 carb, 2 fat
Brands												
Concorde												
Bit-O-Honey Chews	6	186	4	36	NA	0	<1	124	39	NA	1	2 1/2 carb, 1 fat
DeMet's												
Turtles	3 pieces	260	15	130	6	0	5	45	29	1	3	2 carb, 3 fat
Turtles, Sugar Free	3 pieces	150	11	100	6	0	<5	70	20	<1	2	1 carb, 2 fat

Hershey's

	Serving											
5th Avenue Bar	2-oz bar	260	12	110	4.5	0	0	120	37	2	4	2 1/2 carb, 2 fat
Almond Joy	1.6-oz bar	220	13	110	8	0	0	50	26	2	2	2 carb, 3 fat
BreathSavers Mints	1	5	0	0	0	0	0	0	2	0	0	free
Cadbury Chocolate	7 blocks	200	11	100	7	0	10	40	23	<1	3	1 1/2 carb, 2 fat
Cadbury's Caramello Bar	1.6-oz bar	220	10	90	6	0	10	45	29	<1	3	2 carb, 2 fat
Chocolate Candy, Sugar Free	5 pieces	160	13	110	8	0	10	15	24	3	1	1 1/2 carb, 3 fat
Chocolate Kisses	9	230	13	120	8	0	10	35	24	1	3	1 1/2 carb, 3 fat
Cookies & Creme Bar	1.2-oz bar	170	9	80	6	0	5	75	21	0	3	1 1/2 carb, 2 fat
Good & Plenty Licorice	1.4 oz	140	0	0	0	0	0	120	35	0	<1	2 carb
Heath Toffee Bar	1.4-oz bar	210	13	110	7	0	10	135	24	<1	1	1 1/2 carb, 3 fat

CANDY, SWEETS

	Serving	Calories	Fat (g)	Cal. from Fat	Sat. Fat (g)	Trans Fat (g)	Chol. (mg)	Sod. (mg)	Carb. (g)	Fiber (g)	Prot. (g)	Servings/Exchanges
Hershey's 100 Calorie Pretzel Bar	1 bar	100	4.5	40	2.5	0	0	105	13	0	1	1 carb, 1 fat
Hershey's Bliss Milk Chocolate	6 pieces	210	14	120	9	0	5	40	24	1	3	1 1/2 carb, 3 fat
Hershey's Extra Dark Chocolate Bar	3 blocks	210	13	120	8	0	<5	5	20	4	3	1 carb, 3 fat
Hershey's Miniatures	5 pieces	210	13	110	7	0	5	50	25	2	3	1 1/2 carb, 3 fat
Hershey's Nuggets	4 pieces	200	12	110	7	0	10	35	25	1	3	1 1/2 carb, 2 fat
Hershey's Sugar Free Chocolates	5 pieces	160	13	110	8	0	10	15	24	3	1	1 1/2 carb, 3 fat
Hershey's Take 5	1.5-oz bar	200	11	90	5	0	0	180	25	1	4	1 1/2 carb, 2 fat
Jolly Rancher Candy	3 pieces	50	0	0	0	0	0	20	13	0	0	1 carb
Jolly Rancher Hard Candy, Sugar Free	4 pieces	35	0	0	0	0	0	0	13	0	0	1 carb

Kit Kat Bar	1.5-oz bar	210	11	100	7	0	<5	30	28	<1	3	2 carb, 2 fat
Milk Chocolate Bar	1.5-oz bar	210	13	110	8	0	10	35	26	1	3	2 carb, 3 fat
Milk Chocolate Bar, Symphony	1.5-oz bar	220	14	130	8	0	10	65	23	<1	3	1 1/2 carb, 3 fat
Milk Duds	13	170	6	50	3.5	0	0	100	28	0	1	2 carb, 1 fat
Mounds	1.75 oz	230	13	120	10	0	0	55	29	3	2	2 carb, 3 fat
Mr. Goodbar	1.75-oz bar	250	17	140	7	0	<5	65	26	2	5	2 carb, 3 fat
PayDay	2.08-oz bar	240	13	120	2.5	0	0	120	27	2	7	2 carb, 3 fat
Reese's Peanut Butter Cups	1.5 oz 2 pieces	210	13	110	4.5	0	<5	150	24	1	5	1 1/2 carb, 3 fat
Reese's Pieces	1.5 oz	210	10	90	8	0	0	85	26	1	5	2 carb, 2 fat
Reese's Sticks	1.5-oz bar	210	13	110	5	0	0	130	23	1	4	1 1/2 carb, 3 fat

CANDY, SWEETS

	Serving	Calories	Fat (g)	Cal. from Fat	Sat. Fat (g)	Trans Fat (g)	Chol. (mg)	Sod. (mg)	Carb. (g)	Fiber (g)	Prot. (g)	Servings/Exchanges
Reese's 100 Calorie Peanut Butter Wafer	1 bar	100	6	50	2.5	0	0	50	11	0	2	1 carb, 1 fat
Reese's Fast Break	2-oz bar	260	12	100	4.5	0	0	190	35	2	5	2 carb, 2 fat
Reese's NutRageous	1.82-oz bar	260	16	140	5	0	0	100	28	2	6	2 carb, 3 fat
Reese's Peanut Butter Cups, Sugar Free	5 pieces	180	13	110	6	0	<5	120	27	6	3	2 carb, 3 fat
Rolos Caramel	1.7-oz pkg	220	10	80	7	0	5	80	33	0	2	2 carb, 2 fat
Skor Bar	1.4-oz bar	200	12	110	7	0	20	130	25	<1	1	1 1/2 carb, 2 fat
Special Dark Sweet Chocolate Bar	1.5 oz	180	12	110	8	0	<5	15	25	3	2	1 1/2 carb, 3 fat
Tootsie Rolls	6 small	140	3	30	0.5	0	1	15	28	0	1	2 carb, 1 fat

Item	Amount	Cal.	Fat (g)	Cal. Fat	Sat. Fat (g)	Trans Fat (g)	Chol. (mg)	Sodium (mg)	Carb. (g)	Fiber (g)	Prot. (g)	Exchanges/Choices
Twizzlers, Strawberry	4 pieces	160	1	5	0	0	0	95	36	0	1	2 1/2 carb
Twizzlers, Sugar Free	6 pieces	130	1	10	0	0	0	105	33	0	1	2 carb
Whatchamacallit Bar	1.6 oz	230	12	110	9	0	0	140	28	<1	3	2 carb, 2 fat
Whoppers Chocolate Malted Milk Balls	1.5-oz pkg	190	7	60	7	0	<5	115	31	0	1	2 carb, 1 fat
York 100 Calorie Bars	1 bar	100	6	50	4	0	0	10	11	<1	<1	1 carb, 1 fat
York Peppermint Pattie	1 pattie	140	2.5	25	1.5	0	0	10	31	<1	<1	2 carb, 1 fat
York Sugar Free Peppermint Patties	3 pieces	120	8	60	4.5	0	0	5	24	2	1	1 1/2 carb, 2 fat
Zagnut	3 pieces	200	8	70	3	0	0	90	31	1	3	2 carb, 2 fat
Just Born												
Hot Tamales	1.4 oz / 20 pieces	150	0	0	0	0	0	15	36	0	0	2 1/2 carb
Mike and Ike	23 pieces	140	0	0	0	0	0	30	36	0	0	2 1/2 carb
Kraft												
Butter Mints	7 mints	60	0	0	0	0	0	25	14	0	0	1 carb

CANDY, SWEETS

	Serving	Calories	Fat (g)	Cal. from Fat	Sat. Fat (g)	Trans Fat (g)	Chol. (mg)	Sod. (mg)	Carb. (g)	Fiber (g)	Prot. (g)	Servings/Exchanges
Caramels	5	160	3.5	30	2	0	0	95	31	0	2	2 carb, 1 fat
M&M Mars												
3 Musketeers Bar	1.68-oz bar	200	6	60	4	0	5	85	36	1	1	2 1/2 carb, 1 fat
Dove Bar	1 bar	80	4.5	40	3	0	0	10	9	NA	1	1/2 carb, 1 fat
M&M's, Chocolate	1.7 oz	260	11	80	7	0	5	35	37	1	2	2 1/2 carb, 2 fat
M&M's, Peanut	1.75 oz	250	13	120	5	0	5	25	30	2	5	2 carb, 3 fat
Milky Way Bar	2.05-oz bar	270	10	90	7	0	5	95	41	1	2	2 1/2 carb, 2 fat
Munch Bar	1 bar	220	15	130	3.5	0	10	140	17	2	6	1 carb, 3 fat
Skittles	1 bag	230	2.5	20	2.5	0	0	10	51	0	0	3 1/2 carb, 1 fat
Snickers Bar	2.07-oz bar	280	14	130	5	0	5	140	36	1	4	2 1/2 carb, 3 fat
Starburst Fruit Chews	1 pkg	240	5	45	4.5	0	0	0	48	0	0	3 carb, 1 fat

Food	Serving											Exchanges
Twix Caramel Cookie Bar	2-oz bar	280	14	130	11	0	5	115	37	1	3	2 1/2 carb, 3 fat
Nestlé												
100 Grand Bar	1.5-oz bar	190	8	70	5	0	10	90	30	0	1	2 carb, 2 fat
Baby Ruth Bar	2.1-oz bar	280	14	120	8	0	0	130	39	1	4	2 1/2 carb, 3 fat
Butterfinger Bar	2.1-oz bar	270	11	100	6	0	0	135	43	1	4	3 carb, 2 fat
Chunky Bar	1.4-oz bar	190	11	100	5	0	<5	15	24	1	3	1 1/2 carb, 2 fat
Crunch Bar	1.4-oz bar	220	11	100	7	0	10	60	30	1	2	2 carb, 2 fat
Goobers Chocolate-Covered Peanuts	1.5-oz bag	210	14	120	5	0	5	15	22	2	5	1 1/2 carb, 3 fat
Raisinets	3.5-oz box	190	8	70	5	0	5	15	32	1	2	2 carb, 2 fat

CANDY, SWEETS

	Serving	Calories	Fat (g)	Cal. from Fat	Sat. Fat (g)	Trans Fat (g)	Chol. (mg)	Sod. (mg)	Carb. (g)	Fiber (g)	Prot. (g)	Servings/Exchanges
Sno Caps	3.1-oz box	180	8	70	5	0	<5	0	30	2	1	2 carb, 2 fat
Russell Stover												
Mint Patties, Sugar Free	3 pieces	180	12	110	8	0	<5	20	26	2	2	2 carb, 2 fat
Pecan Delights, Sugar Free	3 pieces	190	15	130	7	0	<5	45	23	3	3	1 1/2 carb, 3 fat
Toffee Squares, Sugar Free	3	190	15	130	7	0	0	45	23	2	3	1 1/2 carb, 3 fat
Storck												
Swedish Fish	7 pieces	150	0	0	0	0	0	30	38	0	0	2 1/2 carb
Tootsie												
Dots	11	130	0	0	0	0	0	15	33	0	0	2 carb
Junior Mints	16 (1.4 oz)	170	3	30	2.5	0	0	30	35	1	1	2 carb, 1 fat

Sugar Babies	30 (1.6 oz)	180	1.5	15	0	0	0	40	41	0	0	2 1/2 carb
Weight Watchers by Whitman's												
Coconut Covered Milk Chocolate	3 pieces	150	9	80	7	0	5	50	23	11	2	1 1/2 carb, 2 fat
Pecan Crowns	3 pieces	160	10	90	6	0	<5	20	24	9	2	1 1/2 carb, 2 fat
Werther's												
Caramel Candies	4 pieces	70	1	10	0.5	0	<5	30	15	0	0	1 carb
Caramel Candies, Sugar Free	5 pieces	40	1	10	0.5	0	<5	55	15	0	0	1 carb

CHEESE, COTTAGE CHEESE, CREAM CHEESE

	Serving	Calories	Fat (g)	Cal. from Fat	Sat. Fat (g)	Trans Fat (g)	Chol. (mg)	Sod. (mg)	Carb. (g)	Fiber (g)	Prot. (g)	Servings/Exchanges
American	1 oz	106	9	80	6	0	27	406	<1	0	6	1 high-fat meat
American, Fat Free	3/4-oz slice	30	0	0	0	0	3	270	2	0	5	1 lean meat
American, Reduced Fat	1 oz	68	4	35	2.5	0	14	379	1	0	5	1 lean meat
Blue or Roquefort	1 oz	100	8	70	5	0	21	396	<1	0	6	1 high-fat meat
Brick	1 oz	105	8	70	5	0	27	159	1	0	7	1 high-fat meat
Brie	1 oz	95	8	70	5	0	28	178	0	0	6	1 high-fat meat
Camembert	1 oz	85	7	65	4	0	20	239	0	0	6	1 med-fat meat
Cheddar	1 oz	114	9	80	6	0	30	176	<1	0	7	1 high-fat meat
Cheddar/Colby, Fat Free	1 oz	45	0	0	0	0	3	296	2	0	9	1 lean meat
Cheddar/Colby, Reduced Fat	1 oz	80	5	45	4	0	15	230	1	0	7	1 lean meat
Cheese Spread	1 oz	82	6	55	4	0	16	381	3	0	5	1 med-fat meat

Food	Serving											
Cheshire	1 oz	110	9	80	6	0	29	198	1	0	7	1 high-fat meat
Cottage Cheese, 1% Milkfat, Low Fat	1/4 cup	41	<1	0	<1	0	2	229	2	0	7	1 lean meat
Cottage Cheese, Creamed, 4.5% Milkfat	1/4 cup	54	2	20	1	0	8	210	1	0	7	1 lean meat
Cottage Cheese, Nonfat	1/4 cup	40	0	0	0	0	3	205	2.5	0	7	1 lean meat
Edam	1 oz	101	8	70	5	0	25	274	0	0	7	1 high-fat meat
Feta	1 oz	75	6	55	4	0	25	317	1	0	4	1 med-fat meat
Feta, Fat Free, Plain	1 oz	30	0	0	0	0	0	449	2	0	6	1 lean meat
Fontina	1 oz	110	9	80	5	0	33	227	0	0	7	1 high-fat meat
Gjetost	1 oz	132	8	70	5	0	27	170	12	0	3	1 high-fat meat
Goat Cheese, Hard	1 oz	127	10	90	7	0	30	98	<1	0	9	1 high-fat meat
Gouda	1 oz	101	8	70	5	0	32	232	1	0	7	1 high-fat meat
Gruyere	1 oz	117	9	80	5	0	31	95	0	0	8	1 high-fat meat
Limburger	1 oz	93	8	70	5	0	26	227	0	0	6	1 high-fat meat

CHEESE, COTTAGE CHEESE, CREAM CHEESE

	Serving	Calories	Fat (g)	Cal. from Fat	Sat. Fat (g)	Trans Fat (g)	Chol. (mg)	Sod. (mg)	Carb. (g)	Fiber (g)	Prot. (g)	Servings/Exchanges
Mexican, Reduced Fat	1 oz	81	6	55	3	0	20	201	0	0	8	1 med-fat meat
Monterey Jack	1 oz	106	9	80	5	0	25	152	0	0	7	1 high-fat meat
Monterey Jack, Reduced Fat	1 oz	80	6	55	3.5	0	20	240	1	0	7	1 med-fat meat
Mozzarella, Fat Free	1 oz	45	0	0	0	0	4	335	1	0	8	1 lean meat
Mozzarella, Part Skim	1 oz	72	5	45	3	0	18	175	<1	0	7	1 med-fat meat
Mozzarella, Reduced Fat	1 oz	70	4	35	3	0	15	200	<1	0	8	1 lean meat
Muenster	1 oz	105	9	80	5	0	27	178	0	0	7	1 high-fat meat
Parmesan, Grated	2 Tbsp	43	3	30	2	0	9	153	0	0	4	1 lean meat
Port du Salut	1 oz	100	8	70	5	0	35	151	0	0	7	1 high-fat meat
Provolone	1 oz	100	8	70	5	0	20	248	1	0	7	1 high-fat meat
Ricotta, Fat Free	1/4 cup	45	0	0	0	0	20	50	3	0	8	1 lean meat
Ricotta, Part Skim	1/4 cup	85	5	45	3	0	19	76	3	0	7	1 med-fat meat

Romano	1 oz	110	8	5	0	29	340	1	0	9	1 high-fat meat
String Cheese	1	83	5	3.5	0	18	236	<1	0	7	1 med-fat meat
Swiss	1 oz	108	8	5	0	26	55	1.5	0	8	1 high-fat meat
Swiss, Fat Free	1 oz	41	0	0	0	7	352	3	0	7	1 lean meat
Swiss, Reduced Fat	1 oz	70	3.5	2	0	10	130	0	0	9	1 med-fat meat
Tilsit	1 oz	96	7	5	0	29	213	1	0	7	1 med-fat meat
Brands											
Alpine Lace											
American, White, Reduced Fat, Reduced Sodium	3/4-oz slice	70	5	3	0	15	310	1	0	5	1 med-fat meat
American, Yellow, Reduced Fat, Reduced Sodium	3/4-oz slice	70	5	3	0	15	310	1	0	5	1 med-fat meat
Cheddar, Reduced Fat	3/4-oz slice	70	5	3.5	0	15	135	0	0	6	1 med-fat meat

CHEESE, COTTAGE CHEESE, CREAM CHEESE

	Serving	Calories	Fat (g)	Cal. from Fat	Sat. Fat (g)	Trans Fat (g)	Chol. (mg)	Sod. (mg)	Carb. (g)	Fiber (g)	Prot. (g)	Servings/Exchanges
CO-JACK Semisoft Cheese, Reduced Fat	3/4-oz slice	70	5	50	3.5	0	15	150	0	0	5	1 med-fat meat
Mozzarella, Low Moisture, Reduced Fat	3/4-oz slice	60	4	35	2.5	0	15	160	1	0	5	1 med-fat meat
Muenster, Reduced Sodium	3/4-oz slice	90	7	60	4.5	0	15	110	1	0	6	1 med-fat meat
Provolone, Reduced Fat	3/4-oz slice	70	4.5	40	3	0	10	135	1	0	6	1 med-fat meat
Swiss, Reduced Fat	3/4-oz slice	70	4.5	40	3	0	15	95	1	0	7	1 med-fat meat
Athenos												
Blue Cheese	3 Tbsp	110	9	80	6	0	30	430	2	<1	7	1 high-fat meat
Gorgonzola	3 Tbsp	110	9	80	6	0	30	400	2	<1	7	1 high-fat meat
Traditional Feta	1/4 cup	90	7	60	4	0	25	390	2	<1	7	1 med-fat meat

Breakstone's

Cottage Cheese, 2% Low Fat, Small Curd	1/2 cup	90	2.5	15	1.5	0	15	400	6	0	12	2 lean meat
Cottage Cheese, 4% Milkfat, Large Curd	1/2 cup	120	5	45	3	0	25	430	6	0	12	2 lean meat
Cottage Cheese, 4% Milkfat, Small Curd	1/2 cup	120	5	45	3	0	25	430	6	0	12	2 lean meat
Cottage Cheese, Fat Free, Small Curd	1/2 cup	80	0	0	0	0	10	450	8	0	12	2 lean meat

DiGiorno

Parmesan, Shredded	1/4 cup	110	8	70	4.5	0	25	430	0	0	1	1 high-fat meat
Romano, Grated	2 tsp	20	2	20	1	0	5	75	0	0	2	free

Knudsen

Cottage Cheese, 2% Lowfat, Small Curd	1/2 cup	100	2.5	20	1.5	0	15	440	6	0	14	2 lean meat
Cottage Cheese, Nonfat	1/2 cup	80	0	0	0	0	5	430	7	0	13	2 lean meat

CHEESE, COTTAGE CHEESE, CREAM CHEESE

	Serving	Calories	Fat (g)	Cal. from Fat	Sat. Fat (g)	Trans Fat (g)	Chol. (mg)	Sod. (mg)	Carb. (g)	Fiber (g)	Prot. (g)	Servings/Exchanges
Cottage Doubles, Blueberry	5.6 oz	140	2.5	20	1.5	0	15	400	18	1	11	1 carb, 1 lean meat
Cottage Doubles, Peach	5.6 oz	140	2.5	20	1.5	0	15	390	17	0	11	1 carb, 1 lean meat
Creamed Cottage Cheese, Small Curd	1/2 cup	120	5	45	3	0	25	430	5	0	13	2 lean meat
LiveActive Cottage Cheese	4 oz	90	2	20	1.5	0	15	380	8	3	10	1/2 carb, 1 lean meat
Kraft												
Cheddar & Monterey Jack, Natural 2% Reduced Fat Cubes	7 pieces	90	6	60	4	0	20	260	<1	0	8	1 med-fat meat
Cheddar Cheese Sticks, Mild Cheddar	1 oz	120	10	90	6	0	30	180	0	0	6	1 high-fat meat
Cheddar, 2% Reduced Fat, Mild, Shredded	1 oz	90	7	60	4.5	0	20	220	<1	0	7	1 med-fat meat

Food											
Cheddar, Fat Free, Shredded	1/4 cup	45	0	0	0	<5	280	2	0	9	1 lean meat
Cheddar, Natural	1 oz	120	10	6	90	30	180	0	0	6	1 high-fat meat
Cheddar, Sharp, Cheese Sticks	1 oz	90	6	3.5	50	20	240	1	0	7	1 med-fat meat
Cheddar, Shredded	1 oz	110	9	6	80	25	190	1	0	6	1 high-fat meat
Cheese Cubes, Natural, 2% Reduced Fat	1.5 oz	160	13	9	120	40	280	1	0	10	2 high-fat meat
Cheese Spread, Pimento	2 Tbsp	80	6	4	60	20	170	3	0	2	1 med-fat meat
Cheez Whiz Cheese Dip	2 Tbsp	90	7	4.5	60	30	490	4	0	3	1 med-fat meat
Cheez Whiz Cheese Dip, Light	2 Tbsp	80	3.5	2	30	20	500	6	0	6	1 med-fat meat
Classic Melts Four Cheese Shredded Cheese	1 oz	120	7	7	90	30	310	1	0	7	1 med-fat meat

CHEESE, COTTAGE CHEESE, CREAM CHEESE

	Serving	Calories	Fat (g)	Cal. from Fat	Sat. Fat (g)	Trans Fat (g)	Chol. (mg)	Sod. (mg)	Carb. (g)	Fiber (g)	Prot. (g)	Servings/Exchanges
Colby & Monterey Jack, 2% Reduced Fat, Natural	1/4 cup	80	5	70	3.5	0	15	220	<1	0	7	1 med-fat meat
Colby & Monterey Jack, Shredded	1 oz	100	8	70	5	0	25	190	1	0	6	1 high-fat meat
Colby, Natural	1 oz	110	9	80	6	0	30	180	1	0	6	1 high-fat meat
Cracker Barrel, Spreadable Sharp Cheddar	2 Tbsp	80	8	70	5	0	20	180	<1	0	3	1 high-fat meat
Cream Cheese, Neufchatel, Philadelphia	1 oz	70	6	60	4	0	20	120	1	0	2	1 med-fat meat
Cream Cheese, Philadelphia Brick	1 oz	100	9	80	6	0	35	105	1	0	2	2 fat
Cream Cheese, Philadelphia Brick, Fat Free	1 oz	30	0	0	0	0	5	200	2	0	4	1 lean meat

Food	Serving											Exchanges
Cream Cheese, Philadelphia Soft	2 Tbsp	90	9	80	5	0	35	125	2	0	2	2 fat
Cream Cheese, Philadelphia Soft, Cheesecake	2 Tbsp	100	8	70	5	0	30	115	5	0	1	2 fat
Cream Cheese, Philadelphia Soft, Fat Free	2 Tbsp	30	0	0	0	0	5	200	1	0	5	1 lean meat
Cream Cheese, Philadelphia Soft, Honey Nut	2 Tbsp	90	8	70	4.5	0	30	110	4	0	1	2 fat
Cream Cheese, Philadelphia Soft, Light	2 Tbsp	70	5	45	3	0	20	140	2	0	2	1 fat
Cream Cheese, Philadelphia Soft, Pineapple	2 Tbsp	90	7	70	4.5	0	30	110	4	0	1	1 fat

CHEESE, COTTAGE CHEESE, CREAM CHEESE

	Serving	Calories	Fat (g)	Cal. from Fat	Sat. Fat (g)	Trans Fat (g)	Chol. (mg)	Sod. (mg)	Carb. (g)	Fiber (g)	Prot. (g)	Servings/Exchanges
Cream Cheese, Philadelphia Soft, Salmon	2 Tbsp	90	8	70	5	0	30	210	2	0	2	2 fat
Cream Cheese, Philadelphia Soft, Strawberry	2 Tbsp	90	8	70	4.5	0	30	110	5	0	1	2 fat
Cream Cheese, Philadelphia Whipped	2 Tbsp	60	6	50	3.5	0	20	90	1	0	1	1 fat
Easy Cheese Cheddar Cheese Snack	2 Tbsp	90	6	60	3	0	20	410	2	0	5	1 med-fat meat
Easy Cheese Cheddar 'n Bacon Cheese Snack	2 Tbsp	90	7	60	4.5	0	25	400	2	0	5	1 med-fat meat
Mexican Four Cheese, Shredded, Natural	1 oz	100	8	70	5	0	25	180	1	0	6	1 high-fat meat

Food	Serving											Exchange
Mexican Style, 2% Milk Reduced Fat, Natural Crumbles	1/4 cup	80	5	50	3	0	15	220	<1	0	7	1 med-fat meat
Monterey Jack & Jalapeño Pepper, Natural	1 oz	110	9	80	5	0	25	190	1	0	6	1 high-fat meat
Monterey Jack, Natural	1 oz	110	9	80	6	0	30	190	0	0	6	1 high-fat meat
Mozzarella, Part-Skim, Natural	1 oz	80	6	50	3.5	0	20	220	1	0	7	1 med-fat meat
Mozzarella, Part-Skim, Shredded	1 oz	80	4	50	3.5	0	20	200	1	0	7	1 med-fat meat
Parmesan, Grated	2 tsp	20	1.5	15	1	0	5	85	0	0	2	free
Romano, Grated	2 tsp	20	1.5	15	1	0	5	85	0	0	2	free
Singles American, Fat Free	2/3-oz slice	45	0	0	0	0	<5	250	2	0	4	1 lean meat
Singles, American	2/3-oz slice	60	4.5	40	2.5	0	15	250	1	0	3	1 med-fat meat

CHEESE, COTTAGE CHEESE, CREAM CHEESE

	Serving	Calories	Fat (g)	Cal. from Fat	Sat. Fat (g)	Trans Fat (g)	Chol. (mg)	Sod. (mg)	Carb. (g)	Fiber (g)	Prot. (g)	Servings/Exchanges
Singles, American, 2% Milk	2/3-oz slice	45	2.5	20	1.5	0	10	280	2	0	4	1 lean meat
Singles, Sharp Cheddar, Fat Free	2/3-oz slice	25	0	0	0	0	<5	280	2	0	5	1 lean meat
Singles, Swiss	2/3-oz slice	45	2.5	20	1.5	0	10	270	2	0	4	1 lean meat
Singles, White American	3/4-oz slice	60	5	40	2.5	0	15	260	2	0	4	1 med-fat meat
Smoky Swiss & Cheddar, Natural	1 oz	100	8	70	5	0	25	380	1	0	5	1 high-fat meat
String-Ums 2% Milk String Cheese	1 oz	80	6	50	3.5	0	20	220	1	0	7	1 med-fat meat
Swiss Cheese, Shredded	1 oz	110	8	70	5	0	25	60	1	0	7	1 high-fat meat

Velveeta Cheese Spread	1 oz	80	6	50	4	0	25	410	3	0	5	1 med-fat meat
Velveeta Cheese Spread, 2% Milk	1 oz	60	3	25	1.5	0	10	410	4	0	5	1 lean meat
Velveeta Cheese Spread, Mexican, Mild or Hot	1 oz	90	6	60	4	0	25	430	3	0	5	1 med-fat meat

Lifetime

Cheddar, Fat Free, Shredded	1/3 cup	45	0	0	0	0	<5	310	2	0	8	1 lean meat
Cheddar, Low Fat	1 oz	40	0	0	0	0	<5	220	1	1	8	1 lean meat

Sargento Blends

Cheddar, Medium, Reduced Fat Slices	1 slice	60	4	35	2.5	0	15	135	0	0	6	1 med-fat meat
Cheddar, Mild, Reduced Fat Shredded	1/4 cup	80	6	50	4	0	20	180	<1	0	7	1 med-fat meat
Four Cheese Italian, Reduced Fat Shredded	1/4 cup	80	4.5	40	3	0	15	220	1	0	8	1 med-fat meat

CHEESE, COTTAGE CHEESE, CREAM CHEESE

	Serving	Calories	Fat (g)	Cal. from Fat	Sat. Fat (g)	Trans Fat (g)	Chol. (mg)	Sod. (mg)	Carb. (g)	Fiber (g)	Prot. (g)	Servings/Exchanges
Mozzarella, Light String	1 piece	50	2.5	25	1.5	0	10	160	1	0	6	1 med-fat meat
Swiss, Reduced Fat Slices	1 slice	60	4	35	2	0	10	30	1	0	7	1 med-fat meat
Shamrock												
Cottage Cheese, 2% Lowfat	1/2 cup	100	2	20	1.5	0	15	440	5	0	13	2 lean meat
Cottage Cheese, 4% Original	1/2 cup	110	5	45	4.5	0	40	370	5	0	13	2 lean meat
Smart Balance												
Cheese Product Shreds	1 oz	80	5	50	1.5	0	5	260	<1	0	7	1 med-fat meat
Creamy Cheddar-Flavor Slices	2/3-oz slice	40	2	20	0.5	0	<5	290	2	0	4	1 lean meat
Smart Beat Fat Free Slices	1 slice	25	0	0	0	0	0	170	3	0	3	1 lean meat

COMBINATION FOODS, ENTRÉES, SALADS

	Serving	Calories	Fat (g)	Cal. from Fat	Sat. Fat (g)	Trans Fat (g)	Chol. (mg)	Sod. (mg)	Carb. (g)	Fiber (g)	Prot. (g)	Servings/Exchanges
Beef Burgundy	1 cup	285	11	100	3	NA	91	110	10	2	34	1/2 carb, 5 lean meat
Beef Stroganoff & Noodles	1 cup	342	20	180	8	NA	73	454	21	2	20	1 1/2 carb, 2 med-fat meat, 2 fat
Beef with Macaroni & Tomato Sauce, Homemade	1 cup	254	10	90	4	NA	39	862	26	3	16	2 carb, 2 med-fat meat
Burrito, Bean	1	224	7	65	4	NA	2	493	36	4	7	2 1/2 carb, 1 fat
Burrito, Beef	1	262	11	100	6	NA	32	746	30	<1	13	2 carb, 1 med-fat meat, 1 fat
Cabbage Rolls, Stuffed	8 oz	179	6	55	1	NA	11	551	23	4	8	1 1/2 carb, 1 med-fat meat, 1 fat
Chicken & Noodles, Homemade	1 cup	367	19	170	6	NA	96	600	26	2	22	2 carb, 2 med-fat meat, 2 fat

COMBINATION FOODS, ENTRÉES, SALADS

	Serving	Calories	Fat (g)	Cal. from Fat	Sat. Fat (g)	Trans Fat (g)	Chol. (mg)	Sod. (mg)	Carb. (g)	Fiber (g)	Prot. (g)	Servings/Exchanges
Chicken à la King, Homemade	1 cup	468	34	310	13	NA	186	760	12	1	27	1 carb, 3 med-fat meat, 4 fat
Chicken Tetrazzini	1 cup	372	20	180	7	NA	50	813	28	2	19	2 carb, 2 med-fat meat, 2 fat
Chiles Rellenos	1	425	35	315	17	NA	165	620	7	1	23	1/2 carb, 3 med-fat meat, 4 fat
Chili Con Carne with Beans & Rice	1 cup	297	8	70	4	NA	25	1162	46	6	11	3 carb, 2 fat
Chili Con Carne, No Beans	1 cup	350	19	170	7	NA	81	1407	21	4	25	1 1/2 carb, 3 med-fat meat, 1 fat
Chimichanga, Beef & Bean	1	249	12	110	3	NA	24	242	26	3	11	2 carb, 1 med-fat meat, 1 fat
Chop Suey, Beef, with Noodles	1 cup	425	25	225	5	NA	46	818	31	3	22	2 carb, 2 med-fat meat, 3 fat

Food	Serving											Exchanges
Chop Suey, Shrimp, with Noodles	1 cup	277	12	110	2	NA	122	937	22	2	21	1 1/2 carb, 2 med-fat meat
Chow Mein, Beef, No Noodles	1 cup	275	16	145	4	NA	54	774	12	2	22	1 carb, 3 med-fat meat
Chow Mein, Shrimp, with Noodles	1 cup	277	12	110	2	NA	122	937	22	2	21	1 1/2 carb, 2 med-fat meat
Corndog	1	460	19	170	5	NA	79	973	56	NA	17	4 carb, 1 med-fat meat, 3 fat
Corned Beef Hash, Canned	1 cup	398	25	225	12	NA	73	1188	24	1	19	1 1/2 carb, 2 med-fat meat, 3 fat
Curry, Beef	1 cup	437	32	290	7	NA	70	1323	13	3	27	1 carb, 3 med-fat meat, 3 fat
Eggplant Parmesan	1 cup	320	22	200	10	NA	57	683	17	3	15	1 carb, 2 med-fat meat, 2 fat
Enchilada, Beef & Cheese	1	323	18	160	9	NA	40	1319	31	NA	12	2 carb, 1 med-fat meat, 3 fat

COMBINATION FOODS, ENTRÉES, SALADS

	Serving	Calories	Fat (g)	Cal. from Fat	Sat. Fat (g)	Trans Fat (g)	Chol. (mg)	Sod. (mg)	Carb. (g)	Fiber (g)	Prot. (g)	Servings/Exchanges
Enchilada, Chicken	1	195	9	80	4	NA	36	312	16	2	13	1 carb, 2 med-fat meat
Fajita, Chicken	1	405	13	120	3	NA	41	439	50	4	22	3 carb, 2 med-fat meat, 1 fat
Goulash, Beef, with Noodles	1 cup	341	14	125	4	NA	88	457	23	2	30	1 1/2 carb, 3 med-fat meat
Lasagna	8 oz	302	12	110	NA	NA	34	885	27	NA	22	2 carb, 2 med-fat meat
Macaroni & Cheese	1 cup	228	10	90	4	NA	NA	730	26	NA	9	2 carb, 2 med-fat meat
Meat Loaf, Beef & 1/3 Pork	1 slice	205	14	125	5	NA	84	381	5	<1	15	2 med-fat meat, 1 fat
Meat Tamale	1	183	10	90	4	NA	24	229	16	3	7	1 carb, 1 med-fat meat, 1 fat
Meat Tortellini	1 cup	372	15	135	5	NA	238	797	33	1	25	2 carb, 3 med-fat meat
Moo Goo Gai Pan	1 cup	281	20	180	5	NA	39	327	12	3	15	2 vegetable, 2 med-fat meat, 2 fat

Food	Serving											Exchanges/Choices
Pepper, Stuffed Green Bell	1	229	12	110	5	NA	34	201	20	2	11	1 carb, 1 vegetable, 2 med-fat meat, 2 fat
Pizza, Cheese, Thin Crust	1/4 of 10-inch	317	17	155	7	NA	20	770	28	NA	14	2 carb, 2 med-fat meat, 1 fat
Pizza, Meat, Thin Crust	1/4 of 10-inch	368	21	190	7	NA	29	1000	29	NA	15	2 carb, 2 med-fat meat, 2 fat
Pot Pie	7 oz	450	28	250	NA	NA	34	778	35	NA	13	2 carb, 2 med-fat meat, 4 fat
Quesadilla	1	199	10	90	4	NA	14	255	21	1	6	1 1/2 carb, 2 fat
Quiche Lorraine	1/8 pie	508	39	350	18	NA	205	549	20	<1	20	1 carb, 3 med-fat meat, 5 fat
Ravioli, Cheese with Tomato Sauce	1	336	14	125	6	NA	160	1541	38	2	14	2 1/2 carb, 1 med-fat meat, 2 fat
Salad, Carrot Raisin	1/2 cup	202	14	125	2	NA	10	117	21	2	1	1/2 fruit, 2 vegetable, 3 fat
Salad, Chef Style	1 1/2 cup	267	16	145	8	NA	140	743	5	NA	26	1 vegetable, 3 med-fat meat

COMBINATION FOODS, ENTRÉES, SALADS

	Serving	Calories	Fat (g)	Cal. from Fat	Sat. Fat (g)	Trans Fat (g)	Chol. (mg)	Sod. (mg)	Carb. (g)	Fiber (g)	Prot. (g)	Servings/Exchanges
Salad, Egg	1/2 cup	293	28	250	6	NA	287	333	2	0	8	1 med-fat meat, 5 fat
Salad, Potato, No Egg	1/2 cup	134	7	65	1	NA	5	345	16	2	2	1 carb, 1 fat
Salad, Seafood	1/2 cup	166	12	110	2	NA	64	274	3	<1	13	2 med-fat meat
Salad, Shrimp	1/2 cup	141	9	80	2	NA	103	196	3	<1	13	2 med-fat meat
Salad, Three Bean	1/2 cup	70	4	35	<1	NA	0	257	7	2	2	1/2 carb, 1 fat
Salad, Tuna	1/2 cup	192	10	90	2	NA	13	412	10	0	16	1/2 carb, 2 med-fat meat
Salad, Waldorf	1/2 cup	201	20	180	2	NA	10	118	6	1	2	1/2 fruit, 4 fat
Salmon Patty or Cake	4.5 oz	261	16	145	4	NA	57	657	14	1	16	1 carb, 2 med-fat meat, 1 fat
Shepherd's Pie, Beef	1 cup	287	10	90	3	NA	41	702	31	3	18	2 carb, 2 med-fat meat
Shrimp with Noodles & Cheese Sauce	1 cup	350	15	135	6	NA	220	698	24	2	28	1 1/2 carb, 3 med-fat meat
Shrimp, Stuffed	1 cup	276	14	125	3	NA	221	694	9	<1	28	1/2 carb, 4 lean meat

Food	Serving											Exchanges
Sloppy Joe Gravy/Sauce, Beef	1 cup	380	23	205	9	NA	81	1246	24	3	21	1 1/2 carb, 2 med-fat meat, 3 fat
Soufflé, Cheese, Homemade	1 cup	197	14	125	6	NA	194	299	6	<1	12	2 med-fat meat, 1 fat
Soufflé, Spinach	1 cup	219	18	160	7	NA	184	763	3	3	12	2 med-fat meat, 2 fat
Spaghetti with Meatballs	1 cup	258	10	90	2	NA	NA	1220	29	NA	12	2 carb, 2 med-fat meat
Sukiyaki	1 cup	175	8	70	3	NA	154	762	6	1	19	1/2 carb, 3 lean meat
Swedish Meatballs with Cream Sauce	1 cup	404	23	205	10	NA	162	1157	17	<1	31	1 carb, 4 med-fat meat, 1 fat
Sweet & Sour Pork with Rice	1 cup	269	6	55	2	NA	29	906	40	1	13	2 1/2 carb, 1 med-fat meat
Taco, Chicken	1	173	8	70	3	NA	45	106	9	1	15	1/2 carb, 2 med-fat meat
Tostada, Bean & Cheese	1	223	10	90	5	NA	30	543	27	7	10	2 carb, 1 med-fat meat, 1 fat
Tostada, Bean & Chicken	1	248	11	100	5	NA	53	434	18	3	20	1 carb, 2 med-fat meat

COMBINATION FOODS, ENTREES, SALADS

	Serving	Calories	Fat (g)	Cal. from Fat	Sat. Fat (g)	Trans Fat (g)	Chol. (mg)	Sod. (mg)	Carb. (g)	Fiber (g)	Prot. (g)	Servings/Exchanges
Tuna-Noodle Casserole	9 oz	259	8	70	NA	NA	NA	1043	34	NA	13	2 carb, 2 med-fat meat
Turkey-Noodle Casserole	1 cup	326	13	115	4	NA	84	732	29	2	23	2 carb, 2 med-fat meat, 2 fat
Veal Parmigiana	1 cup	350	20	180	8	NA	138	755	15	1	27	1 strch, 3 med-fat meat
Armour LunchMakers												
Cracker Crunchers, Bologna	1	250	16	140	7	0	35	740	22	1	9	1 1/2 carb, 1 med-fat meat, 2 fat
Loco Nachos	1	400	14	130	3	1.5	10	760	69	4	4	4 1/2 carb, 3 fat
Pepperoni Pizza	1	370	9	80	5	0	15	530	65	5	8	4 carb, 2 fat
Betty Crocker												
Bowl Appetit! Cheddar Broccoli Pasta	1 bowl	310	7	60	2.5	1.5	10	960	52	2	10	3 1/2 carb, 1 fat
Bowl Appetit! Parmesan Pasta	1 bowl	310	8	70	2.5	2.5	<5	1010	51	1	9	3 1/2 carb, 2 fat

Food	Serving	Cal.	Fat (g)	Cal. from Fat	Sat. Fat (g)	Trans Fat (g)	Chol. (mg)	Sod. (mg)	Carb. (g)	Fiber (g)	Sugars (g)	Pro. (g)	Choices/Exchanges
Bowl Appetit! Teriyaki Rice	1 bowl	250	1	5	0	0	0	940	57	2	<1	5	4 carb
Chicken Helper, Cheesy Chicken Enchilada	1 cup	330	7	65	2	0.5	60	820	42	<1	2	25	3 carb, 2 lean meat
Chicken Helper, Chicken Fried Rice	1 cup	250	9	80	2	0	115	550	22	1	1	22	1 1/2 carb, 3 lean meat
Chicken Helper, Creamy Chicken & Noodles	1 cup	280	9	80	2.5	1	60	750	24	<1	1	25	1 1/2 carb, 3 lean meat
Chicken Helper, Fettuccine Alfredo	1 cup	330	11	100	3.5	1.5	60	810	31	1	1	26	2 carb, 3 lean meat
Hamburger Helper, Beef Pasta	1 cup	280	11	100	4.5	0.5	55	760	23	1	1	21	1 1/2 carb, 2 med-fat meat
Hamburger Helper, Cheeseburger Macaroni	1 cup	310	12	110	5	0	60	910	27	<1	<1	22	2 carb, 2 med-fat meat
Hamburger Helper, Cheesy Hashbrowns	1 cup	400	19	170	6	0	55	990	38	2	2	20	2 1/2 carb, 2 med-fat meat, 2 fat

COMBINATION FOODS, ENTREES, SALADS

	Serving	Calories	Fat (g)	Cal. from Fat	Sat. Fat (g)	Trans Fat (g)	Chol. (mg)	Sod. (mg)	Carb. (g)	Fiber (g)	Prot. (g)	Servings/Exchanges
Hamburger Helper, Crunchy Taco	1 cup	340	14	125	5	1	55	870	33	1	20	2 carb, 2 med-fat meat, 1 fat
Hamburger Helper, Double Cheese Enchilada	1 cup	350	13	115	5	1	55	840	40	<1	21	2 1/2 carb, 2 med-fat meat, 1 fat
Hamburger Helper, Italian Sausage	1 cup	290	11	100	4	0.5	55	860	29	1	20	2 carb, 2 med-fat meat
Hamburger Helper, Lasagna	1 cup	280	11	100	4	0.5	55	900	27	<1	19	2 carb, 2 med-fat meat
Hamburger Helper, Philly Cheesesteak	1 cup	320	13	115	5	1	55	750	28	1	22	2 carb, 2 med-fat meat, 1 fat
Hamburger Helper, Potato Stroganoff	1 cup	290	14	125	5	1	60	790	26	1	21	2 carb, 2 med-fat meat, 1 fat
Hamburger Helper, Tomato Basil Penne	1 cup	300	11	100	4	1	55	710	26	1	23	2 carb, 3 lean meat

	Serving	Cal.	Fat (g)	Cal. from Fat	Sat. Fat (g)	Trans Fat (g)	Chol. (mg)	Sod. (mg)	Carb. (g)	Fiber (g)	Prot. (g)	Exchanges/Choices
Suddenly Salad, Caesar	1 cup	310	14	130	2	0	0	640	38	1	6	2 1/2 carb, 3 fat
Suddenly Salad, Chipotle Ranch	1 cup	290	16	140	2	0	15	450	32	2	6	2 carb, 3 fat
Suddenly Salad, Ranch & Bacon	3/4 cup	290	16	140	2	0	15	450	32	1	6	2 carb, 3 fat
Tuna Helper, Creamy Broccoli	1 cup	290	12	110	3	1.5	20	870	34	2	14	2 carb, 1 med-fat meat, 1 fat
Tuna Helper, Fettuccine Alfredo	1 cup	280	12	110	3.5	1.5	20	970	31	1	13	2 carb, 1 med-fat meat, 1 fat
Tuna Helper, Tetrazzini	1 cup	280	11	100	3	0	10	910	31	1	15	2 carb, 2 med-fat meat
Tuna Helper, Tuna Melt	1 cup	300	10	90	3	1.5	20	1050	39	<1	14	2 1/2 carb, 1 med-fat meat, 1 fat
Campbell's SpaghettiOs												
RavioliOs, Beef in Meat Sauce	1 cup	270	8	70	3.5	0	20	1090	38	<1	11	2 1/2 carb, 1 med-fat meat, 1 fat
SpaghettiOs Meatballs	1 cup	240	8	70	3.5	0	15	600	32	4	11	2 carb, 2 fat

COMBINATION FOODS, ENTREES, SALADS

	Serving	Calories	Fat (g)	Cal. from Fat	Sat. Fat (g)	Trans Fat (g)	Chol. (mg)	Sod. (mg)	Carb. (g)	Fiber (g)	Prot. (g)	Servings/Exchanges
SpaghettiOs Original	1 cup	200	1.5	15	0.5	0	5	950	40	3	7	2 1/2 carb
SpaghettiOs with Meat Sauce	1 cup	180	2	20	1	0	10	890	32	3	8	2 carb
Chef Boyardee												
Beef Ravioli	1 cup	240	8	70	3	0	15	900	35	3	8	2 carb, 2 fat
Beefaroni	1 cup	260	10	90	4.5	0	25	990	33	3	10	2 carb, 1 med-fat meat, 1 fat
Cheese Nacho Twistaroni	1 cup	220	7	60	3.5	0	15	950	32	2	8	2 carb, 1 fat
Lasagna	1 cup	270	10	90	5	0	25	830	36	2	9	2 1/2 carb, 2 fat
Healthy Choice Fresh Mixers												
Chicken Cacciatore	1 pkg	310	4	35	1	0	30	600	49	6	20	3 carb, 2 lean meat
Sesame Teriyaki Chicken	1 pkg	380	6	50	1.5	0	20	600	69	3	13	4 1/2 carb, 1 fat

Food	Serving											Exchanges
Steak Portobello	1 pkg	290	6	50	1.5	0	15	600	42	5	16	3 carb, 1 med-fat meat
Sweet & Sour Chicken	1 pkg	390	3	25	1	0	25	400	78	5	12	5 carb, 1 fat
Sweet Hickory BBQ Chicken	1 pkg	370	3	25	1	0	35	600	70	5	16	4 1/2 carb, 1 med-fat meat
Tuscan Style Chicken	1 pkg	320	5	45	1.5	0	25	540	50	6	18	3 carb, 1 med-fat meat
Hormel												
Hormel Compleats, Beef Pot Roast	10 oz	270	6	55	3	0	50	1470	29	3	24	2 carb, 3 lean meat
Hormel Compleats, Beef Steak Tips	10 oz	270	9	80	4	0	45	800	29	2	17	2 carb, 2 med-fat meat
Hormel Compleats, Chicken & Dumplings	10 oz	260	8	70	2	0	40	990	34	1	13	2 carb, 1 med-fat meat, 1 fat
Hormel Compleats, Chicken & Noodles	10 oz	240	8	70	4	0	60	990	27	2	15	2 carb, 1 med-fat meat, 1 fat
Hormel Compleats, Lasagna	10 oz	280	7	65	2	0	50	1100	42	3	13	3 carb, 1 med-fat meat

COMBINATION FOODS, ENTREES, SALADS

	Serving	Calories	Fat (g)	Cal. from Fat	Sat. Fat (g)	Trans Fat (g)	Chol. (mg)	Sod. (mg)	Carb. (g)	Fiber (g)	Prot. (g)	Servings/Exchanges
Microcup Beef Stew	7.5 oz	150	6	55	3	0	25	890	15	2	10	1 carb, 1 med-fat meat
Microcup Spaghetti with Meat Sauce	7.5 oz	210	5	45	2.5	0	15	750	31	3	10	2 carb, 1 med-fat meat
Marie Callender's Home-Style Creations												
Classic Stroganoff	1 pkg	310	10	90	3.5	0	35	860	39	3	17	2 1/2 carb, 1 med-fat meat, 1 fat
Creamy Parmesan Chicken	1 pkg	490	23	210	10	0.5	65	980	43	4	27	3 carb, 3 med-fat meat, 2 fat
Garlic Herb Chicken	1 pkg	340	10	90	3.5	0	30	960	47	4	16	3 carb, 1 med-fat meat, 1 fat
Meatball Lasagna	1 pkg	310	9	80	3	0	20	760	43	6	14	3 carb, 1 med-fat meat, 1 fat
Oscar Mayer Deli Creations												
Flatbread Sandwich, Chicken Bacon Ranch	1 pkg	320	13	120	4.5	0	55	600	29	<1	22	2 carb, 2 med-fat meat, 1 fat

Hot Sandwich Melts, Ham & Cheddar	1 pkg	430	16	140	6	0	55	1540	47	5	28	3 carb, 3 med-fat meat
Hot Sandwich Melts, Steakhouse Cheddar	1 pkg	450	16	140	6	0.5	60	1410	51	3	28	3 1/2 carb, 3 med-fat meat
Hot Sandwich Melts, Turkey Monterey	1 pkg	450	17	160	6	0.5	55	1170	51	4	25	3 1/2 carb, 2 med-fat meat, 1 fat

Oscar Mayer Lunchables

Lunchables, Chicken Dunks	1	320	6	50	1.5	0	30	550	55	0	12	3 1/2 carb, 1 med-fat meat
Lunchables, Deep Dish Cheese Pizza	1	370	11	90	3.5	0	15	500	60	5	10	4 carb, 2 fat
Lunchables, Ham & American Cracker Stackers	1	370	16	140	8	0.5	35	850	40	<1	15	2 1/2 carb, 1 med-fat meat, 2 fat
Lunchables, Mini Hot Dogs	1	380	11	100	3.5	0	20	690	62	1	10	4 carb, 2 fat

COMBINATION FOODS, ENTREES, SALADS

	Serving	Calories	Fat (g)	Cal. from Fat	Sat. Fat (g)	Trans Fat (g)	Chol. (mg)	Sod. (mg)	Carb. (g)	Fiber (g)	Prot. (g)	Servings/Exchanges
Lunchables, Nachos, Cheese Dip & Salsa	1	380	21	190	6	0	15	880	41	<1	7	2 1/2 carb, 4 fat
Lunchables, Pepperoni Pizza	1	410	11	100	5	0	30	630	64	3	16	4 carb, 1 med-fat meat, 1 ft
Lunchables, Turkey & Cheddar Cracker Stackers	1	380	13	110	5	0.5	30	780	53	3	13	3 1/2 carb, 3 fat

COOKING OILS, FATS

Oils

	Serving	Calories	Fat (g)	Cal. from Fat	Sat. Fat (g)	Trans Fat (g)	Chol (mg)	Sod. (mg)	Carb. (g)	Fiber (g)	Prot. (g)	Servings/Exchanges
Avocado Oil	1 tsp	41	4.5	40	<1	0	0	0	0	0	0	1 fat
Canola Oil	1 tsp	40	4.5	40	<1	0	0	0	0	0	0	1 fat
Cocoa Butter Oil	1 tsp	40	4.5	40	3	0	0	0	0	0	0	1 fat
Coconut Oil	1 tsp	39	4.5	40	4	0	0	0	0	0	0	1 fat
Cod Liver/Fish Oil	1 tsp	41	4.5	40	1	0	0	0	0	0	0	1 fat
Corn Oil	1 tsp	40	4.5	40	<1	0	0	0	0	0	0	1 fat
Cottonseed Oil	1 tsp	40	4.5	40	1	0	0	0	0	0	0	1 fat
Flaxseed Oil	1 tsp	40	4.5	40	<1	0	0	0	0	0	0	1 fat
Grapeseed Oil	1 tsp	40	4.5	40	<1	0	0	0	0	0	0	1 fat
Hazelnut Oil	1 tsp	40	4.5	40	<1	0	0	0	0	0	0	1 fat
Olive Oil	1 tsp	40	4.5	40	0.5	0	0	0	0	0	0	1 fat

COOKING OILS, FATS

	Serving	Calories	Fat (g)	Cal. from Fat	Sat. Fat (g)	Trans Fat (g)	Chol (mg)	Sod. (mg)	Carb. (g)	Fiber (g)	Prot. (g)	Servings/Exchanges
Palm Kernel Oil	1 tsp	39	4.5	40	3.5	0	0	0	0	0	0	1 fat
Palm Oil	1 tsp	40	4.5	40	2	0	0	0	0	0	0	1 fat
Peanut Oil	1 tsp	40	4.5	40	1	0	0	0	0	0	0	1 fat
Safflower Oil	1 tsp	44	4.5	40	<1	0	0	0	0	0	0	1 fat
Sardine/Fish Oil	1 tsp	41	4.5	40	1	0	0	32	0	0	0	1 fat
Sesame Oil	1 tsp	40	4.5	40	<1	0	0	0	0	0	0	1 fat
Soybean & Canola Oil	1 tsp	40	4.5	40	<1	0	0	0	0	0	0	1 fat
Soybean Oil	1 tsp	44	4.5	40	<1	0	0	0	0	0	0	1 fat
Sunflower Oil	1 tsp	40	4.5	40	<1	0	0	0	0	0	0	1 fat
Fats												
Chitterlings, Boiled	2 Tbsp	38	3	25	1.5	0	44	3	0	0	2	1 fat
Lard	1 tsp	39	4	35	2	0	4	0	0	0	0	1 fat
Salt Pork, Raw, Cured	.25 oz	51	5	45	2	0	6	91	0	0	<1	1 fat
Shortening	1 tsp	38	4	35	1	0	0	0	0	0	0	1 fat

DESSERTS, CAKE, PIE, CHEESECAKE, COOKIES, BROWNIES

	Serving	Calories	Fat (g)	Cal. from Fat	Sat. Fat (g)	Trans Fat (g)	Chol. (mg)	Sod. (mg)	Carb. (g)	Fiber (g)	Prot. (g)	Servings/Exchanges
Angel Food Cake	1 piece	128	0	0	0	0	0	254	29	<1	3	2 carb
Apple Turnover	1	284	16	145	4	0	0	176	31	2	4	2 carb, 3 fat
Brownie	1 small	115	5	45	1	5	15	88	18	<1	1	1 carb, 1 fat
Cake, Chocolate with Chocolate Icing	1 piece	352	14	125	5	0	55	299	51	2	5	3 1/2 carb, 3 fat
Cake, Frosted	2-inch square	175	6	55	2	0	18	194	29	1	2	2 carb, 1 fat
Cake, Pound with Butter	1 piece	109	6	55	3	0	62	111	14	0	2	1 carb, 1 fat
Cake, Unfrosted	2-inch square	97	3	30	1	0	18	168	17	<1	2	1 carb, 1 fat
Cake, White with Vanilla Icing	1 piece	239	9	90	2	0	35	220	38	0	2	2 1/2 carb, 2 fat
Cake, Yellow with Chocolate Icing	1 piece	243	11	100	3	0	35	216	36	1	2	2 1/2 carb, 2 fat

DESSERTS, CAKE, PIE, CHEESECAKE, COOKIES, BROWNIES

	Serving	Calories	Fat (g)	Cal. from Fat	Sat. Fat (g)	Trans Fat (g)	Chol. (mg)	Sod. (mg)	Carb. (g)	Fiber (g)	Prot. (g)	Servings/Exchanges
Cheesecake	1/12 cake	271	13	117	7	0	29	376	35	2	5	2 carb, 3 fat
Cobbler, Apple	1/2 cup	225	6	55	1	0	2	109	42	1	3	3 carb, 1 fat
Cookies, Chocolate Chip	1	78	5	45	1	0	5	58	9	<1	<1	1/2 carb, 1 fat
Cookies, Fortune	2	60	<1	0	<1	0	2	44	13	<1	<1	1 carb
Cookies, Gingersnaps	3	87	2	20	0.5	0	0	137	16	<1	2	1 carb
Cookies, Lady Fingers	4	161	4	35	1	0	161	65	26	<1	5	2 carb, 1 fat
Cookies, Macaroons	1	97	3	30	3	0	0	59	17	<1	1	1 carb, 1 fat
Cookies, Oatmeal	1	67	3	30	<1	0	5	90	10	NA	1	1/2 carb, 1 fat
Cookies, Peanut Butter	1	95	5	45	<1	0	6	104	12	NA	2	1 carb, 1 fat
Cookies, Sandwich with Creme Filling	2	93	4	45	<1	1	0	97	14	<1	1	1 carb, 1 fat
Cookies, Shortbread	4	161	8	70	2	0	6	146	21	<1	2	1 1/2 carb, 2 fat
Cookies, Soft Raisin	1	60	2	20	<1	0	<1	51	10	<1	<1	1/2 carb

Food	Serving											Exchanges
Cookies, Sugar	1	72	3	30	2	0	0	8	54	10	<1	<1	1/2 carb, 1 fat
Cookies, Sugar-free	3	141	7	65	2	0	0	0	1	20	2	2	1 carb, 1 fat
Cookies, Vanilla Wafers	5	88	3	30	<1	0	0	10	70	15	<1	1	1 carb, 1 fat
Crisp, Apple	1/2 cup	227	5	45	1	0	0	0	495	44	2	2	3 carb, 1 fat
Cupcake, Frosted	1	174	6	65	1	0	0	8	186	29	0	2	2 carb, 1 fat
Pie, Fruit, 2-Crust	1/6	284	13	115	2	0	0	0	300	42	2	2	3 carb, 3 fat
Pie, Pumpkin or Custard	1/8	168	8	70	1	0	0	16	226	22	2	3	1 1/2 carb, 2 fat

CAKE/PIE/CHEESECAKE

Betty Crocker

Food	Serving											Exchanges
Angel Food Mix	1/12 recipe	140	0	0	0	0	0	0	310	32	0	2	2 carb
Brownie Mix, Chocolate Fudge	1/20 recipe	170	9	80	1.5	0		20	95	23	1	2	1 1/2 carb, 2 fat
Brownie Mix, Low-Fat Fudge	1/16 recipe	140	2.5	25	1	0.5		10	130	28	1	2	2 carb, 1 fat
Cake Mix, Super Moist Chocolate Fudge	1/12 recipe	260	12	110	2.5	0		55	380	35	1	3	2 carb, 2 fat

DESSERTS, CAKE, PIE, CHEESECAKE, COOKIES, BROWNIES

	Serving	Calories	Fat (g)	Cal. from Fat	Sat. Fat (g)	Trans Fat (g)	Chol. (mg)	Sod. (mg)	Carb. (g)	Fiber (g)	Prot. (g)	Servings/Exchanges
Cake Mix, Super Moist French Vanilla	1/12 recipe	230	9	80	2	0	55	300	35	0	1	2 carb, 2 fat
Dessert Bar Mix	1/16 recipe	140	4	40	1	1	40	90	24	0	2	1 1/2 carb, 1 fat
Frosting, Rich & Creamy Butter Cream	2 Tbsp	140	5	45	1	2	0	70	23	0	0	1 1/2 carb, 1 fat
Frosting, Rich & Creamy Chocolate	2 Tbsp	130	5	45	1.5	2	0	95	21	<1	0	1 1/2 carb, 1 fat
Pound Cake Mix	1/8 recipe	260	8	70	3	1.5	55	210	45	0	4	3 carb, 2 fat
Claim Jumper												
Chocolate Motherlode 6-layer Cake	1 slice	500	24	210	8	2.5	45	430	71	2	6	4 1/2 carb, 5 fat
Original Carrot Cake	1/6 cake	460	25	230	8	2	60	510	54	2	5	3 1/2 carb, 5 fat

Comstock

Pie Filling, Cherry, No Sugar Added	1/3 cup	35	0	0	0	0	10	8	0	0	1/2 carb
Pie Filling, Country Cherry	1/3 cup	90	0	0	0	0	25	23	1	0	1 1/2 carb
Pie Filling, More Fruit, Apple	1/3 cup	80	0	0	0	0	40	20	1	0	1 carb
Pie Filling, More Fruit, Blueberry	1/3 cup	100	0	0	0	0	10	24	1	0	1 1/2 carb
Pie Filling, More Fruit, Cherry	1/3 cup	100	0	0	0	0	15	23	1	0	1 1/2 carb
Pie Filling, More Fruit, Peach	1/3 cup	100	0	0	0	0	15	26	1	1	2 carb
Pie Filling, Premium Strawberry	1/3 cup	100	0	0	0	0	25	23	1	0	1 1/2 carb

Duncan Hines

DESSERTS, CAKE, PIE, CHEESECAKE, COOKIES, BROWNIES

	Serving	Calories	Fat (g)	Cal. from Fat	Sat. Fat (g)	Trans Fat (g)	Chol. (mg)	Sod. (mg)	Carb. (g)	Fiber (g)	Prot. (g)	Servings/Exchanges
Whipped Chocolate Frosting	3 Tbsp	140	7	60	2	1.5	0	70	20	<1	<1	1 carb, 1 fat
Whipped Vanilla Frosting	3 Tbsp	150	7	60	2	1.5	0	60	22	0	0	1 1/2 carb, 1 fat
Edwards												
Boston Cream Pie	1/10 pie	210	10	90	5	0	25	170	31	<1	3	2 carb, 2 fat
Cookies & Crème	1/6 pie	470	27	240	18	0	10	310	53	2	4	3 1/2 carb, 5 fat
Georgia Pecan Pie	1/8 pie	470	25	220	7	0	80	260	60	2	4	4 carb, 5 fat
Hershey's Crème Pie	1/6 pie	450	27	240	17	0	10	330	48	1	5	3 carb, 5 fat
Key Lime Pie	1/8 pie	450	22	200	16	0	50	310	57	<1	6	4 carb, 4 fat
Singles, Apple Pie	1	380	20	180	10	0	10	370	47	1	3	3 carb, 4 fat
Singles, Hot Fudge Brownie	1	340	17	150	8	0	20	200	46	2	4	3 carb, 3 fat
Turtle Pie	1/8 pie	390	22	200	13	1	10	270	46	1	4	3 carb, 4 fat

Entenmann's

	Amount	Calories	Fat (g)	Calories from Fat	Saturated Fat (g)	Trans Fat (g)	Cholesterol (mg)	Sodium (mg)	Carbohydrate (g)	Fiber (g)	Protein (g)	Servings/Exchanges
All Butter Loaf Cake	1/6 cake	220	9	80	5	0	70	270	30	0	3	2 carb, 2 fat
Banana Crunch Cake	1/8 cake	230	10	90	3	0	30	270	33	<1	2	2 carb, 2 fat
Deluxe French Cheesecake	1/6 cake	390	24	220	12	0	40	400	39	<1	6	2 1/2 carb, 5 fat
Fudge Chocolate Cake	1 slice	270	11	100	4	0	25	230	40	2	3	2 1/2 carb, 2 fat
Homestyle Apple Pie	1/6 pie	380	16	140	8	0	0	400	57	2	3	4 carb, 3 fat
Lemon Crunch Cake	1/9 cake	330	14	130	4	0	45	300	49	<1	3	3 carb, 3 fat
Louisana Crunch Cake	1 slice	330	14	130	4	0	45	300	49	<1	3	3 carb, 3 fat
Marble Loaf Cake	1/8 cake	180	8	70	2	0	35	240	26	<1	2	2 carb, 2 fat

Hostess

	Amount	Calories	Fat (g)	Calories from Fat	Saturated Fat (g)	Trans Fat (g)	Cholesterol (mg)	Sodium (mg)	Carbohydrate (g)	Fiber (g)	Protein (g)	Servings/Exchanges
Ding Dongs	2	360	19	170	13	0	10	230	47	1	2	3 carb, 4 fat
Ho Ho's	3	370	17	150	13	0	30	220	54	1	2	3 1/2 carb, 3 fat
Twinkies	1	150	4.5	40	2.5	0	20	220	27	0	1	2 carb, 1 fat

Little Debbie

	Amount	Calories	Fat (g)	Calories from Fat	Saturated Fat (g)	Trans Fat (g)	Cholesterol (mg)	Sodium (mg)	Carbohydrate (g)	Fiber (g)	Protein (g)	Servings/Exchanges
Chocolate Cupcakes	1	210	8	70	2	0	30	170	33	<1	2	2 carb, 2 fat

DESSERTS, CAKE, PIE, CHEESECAKE, COOKIES, BROWNIES

	Serving	Calories	Fat (g)	Cal. from Fat	Sat. Fat (g)	Trans Fat (g)	Chol. (mg)	Sod. (mg)	Carb. (g)	Fiber (g)	Prot. (g)	Servings/Exchanges
Chocolate Marshmallow Pie	1	180	7	60	4	0	0	105	28	0	2	2 carb, 1 fat
Devil Squares	2	260	11	100	6	0	0	160	38	1	2	2 1/2 carb, 2 fat
Marie Callender's												
Apple Crumb Cobbler	1/8 pie	330	17	150	4	4.5	0	160	44	1	2	3 carb, 3 fat
Banana Cream Pie	1/10 pie	290	17	150	8	2	40	210	30	<1	3	2 carb, 3 fat
Cherry Crunch Pie	1/10 pie	350	15	140	3.5	4.5	0	250	51	1	2	3 1/2 carb, 3 fat
Chocolate Satin Pie	1/8 pie	410	29	260	14	4.5	50	200	36	2	4	2 1/2 carb, 6 fat
Coconut Cream Pie	1/10 pie	310	18	170	10	2	35	220	32	<1	3	2 carb, 4 fat
Dutch Apple Pie	1/10 pie	320	15	130	3.5	4	0	170	47	2	2	3 carb, 3 fat
I Love Chocolate Cream Pie	1/8 pie	350	19	170	9	2	40	190	42	2	4	3 carb, 4 fat
Lattice Apple Pie	1/10 pie	330	18	160	4	5	0	160	42	2	2	3 carb, 4 fat
Lattice Peach Pie	1/10 pie	330	18	160	4	5	0	140	38	0	3	2 1/2 carb, 4 fat

Lemon Meringue Pie	1/10 pie	260	9	80	2.5	2	40	190	44	<1	2	3 carb, 2 fat
Peach Cobbler	1/8 pie	330	19	170	4	5	0	160	38	1	3	2 1/2 carb, 4 fat
Razzleberry Pie	1/9 pie	360	18	160	4	4.5	0	300	47	2	3	3 carb, 4 fat
Turtle Pie	1/8 pie	400	27	240	11	4.5	40	210	39	2	4	2 1/2 carb, 5 fat
Pepperidge Farm												
Apple Turnover	1	270	15	135	8	0	0	230	31	1	4	2 carb, 3 fat
Cherry Turnover	1	270	15	135	8	0	0	230	31	1	4	2 carb, 3 fat
Chocolate Fudge 3-Layer Cake	1/8 cake	230	10	90	2	1.5	20	130	33	1	2	2 carb, 2 fat
Coconut 3-Layer Cake	1/8 cake	240	10	90	3	1.5	20	120	35	<1	2	2 carb, 2 fat
Devil's Food Cake	1/8 cake	220	9	80	2	1.5	20	170	34	<1	2	2 carb, 2 fat
German Chocolate Cake	1/8 cake	240	10	90	3	2	15	200	34	<1	2	2 carb, 2 fat
Pillsbury												
Frosting, Chocolate Fudge	2 Tbsp	140	6	50	1.5	2	0	90	21	<1	0	1 1/2 carb, 1 fat
Frosting, Vanilla	2 Tbsp	150	6	50	1.5	2	0	70	24	0	0	1 1/2 carb, 1 fat

DESSERTS, CAKE, PIE, CHEESECAKE, COOKIES, BROWNIES

	Serving	Calories	Fat (g)	Cal. from Fat	Sat. Fat (g)	Trans Fat (g)	Chol. (mg)	Sod. (mg)	Carb. (g)	Fiber (g)	Prot. (g)	Servings/Exchanges
Sweet Moments Caramel Pecan Crumble	1	390	21	190	9	0.5	40	190	46	1	4	3 carb, 4 fat
Sara Lee												
All Butter Pound Cake	1/4 cake	300	16	140	9	0	110	220	35	<1	4	2 carb, 3 fat
Apple Pie	1/8 pie	340	16	140	7	0	0	330	47	2	3	3 carb, 3 fat
Blueberry Pie	1/6 pie	350	16	150	7	0	0	350	50	2	3	3 carb, 3 fat
Cherry Pie	1/8 pie	340	16	150	7	0	0	350	45	2	3	3 carb, 3 fat
Chocolate Dream Pie	1/8 pie	420	24	220	12	3.5	0	270	47	2	4	3 carb, 5 fat
Cinnamon French Apple Pie	1/10 pie	330	13	120	6	0	0	250	51	2	2	3 1/2 carb, 3 fat
Crumb Coffee Cake	1/6 cake	190	9	80	5	0.5	40	200	24	<1	3	1 1/2 carb, 2 fat
Dutch Apple Pie	1/8 pie	340	14	130	6	0	0	290	52	2	3	3 1/2 carb, 3 fat
French Cheesecake	1/5 cake	410	26	230	13	2.5	20	250	39	0	5	2 1/2 carb, 5 fat

Fruits of the Forest Deep Dish Pie	1/9 pie	350	19	180	8	0	0	310	42	2	3	3 carb, 4 fat
Original Cheesecake Bites	25	440	27	240	13	0.5	60	390	44	1	7	3 carb, 5 fat
Original Cheesecake	1/4 cake	320	17	150	8	2	70	250	36	<1	7	2 1/2 carb, 3 fat
Pumpkin Pie	1/8 pie	260	10	90	4	0	40	320	39	2	4	2 1/2 carb, 2 fat
Southern Pecan Pie	1 piece	470	23	210	8	2	75	440	62	2	5	4 carb, 5 fat

Weight Watchers Smart Ones

Brownie à La Mode	1	200	2.5	35	2.5	0	25	160	36	3	5	2 1/2 carb, 1 fat
Chocolate Chip Cookie Dough Sundae	1	170	3	30	1.5	0	5	100	32	1	3	2 carb, 1 fat
Chocolate Éclair	1	140	4	35	1	0	30	180	24	1	3	1 1/2 carb, 1 fat
Chocolate Mousse	1	180	4	40	3.5	0	<5	100	28	3	7	2 carb, 1 fat
Key Lime Pie	1	190	4.5	40	2	0	10	85	33	<1	4	2 carb, 1 fat

COOKIES/BROWNIES

Archway

DESSERTS, CAKE, PIE, CHEESECAKE, COOKIES, BROWNIES

	Serving	Calories	Fat (g)	Cal. from Fat	Sat. Fat (g)	Trans Fat (g)	Chol. (mg)	Sod. (mg)	Carb. (g)	Fiber (g)	Prot. (g)	Servings/Exchanges
Coconut Macaroon	2	160	8	70	7	0	0	85	22	2	1	1 1/2 carb, 2 fat
Date Oatmeal	1	90	3	25	0.5	1	0	75	16	0	1	1 carb, 1 fat
Frosted Lemon	1	110	4.5	40	1.5	1	0	105	18	0	1	1 carb, 1 fat
Ginger Snap	4	140	5	45	1	0	0	105	22	0	1	1 1/2 carb, 1 fat
Ginger Snap, Reduced Fat	4	130	3.5	30	1	0	0	125	23	0	1	1 1/2 carb, 1 fat
Iced Oatmeal	1	110	4.5	40	1	1	<5	100	17	<1	1	1 carb, 1 fat
Oatmeal	1	110	4	35	1	1	<5	105	18	<1	1	1 carb, 1 fat
Windmill	2	160	6	50	1.5	1.5	0	160	25	<1	2	1 1/2 carb, 1 fat
Duncan Hines												
Oven Ready! Homestyle Brownies	1/12 pan	170	8	70	2	1	20	85	23	<1	2	1 1/2 carb, 2 fat
Estee												
Chocolate Chip	4	150	7	63	2	0	0	30	21	0	2	1 1/2 carb, 1 fat

Coconut	4	140	6	54	2	0	0	25	19	0	2	1 carb, 1 fat
Fudge	4	150	7	63	1	0	0	45	19	0	2	1 carb, 1 fat
Lemon	4	140	6	54	0	0	0	25	19	0	2	1 carb, 1 fat
Oatmeal Raisin	4	130	5	45	1	0	0	25	19	1	2	1 carb, 1 fat
Shortbread	4	130	4	36	1	0	0	150	22	0	2	1 1/2 carb, 1 fat
Vanilla Sandwich	3	160	5	45	1	0	0	35	35	0	2	2 carb, 1 fat
Sugar Free Vanilla Crème Wafers	5	155	8	72	2	0	0	10	21	0	1	1 1/2 carb, 2 fat
Famous Amos												
Chocolate Chip	4	150	7	60	3	0	<5	105	20	<1	1	1 1/2 carb, 1 fat
Chocolate Chip & Pecans	4	150	8	70	3	0	0	95	18	1	2	1 carb, 2 fat
Fifty50												
Butter	4	190	9	80	6	0	30	50	24	<1	2	1 1/2 carb, 2 fat
Chocolate Chip	4	170	9	80	2.5	0	0	35	22	1	2	1 1/2 carb, 2 fat
Hearty Oatmeal	4	160	7	60	1.5	0	0	60	24	1	2	1 1/2 carb, 1 fat

DESSERTS, CAKE, PIE, CHEESECAKE, COOKIES, BROWNIES

	Serving	Calories	Fat (g)	Cal. from Fat	Sat. Fat (g)	Trans Fat (g)	Chol. (mg)	Sod. (mg)	Carb. (g)	Fiber (g)	Prot. (g)	Servings/Exchanges
Sugar Free Vanilla Crème Wafers	6	160	9	80	4	0	0	30	22	0	1	1 1/2 carb, 2 fat
Girl Scout												
Do-Si-Dos	2	120	5	45	1.5	0	0	75	16	<1	2	1 carb, 1 fat
Lemon Chalet Cremes	3	170	7	60	2.5	0	0	95	26	<1	1	2 carb, 1 fat
Peanut Butter Patties or Tagalongs	2	140	9	80	5	0	0	95	13	<1	2	1 carb, 2 fat
Samoas	2	150	8	70	6	0	0	50	18	<1	1	1 carb, 2 fat
Sugar Free Chocolate Chip	3	160	9	80	3	0	0	140	22	2	1	1 1/2 carb, 2 fat
Thin Mints	4	160	8	70	5	0	0	115	22	<1	1	1 1/2 carb, 2 fat
Trefoils	5	170	8	70	2.5	0	0	115	23	<1	2	1 1/2 carb, 2 fat
Health Valley Organic												
Mini Chocolate Chip	4	120	6	60	2	0	5	125	16	1	1	1 carb, 1 fat

Oatmeal Raisin	1	90	3.5	30	0	0	0	50	14	1	2	1 carb, 1 fat
Vanilla Sandwich Cremes	2	130	5	45	3	0	0	110	20	0	1	1 carb, 1 fat
Kashi											
Happy Trail Cookies	1	130	5	45	1	0	0	80	21	4	2	1 1/2 carb, 1 fat
Oatmeal Dark Chocolate	1	130	5	45	1.5	0	0	70	21	3	2	1 1/2 carb, 1 fat
Oatmeal Raisin Flax	1	130	5	45	0.5	0	0	75	20	4	2	1 carb, 1 fat
Keebler											
Chips Deluxe Chocolate Lovers	1	80	4.5	65	2	0	0	65	10	<1	<1	1/2 carb, 1 fat
Chips Deluxe Chocolate Peanut Butter	1	80	4.5	40	2	0	0	65	10	<1	1	1/2 carb, 1 fat
Chips Deluxe Coconut	2	160	9	80	4.5	0	0	85	18	1	2	1 carb, 2 fat
Chips Deluxe Original	2	170	9	80	3.5	0	<5	105	19	<1	2	1 carb, 2 fat
Chips Deluxe Soft 'N Chewy	1	80	4.5	30	1.5	0	0	55	11	<1	<1	1 carb, 1 fat

DESSERTS, CAKE, PIE, CHEESECAKE, COOKIES, BROWNIES

	Serving	Calories	Fat (g)	Cal. from Fat	Sat. Fat (g)	Trans Fat (g)	Chol. (mg)	Sod. (mg)	Carb. (g)	Fiber (g)	Prot. (g)	Servings/Exchanges
E.L. Fudge Double Stuffed	2	180	9	80	3.5	0	<5	95	24	1	2	1 1/2 carb, 2 fat
E.L. Fudge Fudge Original	1	90	3.5	30	1.5	0	5	50	13	<1	1	1 carb, 1 fat
Fudge Shoppe Deluxe Grahams	3	140	7	60	4.5	1.5	0	70	17	<1	1	1 carb, 1 fat
Fudge Shoppe Fudge Sticks	3	150	8	70	5	0	0	30	20	0	<1	1 carb, 2 fat
Fudge Shoppe Fudge Stripes	3	150	7	60	4.5	0	0	110	21	<1	1	1 1/2 carb, 2 fat
Fudge Shoppe Grasshopper	4	140	7	60	4.5	1.5	0	75	19	<1	1	1 carb, 1 fat
Sandies Fudge Drops	4	140	7	60	3.5	0	0	60	18	<1	1	1 carb, 1 fat
Sandies Pecan Shortbread	2	160	10	90	3	0	<5	105	18	<1	1	1 carb, 2 fat

Sandies Simply Shortbread	2	160	9	80	4	0	15	90	19	0	2	1 carb, 2 fat
Soft Batch Chocolate Chip	1	80	3.5	30	1.5	0	0	55	11	<1	<1	1 carb, 1 fat
Soft Batch Peanut Butter	1	80	3.5	30	1.5	0	0	50	10	0	<1	1/2 carb, 1 fat
Vienna Fingers	2	150	6	50	2	0	0	95	23	<1	1	1 1/2 carb, 1 fat
Vienna Fingers Reduced Fat	2	140	4.5	40	1.5	0	0	115	24	<1	1	1 1/2 carb, 1 fat
Little Debbie												
Oatmeal Creme Pie	1	170	7	60	2	0	0	170	26	<1	1	2 carb, 1 fat
Mother's												
Chocolate Chip	2	160	7	60	2	1	<5	150	22	<1	2	1 1/2 carb, 1 fat
Circus Animal	6	150	7	70	7	0	0	60	20	<1	1	1 carb, 1 fat
Coconut Cocadas	5	160	8	70	3.5	1.5	<5	140	21	1	2	1 1/2 carb, 2 fat
Double Fudge	2	170	7	60	2.5	2	0	95	27	1	2	2 carb, 1 fat

DESSERTS, CAKE, PIE, CHEESECAKE, COOKIES, BROWNIES

	Serving	Calories	Fat (g)	Cal. from Fat	Sat. Fat (g)	Trans Fat (g)	Chol. (mg)	Sod. (mg)	Carb. (g)	Fiber (g)	Prot. (g)	Servings/Exchanges
English Tea	2	180	7	60	2.5	2	0	100	27	<1	2	2 carb, 1 fat
Iced Lemonade	4	140	7	60	1.5	0	0	75	19	<1	1	1 carb, 1 fat
Iced Oatmeal	4	130	5	45	1	0	0	135	20	<1	1	1 1/2 carb, 1 fat
Macaroons	2	170	11	100	5	2	0	90	17	1	2	1 carb, 2 fat
Oatmeal	2	130	5	45	1	1.5	0	170	19	<1	2	1 carb, 1 fat
Taffy Sandwich	2	180	8	70	4	1.5	0	125	27	<1	1	2 carb, 2 fat
Vanilla Crèmes	2	180	7	70	3	2	0	105	26	<1	2	2 carb, 1 fat
Murray Sugar Free												
Chocolate Chip	3	160	9	80	3.5	0	<5	130	20	1	2	1 carb, 2 fat
Chocolate Sandwich Creme	3	130	7	60	2.5	0	0	55	19	1	1	1 carb, 1 fat
Fudge Dipped Grahams	4	150	8	70	6	0	0	80	19	1	2	1 carb, 2 fat
Oatmeal	3	140	7	60	2.5	0	0	130	21	3	2	1 1/2 carb, 1 fat
Peanut Butter	3	150	9	80	2.5	0	<5	130	16	1	3	1 carb, 2 fat

Shortbread	8	130	5	45	1.5	0	0	140	21	2	2	1 1/2 carb, 1 fat
Vanilla Sandwich Creme	3	130	6	60	2	0	0	55	20	<1	1	1 carb, 1 fat
Vanilla Sugar Wafer	9	130	5	50	1.5	0	0	90	24	2	2	1 1/2 carb, 1 fat
Nabisco												
Barnum's Animals	8	120	3.5	30	1	0	0	140	22	1	2	1 1/2 carb, 1 fat
Biscos Sugar Wafers	8	140	6	50	2.5	0	0	25	21	0	<1	1 1/2 carb, 1 fat
Cameo Creme Sandwich	1 oz	130	5	40	1	0	0	105	21	0	1	1 1/2 carb, 1 fat
Chips Ahoy! Chewy	2	120	6	50	3	0	0	80	18	1	1	1 carb, 1 fat
Chips Ahoy! Chocolate Chip	3	160	8	70	2.5	0	0	105	21	1	2	1 1/2 carb, 2 fat
Chips Ahoy! Chunky Chocolate	1	80	4.5	40	1.5	0	0	55	11	1	1	1 carb, 1 fat
Chips Ahoy! Chunky White Fudge	1	90	4.5	40	1.5	0	0	60	11	0	2	1 carb, 1 fat
Chips Ahoy! Peanut Butter Chunky	1	90	5	45	2.5	0	0	75	10	0	1	1/2 carb, 1 fat

DESSERTS, CAKE, PIE, CHEESECAKE, COOKIES, BROWNIES

	Serving	Calories	Fat (g)	Cal. from Fat	Sat. Fat (g)	Trans Fat (g)	Chol. (mg)	Sod. (mg)	Carb. (g)	Fiber (g)	Prot. (g)	Servings/Exchanges
Chips Ahoy! White Fudge Chewy	1	120	5	50	3	0	0	120	18	1	1	1 carb, 1 fat
Ginger Snaps	4	120	2.5	20	0	0	0	190	23	0	11	1/2 carb, 1 fat
Lorna Doone Shortbread	4	140	7	60	2	0	0	150	20	0	1	1 carb, 1 fat
Mallomars	2	120	5	45	3	0	0	40	18	1	1	1 carb, 1 fat
Newtons, Fig	2	110	2	20	0	0	0	125	22	1	1	1 1/2 carb
Newtons, Fig, 100% Whole Grain	1 oz	110	2	20	0	0	0	115	21	2	1	1 1/2 carb
Newtons, Fig, Fat Free	2	90	0	0	0	0	0	125	22	1	1	1 1/2 carb
Newtons, Fruit Crisps, Apple Cinnamon	2 pieces	100	2	15	0	0	0	90	20	0	<1	1 carb
Newtons, Minis	1 pkg	130	3	30	0.5	0	0	140	26	2	2	2 carb, 1 fat
Newtons, Raspberry	2	100	1.5	15	0	0	0	110	21	0	1	1 1/2 carb

	Amount	Cal.	Fat (g)		Sat. Fat		Chol.	Sod.	Carb.	Fiber		Exchanges
Newtons, Strawberry	2	100	1.5	15	0	0	0	110	21	0	1	1 1/2 carb
Nilla Wafers, Mini	1 oz	140	6	50	1.5	0	5	115	21	0	1	1 1/2 carb, 1 fat
Nilla Wafers, Original	8	140	6	50	1.5	0	5	115	21	0	1	1 1/2 carb, 1 fat
Nilla Wafers, Reduced Fat	8	110	2	2	0	0	0	110	24	0	1	1 1/2 carb
Nutter Butter	2	130	5	45	1	0.5	0	110	20	1	2	1 carb, 1 fat
Nutter Butter Bites	10	120	5	45	2	0	0	90	17	1	2	1 carb, 1 fat
Oreo Cakesters, Golden	1 pkg	220	10	90	2	0	5	135	32	0	2	2 carb, 2 fat
Oreo Cakesters, Original	1 pkg	250	12	100	2.5	0	5	250	36	1	2	2 1/2 carb, 2 fat
Oreo Fun Stix	1 pkg	90	3.5	35	3.5	0	0	50	13	0	<1	1 carb, 1 fat
Oreo Sandwich Cookies, Chocolate	3	160	7	60	2	0	0	160	25	1	1	1 1/2 carb, 1 fat
Oreo Sandwich Cookies, Chocolate Crème	2	150	7	60	2.5	0	0	110	21	1	1	1 1/2 carb, 1 fat
Oreo Sandwich Cookies, Chocolate Fudge Mint Covered	1	90	4	36	1	0	0	70	12	<1	1	1 carb, 1 fat

DESSERTS, CAKE, PIE, CHEESECAKE, COOKIES, BROWNIES

	Serving	Calories	Fat (g)	Cal. from Fat	Sat. Fat (g)	Trans Fat (g)	Chol. (mg)	Sod. (mg)	Carb. (g)	Fiber (g)	Prot. (g)	Servings/Exchanges
Oreo Sandwich Cookies, Golden Original	3	170	4	60	2	0	0	120	25	0	1	1 1/2 carb, 1 fat
Oreo Sandwich Cookies, Reduced Fat, Chocolate	3	150	4.5	40	1	0	0	160	27	1	1	2 carb, 1 fat
Teddy Grahams, Chocolate	24	130	4.5	40	1	0	0	160	22	2	2	1 1/2 carb, 1 fat
Teddy Grahams, Honey	24	130	4	35	1	0	0	150	23	1	2	1 1/2 carb, 1 fat
Nabisco SnackWell's												
Cookie Cake, Black Forest	1/2 oz	50	0.5	5	0	0	0	40	12	0	1	1 carb, 1 fat
Cookie Cakes, Chocolate Mint	1/2 oz	50	0.5	5	0	0	0	40	12	0	1	1 carb
Cookie Cakes, Devil's Food, Fat Free	50	0	0	0	0	0	25	12	0	1	1	1 carb

Creme Sandwich	2	110	3	25	0.5	0	0	130	20	0	1	1 carb, 1 fat
Lemon Creme Sandwich Cookies, Sugar Free	3	130	6	50	2	0	0	135	23	2	1	1 1/2 carb, 1 fat
Shortbread Cookies, Sugar Free	3	130	6	50	1.5	0	5	140	21	2	2	1 1/2 carb, 1 fat
Pepperidge Farm												
Bordeaux	3	130	5	45	3.5	0	10	95	19	<1	2	1 carb, 1 fat
Brussels	3	150	7	65	4	0	5	65	20	1	2	1 carb, 1 fat
Chessmen	3	120	5	45	3	0	20	80	18	<1	2	1 carb, 1 fat
Chewy Granola, Fruit & Nut	1	140	6	55	1.5	0	5	80	20	2	3	1 carb, 1 fat
Chocolate Chunk, Nantucket	1	140	7	65	4	10	0	80	16	0	2	1 carb, 1 fat
Chocolate Chunk, Sausalito	1	140	8	70	3.5	0	10	80	16	0	2	1 carb, 2 fat

DESSERTS, CAKE, PIE, CHEESECAKE, COOKIES, BROWNIES

	Serving	Calories	Fat (g)	Cal. from Fat	Sat. Fat (g)	Trans Fat (g)	Chol. (mg)	Sod. (mg)	Carb. (g)	Fiber (g)	Prot. (g)	Servings/Exchanges
Chocolate Chunk, Tahoe	1	130	6	55	4	0	<5	85	17	<1	1	1 carb, 1 fat
Geneva	3	160	9	80	4	0	0	95	19	1	2	1 carb, 2 fat
Milano, Black & White	1	180	10	90	5	0	<5	85	21	1	2	1 1/2 carb, 2 fat
Milano, Original	3	180	10	90	5	0	10	80	21	<1	2	1 1/2 carb, 2 fat
Milano, Raspberry	1	130	7	65	4.5	0	<5	40	16	<1	1	1 carb, 1 fat
Petite Cinnamon Twists	3	130	4.5	45	2	0	0	100	21	1	2	1 1/2 carb, 1 fat
Pirouette, Chocolate Hazelnut	2	120	5	45	2	0	5	40	19	1	1	1 carb, 1 fat
Shortbread	2	140	7	65	4	0	10	105	16	<1	2	1 carb, 1 fat
Soft Baked, Dark Chocolate Chunk	1	140	7	65	3	0	10	80	18	1	2	1 carb, 1 fat
Soft Baked, Milk Chocolate Caramel	1	140	6	55	3	0	5	75	21	<1	1	1 1/2 carb, 1 fat
Soft Baked, Oatmeal Raisin	1	130	4.5	45	1.5	0	<5	90	23	2	2	1 1/2 carb, 1 fat

Soft Baked, Sugar	1	140	5	45	2.5	0	10	90	22	0	2	1 1/2 carb, 1 fat
Sugar	3	140	6	55	2.5	0	15	90	20	<1	2	1 carb, 1 fat
Tahiti	2	170	10	90	6	0	5	40	17	2	2	1 carb, 2 fat
Verona, Apricot Raspberry	3	140	5	45	2.5	0	10	100	22	<1	2	1 1/2 carb, 1 fat
Verona, Strawberry	3	140	5	45	2.5	0	10	100	22	<1	2	1 1/2 carb, 1 fat
Pillsbury												
Brownie Mix, Traditional Chocolate Fudge	1/12 recipe	150	6	50	1	1.5	0	120	24	<1	2	1 1/2 carb, 1 fat
Milk Chocolate Chip Cookies	3	150	7	60	3	0	5	90	20	0	1	1 carb, 1 fat
Soft Baked Chocolate Chunk	1	190	9	80	4.5	0	15	140	25	0	2	1 1/2 carb, 2 fat

DIPS, SPREADS, SALSA

	Serving	Calories	Fat (g)	Cal. from Fat	Sat. Fat (g)	Trans Fat (g)	Chol (mg)	Sod. (mg)	Carb. (g)	Fiber (g)	Prot. (g)	Servings/Exchanges
Alouette												
Soft Spreadable Cheese, All Varietites	2 Tbsp	60–80	6–8	55–70	3–5	0	15–30	60–160	1	0	1–2	1 fat
Light Soft Spreadable Cheese	2 Tbsp	50	4	35	2.5	0	15	60	2	0	2	1 fat
Athenos												
Hummus, All Varieties	2 Tbsp	50–60	3	25	0	0	0	150–210	4–5	<1	2	1 fat
NeoClassic Hummus, All Varieties	2 Tbsp	80	5–6	45–55	1	0	0	130–200	5	1	2	1 fat
Dean's												
French Onion or Ranch Dip	2 Tbsp	60	5	45	2.5	0	0	170	2	0	1	1 fat

Guacamole Flavored Dip	2 Tbsp	90	9	80	2.5	0	<5	170	2	0	1	2 fat
Skinny Dip Light French Onion	2 Tbsp	35	1.5	15	1	0	5	210	4	0	2	1 fat
No Fat French Onion	2 Tbsp	30	0	0	0	0	0	240	5	0	2	1/2 carb
Veggie Dip	2 Tbsp	60	5	45	2.5	0	0	170	3	0	1	1 fat
Bacon & Horseradish	2 Tbsp	60	5	45	2.5	0	0	240	2	0	1	1 fat
Cheddar Cheese Pretzel Dip	2 Tbsp	90	9	80	2	0	15	200	3	0	1	2 fat
Honey Mustard Pretzel Dip	2 Tbsp	50	1.5	15	0	0	0	190	9	0	0	1/2 carb
Creamy Taco Dip	2 Tbsp	60	5	45	2	0	0	190	4	1	1	1 fat
Fritos												
Chili Cheese Dip	2 Tbsp	45	3	30	1	0	<5	310	3	0	1	1 fat
Hot Bean Dip	2 Tbsp	40	1	10	0	0	0	210	5	1	2	1/2 carb
Jalapeño Cheddar Flavor Cheese	2 Tbsp	45	4	35	1	0	<5	300	4	0	1	1 fat

DIPS, SPREADS, SALSA

	Serving	Calories	Fat (g)	Cal. from Fat	Sat. Fat (g)	Trans Fat (g)	Chol. (mg)	Sod. (mg)	Carb. (g)	Fiber (g)	Prot. (g)	Servings/Exchanges
Original Flavor Bean Dip	2 Tbsp	40	1	10	0	0	0	170	5	1	2	1/2 carb
Guiltless Gourmet												
Mild or Spicy Black Bean Dip	2 Tbsp	40	0	0	0	0	0	100	7	1	2	1/2 carb
Herdez												
Salsa Casera	2 tsp	10	0	0	0	0	0	270	1	0	0	free
Salsa Verde	2 tsp	10	0	0	0	0	0	310	1	0	0	free
Kaukauna/WisPride												
Garden Vegetable Cheese Spread	2 Tbsp	90	8	70	5	0	25	190	2	0	2	2 fat
Lite Smokey Cheddar Cheese Spread	2 Tbsp	70	3.5	30	2	0	15	190	5	0	5	1 lean meat
Port Wine Cheese Spread	2 Tbsp	90	7	60	3.5	0	20	190	4	0	5	1 med–fat meat

Extremely Creamy Horseradish Spread	2 Tbsp	100	8	70	4	0	20	170	3	0	3	2 fat
Extremely Creamy Mozzarella Spread	2 Tbsp	90	9	80	3.5	0	20	220	1	0	2	2 fat
Kraft												
Pimento Cheese Spread	2 Tbsp	70	6	60	4	0	20	220	3	0	2	1 fat
Bacon Cheese Spread	2 Tbsp	90	8	70	5	0	25	570	1	0	5	1 high fat meat
Sharp Old English Spread	2 Tbsp	90	5	70	5	0	25	520	1	0	5	1 med-fat meat
Roka Blue Cheese Spread	2 Tbsp	80	7	60	5	0	20	340	2	0	3	1 med-fat meat
Cheez Whiz Light	2 Tbsp	80	3.5	30	2	0	20	500	6	0	6	1/2 carb, 1 fat
Cheez Whiz Salsa Con Queso	2 Tbsp	90	7	60	4.5	0	30	500	4	0	3	2 fat
Cheeze Whiz Original	2 Tbsp	90	7	60	4.5	0	30	490	4	0	3	2 fat
Creamy Ranch Dip	2 Tbsp	60	4.5	40	3	0	0	190	3	0	1	1 fat

DIPS, SPREADS, SALSA

	Serving	Calories	Fat (g)	Cal. from Fat	Sat. Fat (g)	Trans Fat (g)	Chol. (mg)	Sod. (mg)	Carb. (g)	Fiber (g)	Prot. (g)	Servings/Exchanges
French Onion Dip Onion Dip	2 Tbsp	60	4.5	40	3	0	0	220	3–4	0	1	1 fat
Easy Cheese Cheddar	2 Tbsp	90	6	60	3	0	20	410	2	0	5	1 med–fat meat
Easy Cheese Cheddar 'N Bacon	2 Tbsp	90	7	60	4.5	0	25	400	2	0	5	1 med–fat meat
Pineapple Cheese Spread	2 Tbsp	70	5	50	3.5	0	15	120	4	0	2	1 fat
Blue Cheese Spread	2 Tbsp	80	7	65	4	0	30	290	2	0	3	2 fat
La Victoria												
Salsa (All Varieties)	2 Tbsp	10	0	0	0	0	0	105–190	2	0	0	free
Litehouse												
Avacado Dip	2 Tbsp	140	15	140	2	0	15	210	2	0	1	3 fat
Low Fat Caramel Dip	2 Tbsp	110	0	0	0	0	0	140	27	0	1	2 carb

	Serving	Cal.	Fat (g)	Cal. Fat	Sat. Fat (g)	Trans Fat	Chol. (mg)	Sod. (mg)	Carb. (g)	Fiber (g)	Prot. (g)	Exchanges/Choices
Lite Ranch Veggie Dip	2 Tbsp	60	6	50	0.5	0	10	230	3	0	1	1 fat
Caramel Dip	2 Tbsp	110	1.5	15	1.5	0	25	125	25	0	1	1 1/2 carb
Ranch Veggie Dip	2 Tbsp	130	13	120	1	0	10	230	3	0	1	3 fat
Spinach Parmesan Veggie Dip	2 Tbsp	120	13	110	1.5	0	15	240	2	0	1	3 fat
Chocolate Dip	1.4 oz	100	1.5	15	0	0	0	45	25	4	0	1 1/2 carb
Vanilla Yogurt Fruit Dip	2 Tbsp	60	1.5	15	0	0	0	50	10	0	1	1/2 carb
Chocolate Yogurt Fruit Dip	2 Tbsp	110	6	50	0	0	0	95	14	0	1	1 carb, 1 fat
Strawberry Glaze	3 Tbsp	70	0	0	0	0	0	50	17	0	0	1 carb
Chocolate Caramel Dip	2 Tbsp	120	3	30	2.5	0	0	120	23	0	1	1 1/2 carb, 1 fat
Maria's Dip												
Creamy Dill	2 Tbsp	100	10	90	3	0	15	140	2	0	1	2 fat
Roasted French Onion	2 Tbsp	100	10	90	3	0	15	220	2	0	1	2 fat
Guacamole Dip	2 Tbsp	40	3	30	1.5	0	5	140	3	1	1	1 fat
Lite Buttermilk Ranch	2 Tbsp	60	5	45	1.5	0	10	310	3	0	2	1 fat

DIPS, SPREADS, SALSA

	Serving	Calories	Fat (g)	Cal. from Fat	Sat. Fat (g)	Trans Fat (g)	Chol. (mg)	Sod. (mg)	Carb. (g)	Fiber (g)	Prot. (g)	Servings/Exchanges
Spinach Parmesan	2 Tbsp	90	9	80	3	0	15	200	2	0	2	2 fat
Honey Vanilla Cream	2 Tbsp	60	4.5	40	2.5	0	15	20	5	0	1	1 fat
Newman's Own												
Bandito Salsa	2 Tbsp	10	0	0	0	0	0	105	2	1	0	free
Mango Salsa	2 Tbsp	20	0	0	0	0	0	140	5	2	1	free
Pineapple Salsa	2 Tbsp	15	0	0	0	0	0	90	3	1	0	free
Black Bean & Corn Salsa	2 Tbsp	20	0	0	0	0	0	140	5	2	1	free
Old El Paso												
Thick 'n Chunky Salsa	2 Tbsp	10	0	0	0	0	0	230	3	0	0	free
Cheese 'n Salsa	2 Tbsp	35	3	25	0.5	1	0	280	3	0	0	1 fat
Ortega												
Thick & Chunky Salsa	2 Tbsp	10	0	0	0	0	0	170	2	0	0	free
Salsa Con Queso	2 Tbsp	45	3	25	1	0	0	280	4	0	1	1 fat

Pace

Chunky Salsa	2 Tbsp	10	0	0	0	0	0	230	2	0	0	free
Black Bean & Roasted Corn Salsa	2 Tbsp	25	0	0	0	0	0	150	5	1	1	free
Pineapple Mango Chipotle Salsa	2 Tbsp	20	0	0	0	0	0	130	4	0	0	free
Mexican Four Cheese Con Queso	2 Tbsp	90	7	1.5	0	65	5	430	5	0	2	1 fat

Rojos Salsa

Chunky Salsa	2 Tbsp	10	0	0	0	0	0	230	2	0	0	free

Rondele

Garlic & Herb Spreadable Cheese	2 Tbsp	70	7	5	0	60	20	150	1	0	2	1 fat
Lite Garlic & Herbs Spreadable Cheese	2 Tbsp	60	4.5	3	0	40	15	190	2	0	3	1 fat
Cheddar Horseradish Spreadable Cheese	2 Tbsp	70	7	4.5	0	60	25	150	1	0	2	1 fat

DIPS, SPREADS, SALSA

	Serving	Calories	Fat (g)	Cal. from Fat	Sat. Fat (g)	Trans Fat (g)	Chol. (mg)	Sod. (mg)	Carb. (g)	Fiber (g)	Prot. (g)	Servings/Exchanges
Ruffles												
Sour Cream & Chives Dip	2 Tbsp	60	5	50	0.5	0	<5	240	2	<1	1	1 fat
Smokey Bacon & Cheddar Dip	2 Tbsp	70	8	50	1	0	<5	100	2	<1	2	2 fat
T. Marzetti's												
Blue Cheese Veggie Dip	2 Tbsp	140	15	130	3	0	15	250	1	0	1	3 fat
Dill Veggie Dip	2 Tbsp	120	13	110	3.5	0	20	200	2	0	1	3 fat
Fat Free Ranch Veggie Dip	2 Tbsp	30	0	0	0	0	0	330	6	0	1	1/2 carb
French Onion Veggie Dip	2 Tbsp	120	12	110	3	0	20	220	2	0	1	3 fat
Light Ranch Veggie Dip	2 Tbsp	60	6	50	1	0	5	240	6	0	0	1/2 carb, 1 fat
Light Caramel Apple Dip	2 Tbsp	100	1.5	10	1	0	5	75	26	0	1	2 carb

Chocolate Fruit Dip	2 Tbsp	110	2	15	0.5	0	0	85	23	1	1	1 1/2 carb
Cream Cheese Fruit Dip	2 Tbsp	70	3	30	2	0	15	85	10	0	0	1/2 carb, 1 fat
Garden Hummus Veggie Dip & Spread	2 Tbsp	70	4.5	40	0.5	0	0	170	5	1	2	1 fat
Old Fashioned Caramel Apple Dip	2 Tbsp	140	6	50	3	0	5	75	22	0	0	1 1/2 carb, 1 fat
Peanut Butter Caramel Apple Dip	2 Tbsp	120	5	25	1	0	0	120	17	1	2	1 carb, 1 fat
Ranch Veggie Dip	2 Tbsp	120	12	110	3.5	0	20	210	2	0	1	2 fat
Spinach Veggie Dip	2 Tbsp	130	13	120	3	0	20	250	2	0	1	3 fat
Tostitos												
Chunky Salsa	2 Tbsp	10	0	0	0	0	0	250	2	<1	0	free
Salsa Con Queso	2 Tbsp	40	2.5	25	1	0	<5	280	5	<1	<1	1 fat
Creamy Spinach Dip	2 Tbsp	50	4	35	0	0	<5	200	2	<1	1	1 fat

EGGS, EGG DISHES, EGG PRODUCTS

	Serving	Calories	Fat (g)	Cal. from Fat	Sat. Fat (g)	Trans Fat (g)	Chol. (mg)	Sod. (mg)	Carb. (g)	Fiber (g)	Prot. (g)	Servings/Exchanges
1-Egg Omelet with Cheese & Ham	1	142	11	100	4	0	231	368	<1	0	10	1 med-fat meat, 1 fat
1-Egg Omelet with Chicken	1	149	10	90	3	0	287	222	<1	0	13	2 med-fat meat
1-Egg Omelet with Fish	1	132	9	80	3	0	267	277	<1	0	10	2 med-fat meat
1-Egg Omelet with Mushroom	1	91	7	65	2	0	204	158	1	<1	6	1 med-fat meat
1-Egg Omelet with Onion, Pepper, Tomato & Mushroom	1	125	9	80	2	0	126	251	7	2	5	1 vegetable, 1 med-fat meat, 1 fat
1-Egg Omelet with Sausage & Mushroom	1	172	13	115	4	0	254	454	1	<1	11	2 med-fat meat, 1 fat
1-Egg Omelet with Spinach	1	95	7	65	2	0	201	201	2	<1	7	1 med-fat meat

1-Egg Omelet, Plain	1	96	7	65	2	0	217	98	<1	0	6	1 med-fat meat
Deviled Egg	1/2 egg & filling	63	5	45	1	0	121	94	<1	0	4	1 med-fat meat
Egg, Boiled/Cooked	1 extra large	90	6	55	2	0	246	72	<1	0	7	1 med-fat meat
Egg, Boiled/Cooked	1 jumbo	99	7	65	2	0	271	79	<1	0	8	1 med-fat meat
Egg, Boiled/Cooked	1 large	78	5	45	2	0	212	62	<1	0	6	1 med-fat meat
Egg, Boiled/Cooked	1 medium	68	5	45	1	0	187	55	<1	0	6	1 med-fat meat
Egg, Boiled/Cooked	1 small	57	4	35	1	0	157	46	<1	0	5	1 med-fat meat
Egg, Fried in Margarine	1 large	90	7	65	2	0	210	94	<1	0	6	1 high-fat meat
Egg, Scrambled, Plain	1	102	7	65	2	0	215	171	1	0	7	2 med-fat meat
Egg Substitute	1/4 cup	30	0	0	0	0	0	115	1	0	6	1 lean meat
Egg Whites	2	32	0	0	0	0	0	110	<1	0	7	1 lean meat
Souffle, Cheese	1 cup	197	14	125	6	0	194	299	6	<1	12	1/2 reduced-fat milk, 1 med-fat meat, 1 fat
Souffle, Spinach	1 cup	234	18	165	8	0	160	770	8	1	11	1/2 reduced-fat milk, 1 med-fat meat, 2 fat

EGGS, EGG DISHES, EGG PRODUCTS

	Serving	Calories	Fat (g)	Cal. from Fat	Sat. Fat (g)	Trans Fat (g)	Chol. (mg)	Sod. (mg)	Carb. (g)	Fiber (g)	Prot. (g)	Servings/Exchanges
Brands												
ConAgra												
Egg Beaters, Cheese & Chive	1/4 cup	35	1	10	0.5	0	<5	210	1	0	5	1 lean meat
Egg Beaters, Garden Vegetable	1/4 cup	30	0	0	0	0	0	160	1	0	5	1 lean meat
Egg Beaters, Original	1/4 cup	30	0	0	0	0	0	115	1	0	6	1 lean meat
Egg Beaters, Whites	3 Tbsp	25	0	0	0	0	0	75	1	0	5	1 lean meat
Egg Beaters. Southwestern	1/4 cup	30	0	0	0	0	0	180	1	0	5	1 lean meat
Crystal Farms												
All Whites	1/4 cup	30	0	0	0	0	0	95	1	0	6	1 lean meat
Better'n Eggs	1/4 cup	30	0	0	0	0	0	120	1	0	6	1 lean meat
Better'n Eggs Plus	1/4 cup	35	0	0	0	0	0	105	0	0	6	1 lean meat

ETHNIC FOODS

ALASKA NATIVE

	Serving	Calories	Fat (g)	Cal. from Fat	Sat. Fat (g)	Trans Fat (g)	Chol. (mg)	Sod. (mg)	Carb. (g)	Fiber (g)	Prot. (g)	Servings/Exchanges
Beach Asparagus	1 cup	15	<1	0	NA	0	0	23	2	NA	1	free
Caribou, Cooked	1 oz	47	1	10	<1	0	31	17	0	0	8	1 lean meat
Dried Fish/King Salmon	1/2 oz	60	5	45	NA	0	NA	NA	0	0	7	1 med-fat meat
Fiddlehead Fern, Raw	1 cup	34	<1	0	NA	0	0	84	5	NA	3	1 vegetable
Gumboots/Leathery Chiton	2 oz	46	<1	0	NA	0	NA	NA	0	0	10	1 lean meat
Halibut, Cooked	1 oz	39	<1	0	<1	0	12	20	0	0	8	1 lean meat
Herring Eggs, Plain	1/2 cup	48	<1	0	NA	0	NA	52	4	0	8	1 lean meat
Highbush Cranberries	1 1/4 cup	58	<1	0	NA	0	0	1	15	NA	<1	1 fruit
Hooligan, Smoked	1 oz	86	7	65	NA	0	NA	NA	0	0	6	1 high-fat meat
Huckleberries	1 cup	56	<1	0	NA	0	0	15	13	NA	<1	1 fruit
Moose, Cooked	1 oz	38	<1	0	<1	0	22	19	0	0	8	1 lean meat

ETHNIC FOODS

	Serving	Calories	Fat (g)	Cal. from Fat	Sat. Fat (g)	Trans Fat (g)	Chol. (mg)	Sod. (mg)	Carb. (g)	Fiber (g)	Prot. (g)	Servings/Exchanges
Muktuk with Skin and Fat	1x1x2 inches	138	12	110	NA	0	NA	NA	0	0	8	1 high-fat meat, 1 fat
Muskrat, Cooked	1 oz	67	3	25	0	0	34	27	0	0	9	1 lean meat
Pike, Cooked	1 oz	33	<1	0	0	0	14	13	0	0	7	1 lean meat
Pilot Bread	1.4-inch round	104	2	20	NA	0	NA	142	18	NA	2	1 starch
Salmon, Sockeye	1 oz	60	3	25	<1	0	24	18	0	0	8	1 lean meat
Salmonberries	1 1/2 cup	55	<1	0	NA	0	0	52	13	NA	1	1 fruit
Seal Meat, Raw	1 oz	41	<1	0	<1	0	NA	NA	0	0	9	1 lean meat
Seal Oil	1 tsp	45	5	45	<1	0	8	NA	0	0	0	1 fat
Seaweed, Dried Black	1 cup	39	<1	0	NA	0	NA	0	39	40	NA	4 Vegetable
Sour Dock, Cooked	1/2 cup	19	<1	0	NA	0	0	NA	4	NA	1	1 vegetable
Venison, Cooked	1 oz	44	<1	0	<1	0	31	15	0	0	9	1 lean meat
Walrus, Raw	1 oz	56	4	35	<1	0	22	NA	0	0	5	1 lean meat

Food	Serving										Exchanges
Whale, Bonehead, Raw	1 oz	37	<1	0	0	NA	17	0	0	7	1 lean meat
Willow Greens, Cooked	1/2 cup	28	<1	0	0	NA	NA	6	NA	2	1 vegetable
CAJUN & CREOLE											
Alligator, Cooked	1 oz	42	0.5	<1	0	19	22	0	0	9	1 lean meat
Beef Tasso	1 oz	47	1	0.5	0	12	NA	0	0	8	1 lean meat
Cafe au Lait	8 oz	76	4	3	35	17	59	6	0	4	1/2 whole milk
Couche-Couche, No Fat Added	1/2 cup	82	<1	NA	0	0	4	17	1	3	1 starch
Cracklins	1/4 cup	131	11	4	100	19	362	0	0	7	1 high-fat meat, 1 fat
Crawfish, Cooked	2 oz	46	0.5	<1	5	81	107	0	0	10	1 lean meat
Cushaw Squash	1/2 cup	41	0.5	<1	5	0	2	9	3	1	1 vegetable
Dewberries/Blackberries	3/4 cup	60	<1	0	0	0	0	15	6	<1	1 fruit
Dove, Cooked	1 oz	62	4	1	35	33	82	0	0	7	1 med-fat meat
Frog Legs, Steamed	2 legs	45	<1	NA	0	31	36	0	0	10	1 lean meat
Goat, Baked or Roasted	1 oz	45	2	<1	0	38	96	0	0	7	1 lean meat

ETHNIC FOODS

	Serving	Calories	Fat (g)	Cal. from Fat	Sat. Fat (g)	Trans Fat (g)	Chol. (mg)	Sod. (mg)	Carb. (g)	Fiber (g)	Prot. (g)	Servings/Exchanges
Guinea, Flesh Only	1 oz	42	1	9	<1	0	24	26	0	0	8	1 lean meat
Hogshead Cheese	1/4 cup	77	6	55	2	0	29	455	0	0	6	1 med-fat meat
Kumquats	5	60	0	0	0	0	0	6	16	4	1	1 fruit
Lamb, Cooked	1 oz	83	6	55	3	0	28	20	0	0	7	1 med-fat meat
Mirliton/Chayote, Cooked	1/2 cup	24	0.5	5	0	0	0	1	5	3	<1	1 vegetable
Muscadines	17	60	0.5	5	0	0	0	2	15	<1	<1	1 fruit
Passionfruit (Maypops)	3	52	0	0	0	0	0	17	13	1	1	1 fruit
Peas, Crowder, Purple Hull	1/2 cup	92	<1	0	<1	0	0	8	15	4	7	1 starch
Persimmons (Japanese)	1/2 of 2 1/2 inches	59	0	0	0	0	0	1	16	1	0.5	1 fruit
Pickled Pigs Feet	1/2 foot	88	7	65	2	0	40	402	0	0	6	1 high-fat meat

Pork Sausage, Cooked	1 oz	105	9	80	3	0	24	367	0	0	6	1 high-fat meat
Pumpkin, Cooked	1/2 cup	20	0	0	0	0	0	1	5	2	<1	1 vegetable
Remoulade Sauce	1 Tbsp	52	6	50	2	0	7	54	<1	0	<1	1 fat
Salt Pork or Fatback	1/2-inch	45	5	45	2	0	5	80	0	0	<1	1 fat
Satsuma/Mandarin	2 small	62	0	0	0	0	0	1	16	1	<1	1 fruit
Shrimp, Dried	36	55	1	9	<1	0	79	77	0.5	0	11	2 lean meat
Smoked Beef Sausage	1 oz	89	8	70	3	0	19	321	<1	0	4	1 high-fat meat
Smoked Pork Sausage	1 oz	110	9	80	3	0	19	426	0	0	6	1 high-fat meat
Squab, Flesh Only, Cooked	1 oz	60	3	25	<1	0	38	22	0	0	7	1 lean meat
Tongue, Beef, Cooked	1 oz	80	6	55	3	0	30	17	0	0	6	1 med-fat meat
Tripe, Cooked	2 oz	57	1	10	<1	0	54	41	0	0	11	2 lean meat
Turtle, Cooked	1.5 oz	57	2	18	<1	0	26	170	0	0	10	1 lean meat
CHINESE AMERICAN												
Amaranth/Chinese Spinach, Cooked	1/2 cup	14	<1	0	0	0	0	14	3	NA	1	1 vegetable

ETHNIC FOODS

	Serving	Calories	Fat (g)	Cal. from Fat	Sat. Fat (g)	Trans Fat (g)	Chol. (mg)	Sod. (mg)	Carb. (g)	Fiber (g)	Prot. (g)	Servings/Exchanges
Amaranth/Chinese Spinach, Raw	1 cup	7	<1	0	0	0	0	6	1	NA	<1	1 vegetable
Arrowheads/Fresh Corn, Large	1	25	<1	0	NA	0	NA	6	5	NA	1	1 vegetable
Baby Corn, Canned	1/2 cup	13	<1	0	NA	0	0	730	2	NA	2	1 vegetable
Bamboo Shoots, Canned	1/2 cup	13	<1	0	0	0	0	5	2	<1	1	1 vegetable
Beef Jerky	1/2 oz	57	4	35	2	NA	7	310	2	<1	5	1 lean meat
Beef Tongue	1 oz	81	6	55	3	0	30	17	<1	0	6	1 med-fat meat
Bitter Melon/Bitter Gourd/Balsam-Pear Pods	1 cup	16	<1	0	0	0	0	5	3	3	<1	1 vegetable
Bok Choy/Chinese Cabbage/Pakchoi	1/2 cup	9	<1	0	0	0	0	46	2	<1	1	1 vegetable
Carambola/Star Fruit	2	60	<1	0	0	0	0	4	14	5	1	1 fruit

Cellophane/Mung Bean Noodles, Cooked	1/2 cup	67	NA	NA	0	0	0	2	16	<1	NA	1 starch
Cha Shu Bun, Frozen, Steamed	2	360	13	115	5	0	20	410	50	1	8	2 starch, 3 fat
Chayote, Raw	1 cup	32	<1	0	0	0	0	5	7	4	1	1 vegetable
Chinese Banana, Dwarf	1	72	<1	0	NA	0	0	18	18	NA	2	1 fruit
Chinese Celery, Raw	1 cup	26	<1	0	0	0	0	116	5	0	2	1 vegetable
Chinese Eggplant, Purple, Cooked	1/2 cup	17	<1	0	NA	0	0	NA	4	2	<1	1 vegetable
Chinese Eggplant, White, Cooked	1/2 cup	20	<1	0	NA	0	0	NA	5	2	<1	1 vegetable
Chinese Sausage	1 oz	100	8	70	3	NA	NA	246	2	NA	6	1 high-fat meat
Chinese/Black Mushrooms, Dried	2	21	<1	0	0	0	0	1	5	<1	<1	1 vegetable
Chinese/Peking/Pe-tsai/Napa Cabbage, Raw	1 cup	12	<1	0	0	0	0	1	3	<1	<1	1 vegetable

ETHNIC FOODS

	Serving	Calories	Fat (g)	Cal. from Fat	Sat. Fat (g)	Trans Fat (g)	Chol. (mg)	Sod. (mg)	Carb. (g)	Fiber (g)	Prot. (g)	Servings/Exchanges
Choy Sum/Chinese Flowering Cabbage	1 cup	9	NA	NA	NA	0	0	NA	2	NA	1	1 vegetable
Coconut Milk	1 Tbsp	35	4	35	3	0	0	2	<1	<1	2	1 fat
Coriander, Raw	1 cup	3	<1	0	0	0	0	4	<1	<1	<1	free
Dried Mung Beans/ Green Beans, Cooked	1/2 cup	106	<1	0	<1	0	0	2	19	8	7	1 starch, 1 lean meat
Dried Red Beans, Cooked	1/3 cup	99	<1	0	0	0	0	6	19	1	6	1 starch, 1 lean meat
Garland Chrysanthemum, Raw	1 cup	4	0	0	NA	0	NA	13	1	NA	<1	free
Ginger Root, Raw	1/4 cup	17	<1	0	NA	0	NA	3	4	NA	<1	free
Gingko Seeds, Canned	1/2 cup	86	1	10	<1	0	0	238	17	7	2	1 starch
Guava, Medium	1 1/2	69	<1	0	<1	0	0	4	16	7	1	1 fruit
Hairy Melon/Hairy Cucumber, Raw	1 cup	22	NA	NA	NA	0	NA	NA	5	2	1	1 vegetable

Kumquat, Medium	5	30	<1	0	0	0	6	16	6	<1	1 fruit
Leeks, Cooked	1/2 cup	16	<1	0	0	0	5	4	<1	<1	1 vegetable
Litchi/Lychee, Canned	1/2 cup	57	<1	0	0	0	27	15	<1	<1	1 fruit
Litchi/Lychee, Raw	10	63	<1	NA	0	0	1	16	1	<1	1 fruit
Longan, Canned	3/4 cup	68	<1	0	0	0	54	18	NA	<1	1 fruit
Longan, Raw	30	58	<1	0	0	0	0	15	1	1	1 fruit
Lotus Root	10 slices	45	<1	<1	0	0	33	14	4	2	1 starch
Luffa, Angled, Raw	1 cup	30	<1	NA	0	0	2	7	NA	1	1 vegetable
Luffa, Smooth/Sponge, Raw	1 cup	34	<1	NA	0	0	6	8	NA	2	1 vegetable
Mango, Small	1/2 cup	68	<1	<1	0	0	2	18	2	<1	1 fruit
Moon Cake, Plain Lotus Seed Paste	1/4	169	8	NA	70	2	NA	24	<1	2	1 1/2 carb, 2 fat
Mung Bean Sprouts, Seed Attached, Raw	1 cup	31	<1	0	0	0	6	6	2	3	1 vegetable
Mustard Greens, Cooked	1/2 cup	11	0	0	0	0	11	2	1	2	1 vegetable

ETHNIC FOODS

	Serving	Calories	Fat (g)	Cal. from Fat	Sat. Fat (g)	Trans Fat (g)	Chol. (mg)	Sod. (mg)	Carb. (g)	Fiber (g)	Prot. (g)	Servings/Exchanges
Mustard Greens, Salted	2 Tbsp	14	<1	0	NA	0	0	NA	4	NA	<1	free
Oriental Radish/Daikon, Raw	1 cup	16	<1	0	0	0	0	18	4	1	<1	1 vegetable
Papaya, Medium	1/2	59	<1	0	<1	0	0	5	15	3	<1	1 fruit
Peapods/Sugar Peas, Cooked	1/2 cup	34	<1	0	0	0	0	3	6	2	3	1 vegetable
Pepper, Chili, Raw	1 cup	60	<1	0	0	0	0	11	14	2	3	3 vegetables
Persimmon	1/2	59	<1	0	0	0	0	1	16	3	<1	1 fruit
Pummelo	3/4 cup	58	<1	0	NA	0	0	1	14	<1	1	1 fruit
Rice Noodles, Fresh	1/2 cup	99	<1	0	0	0	0	NA	23	NA	1	1 1/2 starch
Rice Vermicelli, Cooked	1/2 cup	56	0	0	0	0	0	NA	13	NA	1	1 starch
Salted Duck Egg	1	137	7	65	NA	NA	NA	NA	<1	0	10	1 high-fat meat
Scallop, Dried, Large	1	44	<1	0	NA	NA	NA	NA	1	NA	9	1 lean meat
Sesame Paste	2 tsp	60	5	45	1	0	0	12	2	<1	2	1 fat

Sesame Seeds, Whole, Dried	1 Tbsp	52	5	45	<1	0	0	0	1	2	1	2	1 fat
Shrimp, Dried, Medium	10	40	<1	0	NA	0	NA	NA	2	4	NA	7	1 lean meat
Soybean Milk, Unsweetened	1 cup	81	5	45	<1	0	0	29	29	4	3	7	1 med-fat meat
Soybean Sprouts, Seed Attached, Raw	1 cup	86	5	45	<1	0	0	10	7	7	<1	9	1 vegetable, 1 med-fat meat
Soybeans, Cooked	3 Tbsp	56	3	25	<1	0	0	0	0	3	2	5	1 lean meat
Squid, Raw	2 oz	52	<1	0	<1	0	132	0	26	2	0	9	1 lean meat
Straw Mushrooms, Canned	1/2 cup	20	<1	0	NA	0	0	172	0	4	NA	2	1 vegetable
Sweet Rice Dough Ball	3	220	10	90	6	NA	0		0	29	1	3	2 carb, 2 fat
Taro, Cooked	1/2 cup	94	<1	0	<1	0	0		10	23	3	<1	1 1/2 starch
Tofu/Soybean Curd	4 oz	91	6	55	<1	NA	0		8	2	1	10	1 med-fat meat
Tripe, Beef, Raw	2 oz	56	2	20	1	0	54		26	0	0	8	1 lean meat
Turnip, Raw	1 cup	35	<1	0	0	0	0		87	8	2	1	1 vegetable

ETHNIC FOODS

	Serving	Calories	Fat (g)	Cal. from Fat	Sat. Fat (g)	Trans Fat (g)	Chol. (mg)	Sod. (mg)	Carb. (g)	Fiber (g)	Prot. (g)	Servings/Exchanges
Water Chestnuts, Chinese	1/2 cup	66	<1	0	0	0	0	9	15	2	<1	1 starch
Watercress, Raw	1 cup	4	0	0	0	0	0	14	<1	<1	<1	free
Winter Melon/Wax Gourd/Chinese Preserving Melon	1 cup	17	<1	0	0	0	0	147	4	4	<1	1 vegetable
Won Ton, Cantonese Style	5	83	<1	0	0	0	0	850	13	2	6	1 starch
Yard-Long Beans, Cooked	1/2 cup	24	<1	0	0	0	0	2	5	NA	1	1 vegetable
Yard-Long Beans, Raw	1 cup	43	<1	0	<1	0	0	4	8	NA	3	1 vegetable
FILIPINO AMERICAN												
Bamboo Shoots, Canned	1/2 cup	13	<1	0	<1	0	0	5	2	1	1	1 vegetable

Food	Serving										Exchange
Banana Sauce	1 tsp	11	NA	NA	NA	0	0	3	0	0	free
Banana Squash, Cooked	1/2 cup	24	<1	0	0	0	2	6	1	<1	1 vegetable
Banana, Native, Small	1	46	<1	0	<1	0	0	12	<1	<1	1 fruit
Beef Shank, Lean, Cooked	1 oz	57	2	20	<1	22	18	0	0	10	1 lean meat
Beef Tongue	1 oz	80	6	55	3	30	17	<1	0	6	1 med-fat meat
Bitter Melon, Cooked	1/2 cup	12	<1	0	NA	0	4	3	NA	<1	1 vegetable
Bottle Gourd, Cooked	1/2 cup	9	<1	0	NA	0	NA	2	<1	<1	free
Cassava Tuber, Cooked	1/2 cup	60	<1	0	<1	0	4	15	0	<1	1 starch
Ceylon Moss Bar, Dried	1/4	8	0	0	0	0	3	2	<1	<1	free
Chayote, Cooked	1/2 cup	19	<1	0	0	0	1	4	<1	<1	1 vegetable
Chicken Gizzard, Cooked	1 oz	43	1	10	<1	55	19	<1	0	8	1 lean meat
Chinese Celery, Raw	1 cup	32	2	20	NA	0	48	5	<1	3	1 vegetable
Chinese Sausage	1 oz	100	8	70	3	30	249	2	NA	6	1 high-fat meat
Chinese Spinach, Raw	1 cup	7	<1	0	<1	0	5	1	NA	<1	free

ETHNIC FOODS

	Serving	Calories	Fat (g)	Cal. from Fat	Sat. Fat (g)	Trans Fat (g)	Chol. (mg)	Sod. (mg)	Carb. (g)	Fiber (g)	Prot. (g)	Servings/Exchanges
Clam, Cooked	1 oz	42	<1	0	<1	0	19	32	2	0	7	1 lean meat
Coconut Milk, Canned	1 Tbsp	35	4	35	3	0	0	2	<1	0	<1	1 fat
Corned Beef, Canned	1 oz	71	4	35	2	0	24	285	0	0	8	1 med-fat meat
Cracklings, Crushed	2 Tbsp	42	3	25	<1	0	9	3	0	0	4	1 fat
Fish Sauce	1 Tbsp	4	<1	0	NA	0	NA	1088	0	0	<1	free
Guava, Raw	1 1/2	61	<1	0	<1	0	0	3	14	7	1	1 fruit
Horseradish Leaves, Cooked	1/2 cup	13	<1	0	NA	0	0	2	2	NA	1	1 vegetable
Indian Sardines, Dried	1 oz	57	1	10	NA	0	NA	NA	0	0	11	1 lean meat
Jicama, Cooked	1/2 cup	19	0	0	0	0	0	2	4	<1	<1	1 vegetable
Long-Jawed Anchovy, Dried	2 Tbsp	64	1	10	NA	0	NA	26	0	0	12	1 lean meat
Mango, Small	1/2	61	<1	0	<1	0	0	2	18	3	<1	1 fruit
Mung Beans, Cooked	1/3 cup	71	<1	0	<1	0	0	1	13	NA	5	1 starch

Food												
Mung Bean Noodles, Cooked	3/4 cup	73	0	0	0	0	0	9	18	NA	0	1 starch
Native Sausage, Raw	1 oz	167	17	155	NA	0	NA	NA	<1	0	3	1 high-fat meat, 1 fat
Oriental Radish/Daikon, Raw	1 cup	16	0	0	0	0	0	9	2	NA	<1	free
Oyster, Cooked, Medium	1	41	1	9	<1	0	38	53	3	0	5	1 lean meat
Papaya, Unripe, Cooked	1/2 cup	20	<1	0	NA	0	0	3	5	<1	1	1 vegetable
Papaya, Yellow, Raw, Cubed	1 cup	54	<1	0	<1	0	0	4	14	2	<1	1 fruit
Peapods, Cooked	1/2 cup	34	<1	0	<1	0	0	3	6	1	3	1 vegetable
Plantain, Cooked, Sliced	1/2 cup	89	<1	0	NA	0	0	4	24	2	<1	1 1/2 starch
Pummelo	3/4 cup	62	<1	0	NA	0	0	0	15	2	1	1 fruit
Rice Sticks/Noodles, Cooked	3/4 cup	91	1	10	NA	0	0	1	19	<1	1	1 starch
Sausage, Simulated	1 oz	72	5	45	<1	NA	0	251	3	0	5	1 med-fat meat
Sesame Seeds, Dried	1 Tbsp	52	5	45	<1	0	<1	1	2	<1	2	1 fat

ETHNIC FOODS

	Serving	Calories	Fat (g)	Cal. from Fat	Sat. Fat (g)	Trans Fat (g)	Chol. (mg)	Sod. (mg)	Carb. (g)	Fiber (g)	Prot. (g)	Servings/Exchanges
Shrimp, Fermented, Small	1 Tbsp	12	<1	0	<1	0	0	734	0	<1	3	free
Soy Bean Curd/Tofu	1/2 cup	94	6	55	<1	0	0	9	2	2	10	1 med-fat meat
Spanish Sausage	1 oz	125	11	100	4	NA	30	367	NA	0	7	1 high-fat meat, 1 fat
Swamp Cabbage, Cooked	1/2 cup	9	<1	0	NA	0	0	63	<1	<1	1	free
Taro, Cooked	1/3 cup	62	<1	0	<1	0	0	6	15	NA	<1	1 starch
Watermelon Seeds, Dried	1 Tbsp	38	3	25	<1	0	0	6	1	<1	2	1 fat
Yard-Long Beans, Cooked	1/2 cup	24	<1	0	<1	0	0	2	5	NA	1	1 vegetable
HMONG												
Asian Pear	1	51	<1	0	0	0	0	0	13	4	<1	1 fruit
Bamboo Shoots, Canned	1/2 cup	13	<1	0	<1	0	0	4	2	<1	1	1 vegetable

Food	Serving											Exchange
Beef Tallow	1 tsp	39	4	35	2	NA	5	0	0	0	0	1 fat
Bitter Melon, Raw	1 cup	16	<1	0	0	0	0	5	3	3	<1	1 vegetable
Cellophane/Mung Bean Noodles, Cooked	1/2 cup	67	NA	NA	0	0	0	2	16	<1	NA	1 starch
Chicken Fat	1 tsp	39	4	35	1	0	4	0	0	0	0	1 fat
Chitterlings, Boiled	2 Tbsp	42	4	35	1	0	20	6	0	0	1	1 fat
Coconut Cream, Canned	1 Tbsp	36	3	35	3	0	0	10	2	<1	<1	1 fat
Coconut Milk, Canned	1 Tbsp	30	3	25	3	0	0	2	<1	0	<1	1 fat
Coconut Milk, Raw	1 Tbsp	35	4	35	3	0	0	2	<1	<1	<1	1 fat
Coconut, Raw	2 Tbsp	35	3	25	3	0	0	2	2	<1	<1	1 fat
Condensed Milk, Sweetened	2 Tbsp	123	3	3	2	0	13	46	21	0	3	1 1/2 carb, 1 fat
Coriander/Chinese Parsely, Raw	1 cup	3	<1	0	0	0	0	4	<1	<1	<1	free
Cucuzzi Squash, Cooked	1/2 cup	23	<1	0	0	0	0	14	5	1	<1	1 vegetable

ETHNIC FOODS

	Serving	Calories	Fat (g)	Cal. from Fat	Sat. Fat (g)	Trans Fat (g)	Chol. (mg)	Sod. (mg)	Carb. (g)	Fiber (g)	Prot. (g)	Servings/Exchanges
Fish Sauce	1 Tbsp	6	0	0	0	0	0	1390	<1	0	<1	free
Guava, Medium	1	69	<1	0	<1	0	0	4	16	7	1	1 fruit
Jackfruit	1/2 cup	78	<1	0	0	0	0	2	20	1	1	1 fruit
Leeks, Cooked	1/2 cup	16	<1	0	0	0	0	6	4	NA	<1	1 vegetable
Luffa Gourd/Squash, Raw	1 cup	30	<1	0	NA	0	0	6	7	NA	2	1 vegetable
Mango, Small	1/2	68	<1	0	<1	0	0	2	18	2	<1	1 fruit
Mung Bean Sprouts with Seeds, Cooked	1/2 cup	13	<1	0	0	0	0	6	3	<1	1	1 vegetable
Mustard Greens	1/2 cup	10	<1	0	0	0	0	11	2	1	2	1 vegetable
Papaya, Medium	1/2	59	<1	0	<1	0	9	4	15	3	<1	1 fruit
Peas, Podded, Cooked	1/2 cup	24	<1	0	0	0	0	3	6	2	3	1 vegetable
Peas, Podded, Raw	1/2 cup	26	<1	0	0	0	0	3	5	2	2	1 vegetable
Pheasant, No Skin, Raw	1 oz	38	1	0	<1	0	19	10	0	0	7	1 lean meat

Food	Serving											Exchanges
Pig's Feet	1/2 foot	68	4	35	1.5	0	35	11	0	0	7	1 med-fat meat
Pork Lard	1 tsp	39	4	35	2	NA	4	0	0	0	0	1 fat
Pork, Ground	1 oz	84	6	55	2	0	27	21	0	0	7	1 high-fat meat
Pumpkin Blossom, Cooked	1 cup	20	<1	0	0	0	0	8	4	1	2	free
Pumpkin, Cooked	1/2 cup	24	<1	0	0	0	0	2	6	1	<1	1 vegetable
Rice Noodles, Fresh	1/2 cup	99	<1	0	0	0	0	NA	23	<1	1	1 starch
Squirrel, Roasted	1 oz	49	1	10	<1	0	34	34	0	0	9	1 lean meat
Tofu/Soybean Curd	4 oz, 1/2 cup	94	6	55	<1	0	0	9	2	2	10	1 med-fat meat
Venison	1 oz	45	<1	0	<1	0	32	15	0	0	9	1 lean meat
Vinespinach, Raw	1 cup	11	<1	0	0	0	0	13	2	0	1	free
Yard-Long Beans, Cooked	1/2 cup	102	<1	0	<1	0	0	4	18	NA	7	1 starch, 1 lean meat

INDIAN & PAKISTANI

Food	Serving											Exchanges
Aviyal	1/2 cup	81	2	20	1	0	NA	412	14	NA	2	1 starch

ETHNIC FOODS

	Serving	Calories	Fat (g)	Cal. from Fat	Sat. Fat (g)	Trans Fat (g)	Chol. (mg)	Sod. (mg)	Carb. (g)	Fiber (g)	Prot. (g)	Servings/Exchanges
Brinjal, Cooked	1/2 cup	13	0	0	0	0	0	1	3	1	0	1 vegetable
Chai Masala	1/2 cup	14	0	0	0	0	0	0	3	NA	1	free
Chicken Tikka	3 1-inch pieces	54	2	20	<1	0	23	156	0	0	9	1 lean meat
Chickpeas, Cooked	1/2 cup	134	2	20	<1	0	0	6	23	4	7	1 1/2 starch, 1 lean meat
Coconut, Fresh, Shredded	3 Tbsp	53	5	45	4	0	0	3	2	1	1	1 fat
Coriander, Fresh	1/2 cup	2	0	0	0	0	0	2	0	<1	0	free
Cucumber Raita	1/2 cup	21	0	0	0	0	0	22	3	NA	1	1 vegetable
Dhakla, Khaman	1-inch square	104	5	45	0	0	NA	539	12	NA	5	1 starch, 1 fat
Dhansak	1/2 cup	104	4	35	0.5	0	NA	137	15	NA	4	1 starch, 1 fat
Fresh Shredded Coconut	3 Tbsp	53	5	45	4	0	0	3	2	1	1	1 fat

Food	Serving												Exchange
Ghee	1 tsp	45	5	45	3	0	20	0	0	0	0	0	1 fat
Ginger, Fresh	1/4 cup	17	<1	0	0	0	0	3	4	0.5	0	0	free
Green Plantain, Cooked	1/3 cup	60	<1	0	0	0	0	3	16	1	0		1 starch
Guava, Medium, Raw	1 1/2	61	<1	0	<1	0	0	3	14	7	1		1 fruit
Idli	3 inches	70	0	0	0	0	0	12	12	NA	2		1 starch
Jheera Pani	1/2 cup	16	0.5	5	0.5	0	NA	104	3	NA	1		free
Karela, Cooked	1/2 cup	12	0	0	0	0	0	4	3	1	1		1 vegetable
Lassi	1 cup	90	0	0	0	0	4	128	13	0	10		1 skim milk
Mango, Small, Raw	1/2	68	<1	0	0	0	0	2	18	2	1		1 fruit
Matki Usual	1/2 cup	104	6	55	4	0	0	192	10	NA	3		1 starch, 1 fat
Mung Bean Sprouts, Cooked	1/2 cup	13	<1	0	<1	0	0	6	3	0.5	1		1 vegetable
Mung Dhal, Cooked	1/2 cup	107	<1	0	<1	0	0	2	19	8	7		1 starch, 1 lean meat
Naan	1/4 of 8 x 2 inches	75	2	20	2	0	9	90	13	<1	2		1 starch
Cooked	1/2 cup	34	<1	0	0	0	0	3	8	3	2		1 vegetable

ETHNIC FOODS

	Serving	Calories	Fat (g)	Cal. from Fat	Sat. Fat (g)	Trans Fat (g)	Chol. (mg)	Sod. (mg)	Carb. (g)	Fiber (g)	Prot. (g)	Servings/Exchanges
Paneer	1 oz	103	3	25	2	0	NA	246	12	0	8	1 2% milk
Pesarattu	9 inches	127	5	45	1	0	NA	372	14	NA	5	1 starch, 1 fat
Phulka/Chappathi	6 inches	68	<1	0	<1	0	0	179	15	2	3	1 starch
Poha	1/2 cup	140	6	55	1	0	NA	405	18	NA	2	1 starch, 1 fat
Puri	5 inches	128	7	65	<1	0	0	1	16	2	3	1 starch, 1 fat
Rasam	1 cup	22	1	10	<1	0	NA	255	2	NA	1	free
Sambar	1/2 cup	88	1	10	0	0	NA	263	16	NA	5	1 starch
Tandoori Chicken	1 oz	75	4	35	1	0	NA	152	2	NA	8	1 med-fat meat
Tomato, Dhal	1/2 cup	132	3	25	2	0	NA	262	18	NA	7	1 starch, 1 lean meat
Toor Dhal, Cooked	1/2 cup	103	<1	0	<1	0	0	4	20	5	6	1 starch, 1 lean meat
JEWISH												
Bagel	1/2	78	<1	0	<1	0	0	151	15	<1	3	1 starch
Beef Brisket	1 oz	52	2	20	<1	0	16	28	1	0	6	1 lean meat
Beef Tongue	1 oz	80	6	55	3	0	30	17	<1	0	6	1 med-fat meat

Food	Serving											Exchanges
Bialy	1/2	69	0	0	0	0	0	167	16	1	7	1 starch
Blintzes	2 1/4 oz	80	2	20	<1	0	118	135	13	0	6	1 carb
Borekas	1/2 pie	114	11	100	5	0	45	191	15	<1	5	1 starch, 2 fat
Borscht	1/2 cup	26	<1	0	<1	0	0	473	5	1	2	1 vegetable
Bulgur, Cooked	1/2 cup	76	<1	0	0	0	0	5	17	4	3	1 starch
Bulke Roll	1/2 roll	78	<1	0	NA	0	0	137	15	<1	4	1 starch
Challah	1 oz	81	2	20	<1	0	15	139	14	<1	3	1 starch
Chicken Liver	1 oz	45	2	20	<1	0	179	15	<1	0	7	1 lean meat
Chickpeas	1/2 cup	135	2	20	<1	0	0	6	23	6	7	1 1/2 starch, 1 lean meat
Corned Beef	1 oz	71	5	45	2	NA	28	321	<1	0	5	1 med-fat meat
Couscous	1/2 cup	88	<1	0	0	0	0	4	18	1	3	1 starch
Cream Cheese	1 Tbsp	51	5	45	3	0	16	43	<1	0	1	1 fat
Farfel	1/2 cup	73	<1	0	0	0	0	0	15	<1	2	1 starch
Flanken, Raw	1 oz	51	3	25	1	0	15	20	0	0	6	1 lean meat
Gefilte Fish	2 pieces	71	2	20	<1	0	25	440	6	0	8	1/2 carb, 1 lean meat

ETHNIC FOODS

	Serving	Calories	Fat (g)	Cal. from Fat	Sat. Fat (g)	Trans Fat (g)	Chol. (mg)	Sod. (mg)	Carb. (g)	Fiber (g)	Prot. (g)	Servings/Exchanges
Herring in Wine Sauce	1/4 cup	90	4	35	1	0	25	420	7	0	5	1/2 carb, 1 med-fat meat
Herring, Pickled	1 oz	74	5	45	<1	0	4	247	3	0	4	1 med-fat meat
Horseradish, Root	1 Tbsp	7	<1	0	0	0	0	47	2	<1	<1	free
Kasha, Cooked	1/2 cup	77	<1	0	<1	0	0	3	17	2	3	1 starch
Kasha, Dry	2 Tbsp	71	<1	0	<1	0	0	2	15	2	2	1 starch
Kichlach	2-3	106	4	35	<1	0	42	13	15	<1	3	1 carb, 1 fat
Knishes	1 1/2 oz	114	5	45	<1	0	35	162	15	1	3	1 starch, 1 fat
Kreplach	2 oz	128	4	35	1	0	62	70	13	<1	10	1 carb, 1 lean meat
Kugel	1/2 cup	113	2	20	<1	0	31	277	17	<1	7	1 carb
Leckach	1 oz	84	2	20	<1	0	13	43	16	<1	1	1 starch
Lentils, Cooked	1/2 cup	115	<1	0	0	0	0	2	20	8	9	1 starch, 1 lean meat
Lox	1 oz	33	1	10	<1	0	7	567	0	0	5	1 lean meat
Matzoh	3/4 oz	84	<1	0	0	0	0	0	18	<1	2	1 starch

Food	Serving										Exchanges
Matzoh Ball	3 balls	212	13	115	4	NA	127	16	<1	6	1 carb, 2 1/2 fat
Matzoh Meal	2 Tbsp	65	<1	0	0	0	0	0	<1	2	1 starch
Pastrami	1 oz	99	8	70	3	NA	26	348	0	5	1 high-fat meat
Pickles, Dill, Large	1 1/2	36	<1	0	<1	0	0	2596	8	1	1 vegetable
Potato Flour	2 Tbsp	71	<1	0	<1	0	0	11	14	1	1 starch
Potato Pancakes, Medium	1	124	7	65	1	0	13	232	13	3	1 starch, 1 fat
Pumpernickel Bread	1 oz	71	<1	0	<1	0	0	190	14	3	1 starch
Rye Bread	1 oz	73	<1	0	<1	0	0	187	14	2	1 starch
Sablefish	1 oz	73	6	55	1	0	18	209	0	5	1 med-fat meat
Salmon, Canned	1 oz	39	2	20	<1	0	16	157	0	6	1 lean meat
Sardines, Medium, in Oil, Drained	2	60	3	25	<1	0	41	145	0	7	1 lean meat
Schmaltz	1 tsp	38	4	35	1	0	4	0	0	0	1 fat
Smelt	1 oz	35	<1	0	<1	0	26	22	0	6	1 lean meat
Sour Cream	2 Tbsp	52	5	45	3	0	11	13	<1	0	1 fat

ETHNIC FOODS

	Serving	Calories	Fat (g)	Cal. from Fat	Sat. Fat (g)	Trans Fat (g)	Chol. (mg)	Sod. (mg)	Carb. (g)	Fiber (g)	Prot. (g)	Servings/Exchanges
Split Peas, Cooked	1/2 cup	116	<1	0	0	0	0	2	21	8	8	1 1/2 starch, 1 lean meat
Sweet Wine	4 oz	173	13	115	0	0	0	0	2	10	0	2
Tzimmes	1/4 cup	88	<1	0	0	0	0	118	21	2	1	1 1/2 starch
Whitefish, Smoked	1 oz	31	<1	0	<1	0	9	289	0	0	7	1 lean meat
MEXICAN AMERICAN												
Avocado, Medium	1/8	40	4	35	<1	0	0	3	2	<1	<1	1 fat
Bolillo, Large	1/4	82	<1	0	<1	0	0	183	16	<1	3	1 starch
Chayote, Boiled, Drained	1/2 cup	19	<1	0	0	0	0	1	4	2	<1	1 vegetable
Chorizo	1 oz	129	11	100	4	NA	25	351	<1	0	7	1 high-fat meat, 1 fat
Corn Tortilla, 6-inch	1	58	<1	0	<1	0	0	42	12	1	2	1 starch
Corn Tortilla, Fat Added, 6-inch	1	102	6	55	<1	NA	0	42	12	1	2	1 starch, 1 fat

Food	Serving											Exchanges
Flour Tortilla, 6-inch	1	104	2	20	<1	0	0	153	18	1	3	1 starch
Flour Tortilla, Fat Added, 6-inch	1	148	7	65	1	NA	0	153	18	1	3	1 starch, 1 fat
Frijoles Cocidos	1/2 cup	117	<1	0	<1	0	0	2	22	7	7	1 starch, 1 lean meat
Frijoles Refritos, Fat Added	1/2 cup	161	5	45	<1	0	0	378	22	7	7	1 starch, 1 lean meat, 1 fat
Jicama, Raw	1 cup	49	<1	0	0	0	0	5	12	6	<1	2 vegetable
Mango, Small, Raw	1/2	68	<1	0	<1	0	0	2	18	2	<1	1 fruit
Menudo	1 cup	170	9	65	4	NA	0	950	1	NA	20	3 lean meat
Nopales, Cooked	1/2 cup	11	0	0	0	0	0	15	3	2	1	1 vegetable
Nopales, Raw	1 cup	14	<1	0	<1	0	0	19	3	2	1	1 vegetable
Pan Dulce, 5-inch	1	458	21	190	NA	NA	NA	389	59	NA	8	4 carb, 4 fat
Papaya, Raw, Cubed	1 cup	55	<1	0	<1	0	0	4	14	3	<1	1 fruit
Peppers, Hot Green Chili, Chopped, Raw	1 cup	60	<1	0	0	0	0	11	14	2	3	2 vegetable
Queso Anejo	1 oz	106	9	80	5	30	0	321	1	0	6	1 high-fat meat

ETHNIC FOODS

	Serving	Calories	Fat (g)	Cal. from Fat	Sat. Fat (g)	Trans Fat (g)	Chol. (mg)	Sod. (mg)	Carb. (g)	Fiber (g)	Prot. (g)	Servings/Exchanges
Queso Asadero	1 oz	101	8	70	5	0	30	186	<1	0	6	1 high-fat meat
Queso Chihuahua	1 oz	106	8	70	5	0	30	175	2	0	6	1 high-fat meat
Queso Fresco	1 oz	83	7	65	4	0	NA	200	NA	0	6	1 med-fat meat
Salsa De Chile	1/4 cup	14	<1	0	0	0	0	166	3	1	<1	free
Taco Shell, 6-inch	2	122	6	55	<1	0	0	95	16	2	2	1 starch, 1 fat
Verdolagas, Cooked	1/2 cup	10	<1	0	0	0	0	26	2	1	<1	1 vegetable
NAVAJO												
Blue Corn Mush	3/4 cup	94	<1	0	NA	0	0	32	21	NA	3	1 starch
Corn Hominy, Steamed	1/2 cup	70	1	10	<1	0	0	18	13	3	2	1 starch
Four Tortilla, 8-inch	1/4	87	<1	0	NA	0	0	211	19	1	3	1 starch
Mutton, Lean and Fat, Cooked	1 oz	96	9	80	NA	0	NA	NA	0	0	4	1 high-fat meat
Mutton, Lean, Cooked	1 oz	55	3	25	1	0	21	10	0	0	8	1 lean meat
Piñon Nuts, in Shell	1 Tbsp	60	6	55	<1	0	0	7	<1	1	1	1 fat

PLAINS INDIAN

Beans, Dried, Cooked	1/2 cup	117	<1	0	<1	0	0	1	22	7	7	1 1/2 starch, 1 lean meat
Beef Fat, Raw	1 tsp	38	4	35	2	0	5	0	0	0	0	1 fat
Biscuit Mix, Dry	1/4 cup	129	5	45	1	0	19	383	19	<1	2	1 starch, 1 fat
Buffalo/Bison	1 oz	40	<1	0	<1	0	23	16	0	0	8	1 lean meat
Chicken with Skin, Fried	1 oz	76	4	35	1	0	26	24	<1	0	8	1 med-fat meat
Commodity Meat, Luncheon	1 oz	97	9	80	NA	NA	NA	420	1	NA	3	1 high-fat meat
Cracklings	1/3 oz	57	5	45	2	0	9	18	0	0	2	1 fat
Dry Meat	1 oz	47	1	10	<1	0	12	984	<1	0	8	1 lean meat
Eggs, Dried Powdered	3 Tbsp	81	7	65	2	0	351	12	0	0	4	1 med-fat meat
Elk, Roasted	1 oz	41	<1	0	<1	0	0	17	0	0	9	1 lean meat
Huckleberries	1 cup	56	<1	0	NA	0	NA	15	13	NA	<1	1 fruit
Indian Corn, Dried	1/4 cup	132	2	20	NA	0	NA	37	26	<1	4	2 starch
Kidney, Raw	1 oz	30	<1	0	<1	0	81	51	<1	0	5	1 lean meat

ETHNIC FOODS

	Serving	Calories	Fat (g)	Cal. from Fat	Sat. Fat (g)	Trans Fat (g)	Chol. (mg)	Sod. (mg)	Carb. (g)	Fiber (g)	Prot. (g)	Servings/Exchanges
Lemon, Raw, Peeled	1	17	<1	0	NA	0	0	1	5	0	<1	free
Liver, Beef	1 oz	46	1	10	<1	0	110	20	1	0	7	1 lean meat
Pheasant, Skinless	1 oz	38	1	10	<1	0	0	10	0	0	7	1 lean meat
Pilot Bread	4-inch piece	104	2	20	NA	0	NA	142	18	NA	2	1 starch
Potatoes, Fried	1/2 cup	163	11	100	4	0	NA	19	17	2	2	1 starch, 2 fat
Short Ribs	1 oz	83	5	45	2	0	0	16	0	0	9	1 med-fat meat
Sweetbreads, Fried	1 oz	108	8	70	3	NA	NA	126	1	0	7	1 high-fat meat
Venison	1 oz	45	<1	0	<1	0	32	15	0	0	9	1 lean meat
White Fish, Dry Heat Cooked	1 oz	49	2	20	<1	0	22	19	0	0	7	1 lean meat
Wild Rice,	1/2 cup	82	<1	0	0	0	0	3	17	<1	3	1 starch
SOUTHERN & SOUL												
Fatback, Raw	1/4 oz	58	6	55	2	0	4	1	0	0	0	1 fat

Food	Serving	Cal										Exchange
Ham Hock	1 oz	90	7	65	2	0	18	383	2	0	6	1 high-fat meat
Hog Jowl	1 oz	54	5	55	2	0	9	7	0	0	2	1 fat
Hog Maw	1 oz	45	3	25	NA	0	55	15	0	0	5	1 lean meat
Hominy	3/4 cup	86	1	10	<1	0	0	252	17	3	2	1 starch
Kale, Cooked	1/2 cup	21	0	0	0	0	0	15	4	1	1	1 vegetable
Lard	1 tsp	38	4	40	2	0	4	0	0	0	0	1 fat
Muscadines	17	60	0.5	5	0	0	0	2	15	1	<1	1 fruit
Opossum	1 oz	63	3	25	NA	0	23	27	0	0	9	1 lean meat
Oxtail	1 oz	72	4	35	1	0	30	20	0	0	9	1 med-fat meat
Pig Ear	1/4 ear	47	3	25	NA	0	26	48	0	0	5	1 lean meat
Pigs Feet	1/2 foot	68	4	35	2	0	35	58	0	0	7	1 med-fat meat
Pig Tail	1 oz or 1/3 tail	113	10	90	4	0	37	48	0	0	5	1 high-fat meat
Poke Salad, Cooked	1/2 cup	16	0	0	0	0	0	NA	3	1	2	1 vegetable
Pork Brains	1 oz	39	3	25	0.5	0	727	26	0	0	4	1 lean meat
Pork Cracklings	1 Tbsp	57	5	45	2	0	9	18	0	0	2	1 fat

ETHNIC FOODS

	Serving	Calories	Fat (g)	Cal. from Fat	Sat. Fat (g)	Trans Fat (g)	Chol. (mg)	Sod. (mg)	Carb. (g)	Fiber (g)	Prot. (g)	Servings/Exchanges
Pork Neck Bones	1 oz	66	4	35	2	0	24	20	0	0	7	1 med-fat meat
Pork Skin (Rind), Fried	1 cup	68	4	35	2	0	17	231	0	0	8	1 med-fat meat
Pork Tongue	1 oz, 1/3 tongue	77	5	45	2	0	42	31	0	0	7	1 med-fat meat
Sousemeat (Headcheese)	1 oz	60	5	45	1	0	23	357	0	0	5	1 med-fat meat
Succotash	1/2 cup	79	1	10	0	0	0	38	17	5	4	1 starch
Tripe	2 oz	56	2	20	1	0	54	26	0	0	8	1 lean meat

FAST FOODS

ARBY'S

Roast Beef Sandwiches

	Serving	Calories	Fat (g)	Cal. from Fat	Sat. Fat (g)	Trans Fat (g)	Chol. (mg)	Sod. (mg)	Carb. (mg)	Fiber (g)	Prot. (g)	Servings/Exchanges
Regular Roast Beef	1	320	14	125	5	0.5	44	953	34	2	21	2 carb, 2 med-fat meat, 1 fat
Super Roast Beef	1	399	19	170	6	1	40	1061	44	2	21	3 carb, 2 med-fat meat, 2 fat
Bacon & Bleu Roastburger	1	466	23	210	9	1	52	1372	44	2	21	3 carb, 2 med-fat meat, 2 fat
Beef 'n Cheddar, Regular	1	440	21	190	6	1	55	1275	43	2	22	3 carb, 2 med-fat meat, 2 fat
Ham & Swiss Melt	1	268	8	70	3	0	25	1042	35	1	17	2 carb, 2 med-fat meat

Chicken

	Serving	Calories	Fat (g)	Cal. from Fat	Sat. Fat (g)	Trans Fat (g)	Chol. (mg)	Sod. (mg)	Carb. (mg)	Fiber (g)	Prot. (g)	Servings/Exchanges
Chicken Bacon & Swiss, Crispy	1	544	25	225	7	0	65	1632	50	2	32	3 carb, 3 med-fat meat, 2 fat

FAST FOOD

	Serving	Calories	Fat (g)	Cal. from Fat	Sat. Fat (g)	Trans Fat (g)	Chol. (mg)	Sod. (mg)	Carb. (g)	Fiber (g)	Prot. (g)	Servings/Exchanges
Chicken Breast Fillet, Roast	1	383	16	145	3	0	51	921	37	2	23	2 1/2 carb, 2 med-fat meat, 1 fat
Popcorn Chicken, Regular	1	363	16	145	3	0	54	930	27	2	24	2 1/2 carb, 2 med-fat meat, 1 fat
Roast Chicken Club	1	498	20	180	7	0	65	1540	65	2	30	3 carb, 3 med-fat meat, 1 fat
Market Fresh Sandwiches												
Corned Beef Reuben	1	590	32	290	9	0.5	77	1685	55	3	32	3 1/2 carb, 3 med-fat meat, 3 fat
Pecan Chicken Salad Sandwich, Grilled	1	870	44	400	6	0	65	1510	88	7	34	6 carb, 4 med-fat meat, 5 fat
Roast Ham & Swiss	1	691	31	280	8	0.5	59	1952	75	5	33	5 carb, 3 med-fat meat, 3 fat
Roast Turkey & Swiss	1	708	30	270	8	0.5	83	1677	74	5	41	5 carb, 4 med-fat meat, 2 fat

Roast Turkey, Ranch & Bacon	1	818	38	340	11	0.5	102	2146	75	5	46	5 carb, 5 med-fat meat, 3 fat
Ultimate BLT	1	779	45	405	11	0.5	51	1571	75	6	23	5 carb, 1 med-fat meat, 8 fat
Toasted Subs												
French Dip & Swiss	1	533	19	170	8	1	54	2169	67	3	29	4 1/2 carb, 2 med-fat meat, 2 fat
Philly Beef	1	610	30	270	9	1	63	1549	62	3	29	4 carb, 2 med-fat meat, 4 fat
Turkey Bacon Club	1	605	34	305	6	0	67	1701	65	3	35	4 carb, 3 med-fat meat, 4 fat
Market Fresh Chopped Salads												
Chopped Italian Salad	1	386	28	250	12	1	78	1420	11	3	21	1 carb, 3 med-fat meat, 3 fat
Chopped Turkey Club Salad	1	230	11	100	6	0.5	54	801	9	3	22	1/2 carb, 3 lean meat

FAST FOOD

	Serving	Calories	Fat (g)	Cal. from Fat	Sat. Fat (g)	Trans Fat (g)	Chol. (mg)	Sod. (mg)	Carb. (g)	Fiber (g)	Prot. (g)	Servings/Exchanges
Farmhouse Chicken Salad, Crispy	1	395	19	170	7	0.5	65	857	25	4	25	1 1/2 carb, 3 med-fat meat, 1 fat
Farmhouse Chicken Salad, Grilled	1	229	11	100	6	0.5	58	579	9	3	20	1/2 carb, 2 med-fat meat
Salad Dressing												
Balsamic Vinaigrette	1 pkg	130	5	45	2	0	0	460	5	0	0	1 fat
Buttermilk Ranch	1 pkg	230	24	215	4	0	10	390	2	0	1	5 fat
Dijon Honey Mustard	1 pkg	180	17	155	3	0	15	240	8	0	1	2 fat
Sides & Sidekickers												
Cheddar Cheese Sauce	1 pkg	25	2	20	2	0	5	182	2	0	0	1 fat
Curly Fries, Large	1 order	604	36	325	7	0.5	0	1413	70	7	8	5 carb, 7 fat
Curly Fries, Medium	1 order	496	29	260	5	0.5	0	1160	58	6	7	4 carb, 5 fat
Curly Fries, Small	1 order	338	20	180	4	0	0	790	39	4	4	2 1/2 carb, 4 fat
Jalapeño Bites, Large	8	486	34	305	14	1.5	45	841	47	3	9	3 carb, 6 fat

Jalapeño Bites, Regular	5	305	21	190	9	1	28	526	29	2	5	2 carb, 4 fat
Mozzarella Sticks, Large	6	637	42	380	19	1.5	68	2047	56	3	27	4 carb, 2 med-fat meat, 6 fat
Mozzarella Sticks, Regular	4	426	28	250	13	1	45	1370	38	2	16	2 1/2 carb, 2 med-fat meat, 3 fat
Onion Petals, Large	1 order	480	33	300	5	1	0	482	51	3	6	3 1/2 carb, 6 fat
Onion Petals, Regular	1 order	248	17	155	3	1	0	249	26	2	3	3 carb, 3 fat
Potato Cakes	2	246	18	160	4	0	0	391	26	2	2	2 carb, 3 fat

Desserts

Apple Turnover	1	380	14	125	7	0.5	0	287	58	3	3	4 carb, 2 fat
Cherry Turnover	1	364	13	115	7	0.5	0	269	58	1	4	4 carb, 2 fat

BOSTON MARKET

Individual Meals

1 Thigh & 1 Drumstick	5 oz	290	17	150	5	0	210	950	0	0	37	5 lean meat
1/2 BBQ Chicken	14.5 oz	730	30	270	9	0	405	2360	28	1	90	2 carb, 12 lean meat
1/4 White BBQ Chicken	9 oz	430	13	115	4	0	200	1400	28	1	52	2 carb, 6 med-fat meat

FAST FOOD

	Serving	Calories	Fat (g)	Cal. from Fat	Sat. Fat (g)	Trans Fat (g)	Chol. (mg)	Sod. (mg)	Carb. (g)	Fiber (g)	Prot. (g)	Servings/Exchanges
1/4 White Rotisserie Chicken	6.5 oz	320	12	110	4	0	200	900	0	0	52	7 lean meat
1/4 White Rotisserie Chicken, No Skin	6.8 oz	240	4	35	1	0	180	890	1	0	50	7 lean meat
3 Piece BBQ Dark Chicken	9 oz	430	13	120	4	0	200	1400	28	1	52	2 carb, 7 lean meat
3 Piece Dark Individual Meal	7.3 oz	390	22	190	6	0	290	1270	1	0	51	7 lean meat
3 Piece Dark Skinless (2 Thighs & Drumstick)	7 oz	350	15	130	4.5	0	280	1210	0	0	52	7 lean meat
BBQ Brisket	6.5 oz	400	20	180	1.5	0	40	760	28	1	26	2 carb, 3 med-fat meat, 1 fat
Beef Brisket	4 oz	280	20	180	1.5	0	40	260	1	0	26	4 med-fat meat
Beef Shepherd's Pie	14 oz	480	25	230	9	0	55	1490	40	5	25	3 carb, 2 med-fat meat, 3 fat

	Amount	Cal.	Fat (g)	Fat Cal.	Sat. Fat (g)	Trans Fat (g)	Chol. (mg)	Sod. (mg)	Carb. (g)	Fiber (g)	Pro. (g)	Exchanges/Choices
Crispy Country Chicken with Gravy	8 oz	480	23	200	4.5	0	80	1150	36	1	33	3 carb, 3 med-fat meat, 2 fat
Half Rotisserie Chicken	12 oz	610	29	260	9	0	405	1860	1	1	89	13 lean meat
Meatloaf	7.6 oz	520	36	320	16	1.5	145	1030	21	0	29	1 1/2 carb, 3 med-fat meat, 4 fat
Pastry Top Chicken Pot Pie	15 oz	800	48	430	18	7	140	1090	59	4	32	4 carb, 3 med-fat meat, 7 fat
Roasted Turkey	4 oz	150	2.5	25	1	0	55	500	0	0	31	4 lean meat
Soups & Sides												
Baked Beans	7.7 oz	270	1.5	15	0	0	0	1000	53	11	11	3 1/2 carb
Beef Gravy	3 oz	35	1.5	15	0.5	0	0	500	4	0	1	1/2 carb
Caesar Salad Dressing	2.5 oz	360	38	340	6	0.5	30	910	4	1	2	8 fat
Caesar Side Salad	3.2 oz	180	17	150	3.5	0	15	410	4	1	4	1 vegetable, 3 fat
Caesar Side Salad, No Dressing	2.2 oz	40	2	20	1.5	0	5	75	3	1	3	1 med-fat meat
Chicken Noodle Soup	14 oz	250	8	70	2.5	0	95	1420	23	2	22	1 1/2 carb, 2 med-fat meat

FAST FOOD

	Serving	Calories	Fat (g)	Cal. from Fat	Sat. Fat (g)	Trans Fat (g)	Chol. (mg)	Sod. (mg)	Carb. (g)	Fiber (g)	Prot. (g)	Servings/Exchanges
Chicken Tortilla Soup with Toppings	12.8 oz	410	26	230	7	0	70	2100	30	2	17	2 carb, 2 med-fat meat, 3 fat
Cinnamon Apples	5.1 oz	210	3	25	0	0	0	15	47	3	0	3 carb, 1 fat
Coleslaw	6.6 oz	300	20	180	4.5	0	15	280	27	4	2	2 carb, 4 fat
Creamed Spinach	6.7 oz	280	23	210	15	0	70	580	12	4	9	1 carb, 1 med-fat meat, 4 fat
Fresh Steamed Vegetables, Lowfat	4.8 oz	60	2	20	0	0	0	40	8	3	2	2 vegetable
Fresh Vegetable Stuffing	4.8 oz	190	8	70	1	0	0	580	25	2	3	1 1/2 carb, 2 fat
Garlic Dill New Potatoes, Lowfat	5.5 oz	140	3	30	1	0	0	120	24	3	3	1 1/2 carb, 1 fat
Garlic Spinach	6 oz	130	9	80	6	0	20	200	9	5	5	2 vegetable, 2 fat
Green Beans	3.2 oz	60	3.5	35	1.5	0	0	180	7	3	2	1 vegetable, 1 fat
Macaroni & Cheese	7.8 oz	300	11	100	7	0	30	1110	35	2	11	2 carb, 1 med-fat meat, 1 fat

Mashed Potatoes	7.8 oz	270	11	100	5	0	25	820	36	4	5	2 1/2 carb, 2 fat
Potato Salad	7 oz	390	29	260	7	0	20	640	26	3	3	2 carb, 6 fat
Poultry Gravy	4 oz	50	2	20	0.5	0	0	690	7	0	0	1/2 carb
Seasoned Fresh Fruit Salad, Lowfat	5 oz	60	0	5	0	0	0	20	15	1	1	1 fruit
Southern Style Squash Casserole	8 oz	300	19	170	7	0	30	1390	23	3	10	1 1/2 carb, 1 med-fat meat, 3 fat
Sweet Corn	6.2 oz	170	4	35	1	0	0	95	37	2	6	2 1/2 carb, 1 fat
Sweet Potato Casserole	7 oz	460	16	140	4.5	0	5	270	77	3	4	6 1/2 carb 3 fat
Sandwiches												
BBQ Brisket Sandwich	12 oz	800	30	270	6	0	60	1840	90	3	43	6 carb, 4 med-fat meat, 2 fat
Boston Sirloin Dip Carver	13 oz	900	46	410	13	2	165	1610	62	3	57	4 carb, 6 med-fat meat, 3 fat
Boston Turkey Carver	12 oz	700	26	240	8	0.5	95	1710	65	3	50	4 carb, 5 med-fat meat
Classic Chicken Salad Sandwich	12.8 oz	800	41	370	7	5	145	1900	65	4	40	4 carb, 4 med-fat meat, 4 fat

FAST FOOD

	Serving	Calories	Cal. from Fat	Fat (g)	Sat. Fat (g)	Trans Fat (g)	Chol. (mg)	Sod. (mg)	Carb. (g)	Fiber (g)	Prot. (g)	Servings/Exchanges
Crispy Country Chicken Carver	14 oz	1020	380	42	7	0	90	2210	114	4	45	7 1/2 carb, 3 med-fat meat, 5 fat
Meatloaf Open-Faced Sandwich	13 oz	670	350	38	17	1.5	145	1760	48	1	34	3 carb, 4 med-fat meat, 4 fat
Roasted Sirloin Open-Faced Sandwich	12 oz	410	140	15	6	1	100	1640	32	1	35	2 carb, 4 lean meat
Rotisserie Chicken Open-Faced Sandwich	10 oz	320	70	8	2.5	0	95	1630	34	1	27	2 carb, 3 lean meat
Salads												
Crispy Country Chicken	3 oz	220	90	11	2	0	40	480	16	1	16	1 carb, 2 med-fat meat
Market Chopped Salad	14 oz	480	360	40	8	1	10	1640	24	7	9	1 1/2 carb, 1 med-fat meat, 7 fat
Roasted Sirloin	3 oz	160	50	6	2	0	75	170	0	0	26	4 lean meat
Rotisserie Chicken	5 oz	180	25	3	0	125	620	0	0	0	39	6 lean meat

Desserts

Item	Serving											
Apple Gallette	4.73 oz	420	22	190	12	0	25	280	54	3	3	4 1/2 carb, 4 fat
Chocolate Chip Fudge Brownie	3 oz	320	13	120	3	0	50	220	49	3	5	3 carb, 3 fat
Chocolate Chunk Cookie	2.75 oz	370	19	170	9	0	20	340	49	2	4	3 carb, 4 fat
Cornbread	2 oz	180	5	45	1.5	1.5	10	320	31	0	2	2 carb, 1 fat
Pecan Pie	5.5 oz	640	36	320	11	0	115	340	74	2	7	5 carb, 7 fat

BURGER KING

WHOPPER Sandwiches

Item	Serving											
WHOPPER	1	670	40	360	11	1.5	75	1020	51	3	29	3 1/2 carb, 3 med-fat meat, 5 fat
WHOPPER with Cheese	1	770	48	430	16	1.5	100	1450	52	3	33	3 1/2 carb, 4 med-fat meat, 6 fat
Double WHOPPER	1	920	58	520	19	2.5	140	1090	51	3	48	3 1/2 carb, 6 med-fat meat, 6 fat

FAST FOOD

	Serving	Calories	Fat (g)	Cal. from Fat	Sat. Fat (g)	Trans Fat (g)	Chol. (mg)	Sod. (mg)	Carb. (g)	Fiber (g)	Prot. (g)	Servings/Exchanges
Double WHOPPER with Cheese	1	1010	66	595	24	2.5	160	1530	53	3	53	3 1/2 carb, 6 med-fat meat, 7 fat
Triple WHOPPER	1	1160	76	685	27	3	205	1170	51	3	68	3 1/2 carb, 8 med-fat meat, 7 fat
Triple WHOPPER with Cheese	1	1250	84	755	32	3.5	225	1600	52	3	73	3 1/2 carb, 9 med-fat meat, 8 fat
WHOPPER JR.	1	370	21	190	6	0.5	40	560	31	2	16	2 carb, 2 med-fat meat, 2 fat
WHOPPER JR. with Cheese	1	420	25	225	8	1	50	780	31	2	18	2 carb, 2 med-fat meat, 3 fat
Flame Broiled Burgers												
Hamburger	1	290	12	110	4.5	0.5	35	550	30	1	15	2 carb, 2 med-fat meat, 1 fat
Cheeseburger	1	340	16	145	7	0.5	45	770	31	1	18	2 carb, 2 med-fat meat, 1 fat

Double Hamburger	1	420	22	200	9	1	65	590	30	1	26	2 carb, 3 med-fat meat, 2 fat
Double Cheeseburger	1	510	29	260	14	1.5	90	1020	31	1	30	2 carb, 3 med-fat meat, 3 fat
BK Double Stacker	1	620	39	350	16	1.5	105	110	32	1	34	2 carb, 4 med-fat meat, 4 fat
BK Triple Stacker	1	820	55	495	23	2	160	1450	33	1	49	2 carb, 6 med-fat meat, 5 fat
BK Quad Stacker	1	1010	70	630	30	3	210	1800	34	1	64	2 carb, 8 med-fat meat, 6 fat
Steakhouse T	1	970	61	550	23	1	135	1930	44	4	42	3 1/2 carb, 5 med-fat meat, 7 fat
Mushroom & Swiss Steakhouse T	1	870	49	440	20	0.5	125	1890	54	4	43	3 1/2 carb, 5 med-fat meat, 5 fat

Chicken, Fish & Veggie

TENDERGRILL Chicken Sandwich	1	490	21	190	4	0	55	1220	51	3	26	3 1/2 carb, 2 med-fat meat, 2 fat

FAST FOOD

	Serving	Calories	Fat (g)	Cal. from Fat	Sat. Fat (g)	Trans Fat (g)	Chol. (mg)	Sod. (mg)	Carb. (g)	Fiber (g)	Prot. (g)	Servings/Exchanges
TENDERCRISP Chicken Sandwich	1	800	46	415	8	0.5	70	1640	68	3	32	4 1/2 carb, 3 med-fat meat, 6 fat
Original Chicken Sandwich	1	630	39	350	7	0.5	65	1390	46	3	24	3 carb, 2 med-fat meat, 6 fat
Chicken Tenders	4 pieces	180	11	100	3	0	30	310	13	0	9	1 carb, 1 med-fat meat, 1 fat
Chicken Tenders	6 pieces	270	16	145	3.5	0	45	460	19	0	14	1 carb, 2 med-fat meat, 1 fat
Chicken Tenders	8 pieces	360	21	190	4	0	60	610	25	0	18	1 1/2 carb, 2 med-fat meat, 2 fat
Kraft Macaroni & Cheese	1 order	160	5	45	1.5	0	10	340	22	1	7	1 1/2 carb, 1 med-fat meat
BK Chicken Fries	9 pieces	380	22	200	4	0	40	1220	24	2	21	1 1/2 carb, 2 med-fat meat, 2 fat

Item												Exchanges
BK BIG FISH Sandwich	1	640	32	290	5	0.5	45	1540	66	3	23	4 1/2 carb, 1 med-fat meat, 5 fat
BK VEGGIE Burger	1	420	16	145	2.5	0	10	1090	46	7	23	3 carb, 2 med-fat meat, 1 fat
Side Orders												
BK Fresh Apple Fries	1 order	25	0	0	0	0	0	0	6	1	0	1/2 fruit
Caramel Sauce	1 order	45	0.5	5	0	0	0	35	10	0	0	1 carb
Cheesy TOTS Potatoes	9 pieces	330	18	160	6	0	20	950	31	3	11	2 carb, 1 med-fat meat, 3 fat
French Fries, Small, Salted	1 order	340	17	155	3.5	0	0	590	44	4	4	3 carb, 3 fat
French Fries, Small, Salt Not Added	1 order	340	17	155	3.5	0	0	380	44	4	4	3 carb, 3 fat
French Fries, Medium, Salted	1 order	480	23	205	5	0	0	820	61	5	5	4 carb, 5 fat
French Fries, Medium, Salt Not Added	1 order	480	23	205	5	0	0	530	61	5	5	4 carb, 5 fat

FAST FOOD

	Serving	Calories	Fat (g)	Cal. from Fat	Sat. Fat (g)	Trans Fat (g)	Chol. (mg)	Sod. (mg)	Carb. (g)	Fiber (g)	Prot. (g)	Servings/Exchanges
French Fries, Large, Salted	1 order	580	28	250	6	0	0	990	74	6	6	5 carb, 6 fat
French Fries, Large, Salt Not Added	1 order	580	28	250	6	0	0	640	74	6	6	5 carb, 6 fat
French Fries, Value, Salted	1 order	220	11	100	2.5	0	0	380	28	2	2	2 carb, 2 fat
Onion Rings, Small	1 order	310	17	155	3	0	0	490	36	3	4	2 1/2 carb, 3 fat
Onion Rings, Medium	1 order	450	24	215	4	0	0	700	52	5	6	3 1/2 carb, 5 fat
Onion Rings, Large	1 order	510	27	245	4.5	0	0	810	60	5	7	4 carb, 5 fat
Dipping Sauces												
BBQ Dipping Sauce	1 oz	40	0	0	0	0	0	310	11	0	0	1 carb
Honey Mustard Dipping Sauce	1 oz	90	6	55	1	0	10	180	8	0	0	1/2 carb, 1 fat
Sweet & Sour Dipping Sauce	1 oz	45	0	0	0	0	0	55	11	0	0	1 carb

Item	Serving										
Ranch Dipping Sauce	1 oz	140	15	135	2.5	0	5	95	1	0	1	3 fat
Buffalo Dipping Sauce	1 oz	80	8	70	1.5	0	5	360	2	0	0	2 fat
Zesty Onion Ring Dipping Sauce	1 oz	150	15	135	2.5	0	15	210	3	1	0	3 fat

BK Salad Collection

Item	Serving										
Side Salad	1	40	2	20	1	0	5	45	2	1	3	1 vegetable
TENDERGRILL Chicken Garden Salad	1	210	7	65	3	0	75	780	8	3	29	1/2 carb, 4 lean meat
TENDERCRISP Chicken Garden Salad	1	410	23	205	6	0	65	1060	27	4	27	2 carb, 3 med-fat meat, 2 fat
Garden Salad, No Chicken	1	70	4	35	2.5	0	10	100	7	3	4	1 vegetable, 1 fat

Salad Dressings & Toppings

Item	Serving										
KEN's Creamy Caesar Dressing	2 oz	210	21	190	4	0	25	610	4	0	3	4 fat
KEN's Honey Mustard Dressing	2 oz	270	23	205	3	0	20	510	15	0	1	1 carb, 5 fat

FAST FOOD

	Serving	Calories	Fat (g)	Cal. from Fat	Sat. Fat (g)	Trans Fat (g)	Chol. (mg)	Sod. (mg)	Carb. (g)	Fiber (g)	Prot. (g)	Servings/Exchanges
KEN's Light Italian Dressing	2 oz	120	11	100	1.5	0	0	440	5	0	0	2 fat
KEN's Ranch Dressing	2 oz	190	20	180	3	0	20	550	2	0	1	4 fat
Desserts												
Dutch Apple Pie	1	320	13	115	5	0	0	290	47	1	2	3 carb, 3 fat
HERSHEY's Sundae Pie	1	310	19	170	12	0	10	220	32	1	3	2 carb, 4 fat
Breakfast												
BK Breakfast Shots, Sausage & Cheese	2 pkg	420	31	280	10	0.5	215	910	18	1	18	1 carb, 2 med-fat meat, 4 fat
BK Breakfast Shots, Ham & Cheese	2 pkg	270	16	145	5	0	190	840	18	1	13	1 carb, 1 med-fat meat, 2 fat
Croissan'wich with Bacon, Egg & Cheese	1	350	19	170	8	0	155	870	27	0	15	2 carb, 1 med-fat meat, 1 fat
Croissan'wich with Ham, Egg & Cheese	1	340	17	155	7	0	160	1200	28	0	18	2 carb, 2 med-fat meat, 1 fat

Item	Amount											Exchanges
Croissan'wich with Sausage, Egg & Cheese	1	470	31	280	11	0.5	175	1030	28	0	20	2 carb, 2 med-fat meat, 4 fat
Croissan'wich with Sausage & Cheese	1	380	24	215	10	0	50	780	26	0	14	2 carb, 1 med-fat meat, 4 fat
Croissan'wich with Egg & Cheese	1	310	16	145	7	0	145	730	27	0	12	2 carb, 1 med-fat meat, 2 fat
Double Croissan'wich with Sausage, Egg & Cheese	1	690	50	450	19	1	220	1560	30	0	30	2 carb, 3 med-fat meat, 8 fat
Double Croissan'wich with Ham, Egg & Cheese	1	420	21	190	10	0.5	190	1890	30	0	26	2 carb, 3 med-fat meat, 1 fat
French Toast Sticks	5 pieces	380	18	160	3	0	0	430	49	2	5	3 carb, 4 fat
Hash Browns, Small	1	420	27	245	6	0	0	680	40	6	3	2 1/2 carb, 5 fat
Hash Browns, Medium	1	610	39	350	8	0	0	980	58	8	5	4 carb, 8 fat

FAST FOOD

	Serving	Calories	Fat (g)	Cal. from Fat	Sat. Fat (g)	Trans Fat (g)	Chol. (mg)	Sod. (mg)	Carb. (g)	Fiber (g)	Prot. (g)	Servings/Exchanges
Drinks												
Mocha BK Joe Iced Coffee	1	360	10	90	6	0	40	290	66	1	6	4 1/2 carb, 1 fat
Chocolate Shake	12 oz	310	11	100	7	0	45	220	53	1	6	3 1/2 carb, 2 fat
Chocolate Shake	22 oz	670	21	190	13	0.5	80	510	119	2	11	8 carb, 4 fat
Chocolate Shake	32 oz	990	31	280	20	1	120	750	178	3	17	12 carb, 6 fat
Vanilla Shake	12 oz	270	11	100	7	0	45	180	42	0	6	3 carb, 2 fat
Vanilla Shake	22 oz	480	20	180	13	0.5	80	320	76	0	11	5 carb, 4 fat
Vanilla Shake	32 oz	720	29	260	19	1	120	480	113	1	16	7 1/2 carb, 6 fat
Oreo BK Sundae Shake, Medium	22 oz	1010	35	315	21	1	95	800	171	3	15	11 carb, 7 fat
CARL'S JR.												
Big Hamburger	1	460	17	160	8	0.5	50	1090	54	3	24	3 1/2 carb, 2 med-fat meat, 1 fat

												Exchanges
Famous Star with Cheese	1	660	39	340	13	1	80	1300	53	3	27	3 1/2 carb, 2 med-fat meat, 6 fat
Super Star with Cheese	1	920	58	510	23	1.5	145	1640	54	3	47	3 1/2 carb, 5 med-fat meat, 7 fat
Chili Cheeseburger	1	780	41	370	19	1.5	105	1650	58	4	41	4 carb, 4 med-fat meat, 5 fat
Double Western Bacon Cheeseburger	1	960	52	470	23	2	140	1750	70	3	52	4 1/2 carb, 5 med-fat meat, 5 fat
Jalapeno Burger	1	720	46	410	15	0.5	85	1340	50	3	27	3 carb, 3 med-fat meat, 6 fat
Western Bacon Cheeseburger	1	710	33	300	13	1	75	1410	69	3	32	4 1/2 carb, 3 med-fat meat, 3 fat
Charbroiled BBQ Chicken Sandwich	1	380	7	60	1.5	0	60	1010	49	2	34	3 carb, 4 lean meat
Charbroiled Chicken Club Sandwich	1	560	27	240	7	0	90	1280	44	2	39	3 carb, 4 med-fat meat, 1 fat

FAST FOOD

	Serving	Calories	Fat (g)	Cal. from Fat	Sat. Fat (g)	Trans Fat (g)	Chol. (mg)	Sod. (mg)	Carb. (g)	Fiber (g)	Prot. (g)	Servings/Exchanges
Charbroiled Sante Fe Chicken Sandwich	1	630	35	310	8	0	95	1410	44	2	36	3 carb, 4 med-fat meat, 3 fat
Bacon Swiss Crispy Chicken Sandwich	1	750	40	360	9	1.5	70	1990	62	4	36	6 carb, 3 med-fat meat, 5 fat
Spicy Chicken Sandwich	1	420	27	230	5	0	25	930	33	2	12	2 carb, 1 med-fat meat, 5 fat
Chicken Strips	3 pieces	370	26	230	6	0	30	620	19	2	14	1 carb, 2 med-fat meat, 3 fat
Carl's Catch Fish Sandwich	1	710	37	330	6	0	40	1280	74	4	20	5 carb, 1 med-fat meat, 6 fat
Low Carb Six Dollar Burger	1	570	43	380	18	2	120	1480	7	1	38	1/2 carb, 5 med-fat meat, 4 fat
Original Six Dollar Burger	1	890	54	480	20	2	130	2040	58	3	45	4 carb, 5 med-fat meat, 6 fat

Western Bacon Six Dollar Burger	1	1020	53	480	22	2.5	130	2520	81	3	53	5 carb, 5 med-fat meat, 6 fat
Kid's Hamburger	1	230	10	90	3.5	0.5	25	550	24	1	9	1 1/2 carb, 1 med-fat meat, 1 fat
Kid's Cheeseburger	1	290	15	140	7	0.5	40	830	24	1	12	1 1/2 carb, 1 med-fat meat, 2 fat

Sides

Natural-Cut French Fries, Kids	1 order	220	11	100	2	0	0	580	29	2	3	2 carb, 2 fat
Natural-Cut Fries, Small	1 order	320	15	140	3	0	0	830	42	4	4	3 carb, 3 fat
Natural-Cut Fries, Medium	1 order	460	22	200	4.5	0	0	1180	60	5	5	4 carb, 4 fat
Natural-Cut Fries, Large	1 order	500	24	210	5	0	0	1290	65	5	6	4 carb, 5 fat
Chicken Stars	6 pieces	320	24	220	6	0	35	460	14	2	12	1 carb, 1 med-fat meat, 4 fat
Chili Cheese Fries	1 order	990	56	510	19	1	70	2380	89	8	28	6 carb, 2 med-fat meat, 9 fat

FAST FOOD

	Serving	Calories	Fat (g)	Cal. from Fat	Sat. Fat (g)	Trans Fat (g)	Chol. (mg)	Sod. (mg)	Carb. (g)	Fiber (g)	Prot. (g)	Servings/Exchanges
CrissCut Fries	1 order	450	29	260	5	0	0	900	42	4	5	3 carb, 6 fat
Fish & Chips	1 order	730	39	350	7	0	25	1630	72	6	22	5 carb, 1 med-fat meat, 7 fat
Fried Zucchini	1 order	330	18	160	3	0	0	610	36	2	6	2 1/2 carb, 4 fat
Onion Rings	1 order	530	28	250	4.5	0	0	590	61	3	8	4 carb, 6 fat
Salads (without Dressing)												
Grilled Chicken Salad	1	200	6	60	3	0	70	610	13	3	24	1 carb, 3 lean meat
Garden Side Salad	1	50	2.5	20	1.5	0	5	75	5	2	3	1 vegetable, 1 fat
Green Burrito Taco Salad	1	970	58	530	19	1.5	85	1850	76	17	42	5 carb, 4 med-fat meat, 8 fat
Salad Dressings												
Blue Cheese Dressing	2-oz pkt	320	34	310	7	0	20	410	1	0	2	7 fat
House Dressing	2-oz pkt	220	22	200	3.5	0	20	440	3	0	1	4 fat
Low Fat Balsamic Dressing	2-oz pkt	35	1.5	15	0	0	0	480	4	0	0	1 fat

Thousand Island Dressing	2-oz pkt	240	23	210	3.5	0	20	460	7	0	0	1/2 carb, 5 fat
Breakfast												
Bacon & Egg Burrito	1	550	32	290	10	0	500	990	37	1	29	2 1/2 carb, 3 med-fat meat, 3 fat
Breakfast Burger	1	780	41	370	15	1	305	1460	64	3	38	4 carb, 4 med-fat meat, 4 fat
Croissant Sunrise Sandwich	1	590	44	390	17	0	285	810	27	1	20	2 carb, 2 med-fat meat, 7 fat
French Toast Dips, No Syrup	5 pieces	460	21	190	4	0	0	570	60	3	9	4 carb, 4 fat
Hash Brown Nuggets	1 order	350	23	210	4	0	0	440	32	3	3	2 carb, 5 fat
Loaded Breakfast Burrito	1	780	49	440	16	0	510	1480	51	3	36	3 carb, 3 med-fat meat, 7 fat
Sourdough Breakfast Sandwich	1	450	21	190	8	0	270	1470	38	1	29	2 1/2 carb, 3 med-fat meat, 1 fat

FAST FOOD

	Serving	Calories	Fat (g)	Cal. from Fat	Sat. Fat (g)	Trans Fat (g)	Chol. (mg)	Sod. (mg)	Carb. (g)	Fiber (g)	Prot. (g)	Servings/Exchanges
Steak & Egg Burrito	1	650	36	330	14	0	535	1750	43	1	41	3 carb, 4 med-fat meat, 3 fat
CHIPOTLE												
Flour Tortilla, Burrito	1	290	9	80	3	0	0	970	44	2	7	3 carb, 2 fat
Flour Tortilla, Taco	1	90	2.5	25	1	0	0	200	13	<1	2	1 carb, 1 fat
Crispy Taco Shell	1	60	2	20	0.5	0	0	10	9	1	<1	1/2 carb
Cilantro-Lime Rice	3 oz	130	3	30	0.5	0	0	150	23	0	2	1 1/2 carb
Black Beans	4 oz	120	1	10	0	0	0	250	23	11	7	1 1/2 carb
Pinto Beans	4 oz	120	1	10	0	0	5	330	22	10	7	1 1/2 carb
Fajita Vegetables	2.5 oz	20	0.5	5	0	0	0	170	4	1	1	1 vegetable
Barbacoa	4 oz	170	7	60	2.5	0	60	510	2	0	24	3 lean meat
Chicken	4 oz	190	6.5	60	2	0	115	370	1	0	32	5 lean meat
Carnitas	4 oz	190	8	70	2.5	0	70	540	1	0	27	4 lean meat
Steak	4 oz	190	6.5	60	2	0	65	320	2	0	30	4 lean meat

Tomato Salsa	3.5 oz	20	0	0	0	0	470	4	<1	1	free
Corn Salsa	3.5 oz	80	1.5	15	0	0	410	15	3	3	1 carb
Red Tomatillo Salsa	2 oz	40	1	10	0	0	510	8	4	2	2 vegetable
Green Tomatillo Salsa	2 oz	15	0	5	0	0	230	3	1	1	free
Cheese	1 oz	100	8.5	80	5	30	180	0	0	8	1 med-fat meat
Sour Cream	2 oz	120	10	90	7	40	30	2	0	2	2 fat
Guacamole	3.5 oz	150	13	120	2	0	190	8	6	2	1/2 carb, 3 fat
Romaine Lettuce, in Salad	2.5 oz	10	0	0	0	0	5	2	1	1	free
Romaine Lettuce, in Taco	1 oz	5	0	0	0	0	0	1	1	0	free
Chips	4 oz	570	27	240	3.5	0	420	73	8	8	4 1/2 carb, 5 fat
Vinaigrette	2 oz	260	24.5	220	4	0	700	12	1	0	1 carb, 5 fat
CINNABON											
Caramel Pecanbon	1	1100	56	505	10	5	600	141	8	16	9 carb, 11 fat
Cinnabon Classic	1	813	32	290	8	5	801	117	4	15	7 1/2 carb, 6 fat

FAST FOOD

	Serving	Calories	Fat (g)	Cal. from Fat	Sat. Fat (g)	Trans Fat (g)	Chol. (mg)	Sod. (mg)	Carb. (g)	Fiber (g)	Prot. (g)	Servings/Exchanges
Cinnabon Stix	5 sticks	379	21	190	6	4	16	413	41	1	6	3 1/2 carb, 4 fat
Minibon	1	339	13	115	3	2	27	337	49	2	6	3 carb, 3 fat
DUNKIN DONUTS												
Donuts												
Apple Crumb	1	460	14	130	8	0	0	330	80	2	4	5 carb, 3 fat
Bavarian Crème	1	250	12	110	5	0	0	330	31	1	3	2 carb, 2 fat
Blueberry Cake	1	330	18	160	8	0	25	460	38	1	3	2 1/2 carb, 4 fat
Boston Kreme	1	280	12	110	5	0	0	350	38	1	3	2 1/2 carb, 2 fat
Chocolate Frosted Cake	1	340	19	170	8	0	25	330	38	1	3	2 1/2 carb, 4 fat
Chocolate Glazed Cake	1	280	15	140	7	0	0	400	33	1	3	2 carb, 3 fat
Chocolate Kreme Filled	1	310	16	140	7	0	0	340	37	1	4	2 1/2carb, 3 fat
Glazed	1	220	9	80	4	0	0	320	31	1	3	2 carb, 2 fat
Glazed Cake	1	320	18	160	8	0	25	310	37	1	3	2 1/2 carb, 4 fat
Jelly Filled	1	260	11	100	5	0	0	330	36	1	3	2 1/2carb, 2 fat

Maple Frosted	1	230	10	90	4	0	0	330	33	1	3	2 carb, 2 fat
Old Fashioned Cake	1	280	18	160	8	0	25	310	27	1	3	2 carb, 1 fat
Powdered Cake	1	300	18	160	8	0	25	310	30	1	3	2 carb, 4 fat
Sugar Raised	1	190	9	80	4	0	0	320	22	1	3	1 1/2 carb, 2 fat
Toffee for Your Coffee	1	400	24	220	11	0	10	330	42	1	4	3 carb, 5 fat
Vanilla Kreme Filled	1	320	17	160	8	0	0	340	37	1	3	2 1/2 carb, 3 fat
Fancies												
Apple Fritter	1	400	15	130	6	0	0	530	63	2	5	4 carb, 3 fat
Coffee Roll	1	370	18	160	7	0	0	510	49	2	5	3 carb, 4 fa
Éclair	1	350	14	120	5	0	0	460	53	1	4	3 1/2 carb, 3 fat
Glazed Fritter	1	400	15	130	6	0	0	530	63	2	5	4 carb, 3 fat
Maple Frosted Coffee Roll	1	380	18	160	8	0	0	520	50	2	5	3 carb, 4 fat
Munchkins												
Glazed	1	50	2.5	20	1	0	0	65	7	0	1	1/2 carb, 1 fat
Glazed Cake	1	60	3	30	1.5	5		65	8	0	1	1/2 carb, 1 fat
Jelly Filled	1	60	2.5	20	1	0	0	65	8	0	1	1/2 carb, 1 fat

FAST FOOD

	Serving	Calories	Fat (g)	Cal. from Fat	Sat. Fat (g)	Trans Fat (g)	Chol. (mg)	Sod. (mg)	Carb. (g)	Fiber (g)	Prot. (g)	Servings/Exchanges
Plain Cake	1	50	3	30	1.5	0	5	60	5	0	1	1 fat
Powdered Cake	1	60	3.5	30	1.5	0	5	60	6	0	1	1/2 carb, 1 fat
Sticks												
Cinnamon Cake	1	310	20	180	9	0	25	300	30	1	3	2 carb, 4 fat
Glazed Cake	1	340	20	180	9	0	25	300	38	1	3	2 1/2 carb, 4 fat
Plain Cake	1	300	20	180	9	0	25	300	26	1	3	2 1/2 carb, 4 fat
Muffins												
Banana Walnut	1	540	23	205	6	0	75	550	73	3	10	5 carb, 5 fat
Blueberry	1	510	16	140	1.5	0	15	490	87	3	6	6 carb, 3 fat
Chocolate Chip	1	630	23	210	6	0	20	520	98	5	8	6 1/2 carb, 5 fat
Coffee Cake	1	620	25	230	7	0	20	530	93	2	7	6 carb, 5 fat
Corn	1	510	17	150	2	0	20	860	84	2	6	5 1/2 carb, 3 fat
Honey Bran Raisin	1	500	14	130	1.5	0	15	450	86	9	7	5 1/2 carb, 3 fat
Reduced Fat Blueberry	1	450	10	90	1.5	0	15	670	86	3	6	5 1/2 carb, 2 fat

Danish

Apple Cheese	1	330	16	150	7	0	0	270	41	1	4	3 carb, 3 fat
Cheese	1	330	17	150	8	0	5	270	39	1	5	2 1/2 carb, 3 fat
Strawberry Cheese	1	320	16	150	7	0	0	260	40	1	4	2 1/2 carb, 3 fat

Bagels

Cinnamon Raisin	1	370	4	35	0.5	0	0	530	72	3	13	5 starch, 1 fat
Everything	1	430	7	65	0.5	0	0	780	75	3	17	5 starch, 1 fat
Garlic	1	350	3.5	30	0.5	0	0	780	76	4	15	5 starch, 1 fat
Plain	1	330	3	30	0.5	0	0	780	71	3	14	4 1/2 starch, 1 fat
Wheat	1	350	4	35	0.5	0	5	650	66	5	13	4 1/2 starch, 1 fat

Cream Cheese

Plain Cream Cheese	1.8 oz	150	15	130	9	0.5	40	250	3	0	3	3 fat
Reduced Fat Cream Cheese	1.8 oz	100	8	70	5	0	25	250	5	0	4	2 fat
Reduced Fat Smoked Salmon Cream Cheese	1.8 oz	140	11	100	7	0	35	260	6	0	4	1/2 carb, 2 fat

FAST FOOD

Oven Toasted Breakfast Sandwiches

	Serving	Calories	Fat (g)	Cal. from Fat	Sat. Fat (g)	Trans Fat (g)	Chol. (mg)	Sod. (mg)	Carb. (g)	Fiber (g)	Prot. (g)	Servings/Exchanges
Bacon, Egg & Cheese Bagel	1	530	18	160	6	0	195	1370	76	3	26	5 starch, 2 med-fat meat, 2 fat
Bacon, Egg & Cheese on English Muffin	1	360	16	150	6	0	195	920	35	2	18	2 starch, 2 med-fat meat, 1 fat
Egg & Cheese on Biscuit	1	430	26	240	13	0	195	1010	36	1	13	2 1/2 starch, 1 med-fat meat, 4 fat
Egg & Cheese on English Muffin	1	320	13	120	5	0	190	730	34	2	14	2 starch, 1 med-fat meat, 2 fat
Ham, Egg & Cheese on Bagel	1	520	17	150	6	0	210	1480	75	3	28	5 starch, 2 med-fat meat, 1 fat
Ham, Egg & Cheese on Croissant	1	510	30	270	12	0	210	1050	39	1	21	2 1/2 starch, 2 med-fat meat, 4 fat
Sausage Biscuit	1	450	28	250	14	0	45	1020	33	1	12	2 starch, 1 med-fat meat, 5 fat

	Serving	Cal	Fat (g)		Sat Fat (g)		Chol (mg)	Sod (mg)	Carb (g)	Fiber (g)	Prot (g)	Exchanges/Choices
Sausage, Egg & Cheese on English Muffin	1	490	28	250	10	0	235	1130	35	2	22	2 starch, 2 med-fat meat, 4 fat
Favorites Sandwiches												
Steak & Cheese	1	470	16	140	6	0	75	2040	50	2	31	3 starch, 3 med-fat meat
Toasted Italian	1	560	25	220	9	0	75	2630	52	3	33	3 1/2 starch, 3 med-fat meat, 2 fat
Tuna Melt	1	770	30	270	7	0	70	1560	57	3	36	4 starch, 3 med-fat meat, 3 fat
Turkey & Bacon Club	1	440	13	110	3	0	45	1800	51	3	35	3 1/2 starch, 3 med-fat meat
Beverages												
Cappucino	10 oz	80	4	35	2.5	0	15	70	7	0	4	1/2 carb, 1 fat
Caramel Swirl Latte	10 oz	230	6	50	3.5	0	25	150	35	0	8	2 carb, 1 fat
Coffee Coolatta with Cream	16 oz	330	23	210	14	0.5	80	60	28	3	3	2 carb, 5 fat

FAST FOOD

	Serving	Calories	Fat (g)	Cal. from Fat	Sat. Fat (g)	Trans Fat (g)	Chol. (mg)	Sod. (mg)	Carb. (g)	Fiber (g)	Prot. (g)	Servings/Exchanges
Coffee Coolatta with Milk	16 oz	170	4	35	2.5	0	15	75	29	0	4	2 carb, 1 fat
Coffee Coolatta with Skim Milk	16 oz	140	0	0	0	0	0	75	30	0	4	2 carb
Espresso	1.75 oz	0	0	0	0	0	0	5	1	0	0	free
Iced Latte	16 oz	120	6	50	3.5	0	25	105	10	0	6	1/2 carb, 1 fat
Iced Mocha Spice Latte	16 oz	220	6	60	4	0	25	95	34	1	7	2 carb, 1 fat
Latte	10 oz	120	6	50	3.5	0	25	105	10	0	6	1/2 carb, 1 fat
Tropicana Orange Coolatta	16 oz	220	0	0	0	0	0	35	52	0	1	3 1/2 carb
Vanilla Bean Coolatta	16 oz	430	6	50	3.5	0	20	170	90	0	3	6 carb, 1 fat
DAIRY QUEEN												
Burgers												
Original Hamburger	1	350	14	130	7	0.5	50	680	33	1	17	2 carb, 2 med-fat meat, 1 fat

Original Cheeseburger	1	400	18	160	7	0.5	65	920	34	1	19	2 carb, 2 med-fat meat, 2 fat
Original Double Cheeseburger	1	640	34	310	18	1	125	1230	34	1	34	2 carb, 4 med-fat meat, 3 fat
Original Bacon Double Cheeseburger	1	730	41	370	21	1	150	1550	35	1	41	2 carb, 5 med-fat meat, 3 fat
Classic GrillBurger	1	470	21	190	8	0.5	50	950	42	2	24	3 carb, 2 med-fat meat, 2 fat
1/4 lb Bacon Cheddar GrillBurger	1	650	35	320	15	1	95	1410	41	2	36	3 carb, 4 med-fat meat, 3 fat
1/2 lb GrillBurger	1	720	40	360	15	1.5	105	1240	42	2	42	3 carb, 5 med-fat meat, 3 fat
1/2 lb GrillBurger with Cheese	1	870	51	460	23	1.5	140	1440	42	2	51	3 carb, 6 med-fat meat, 4 fat
1/2 lb Flame Thrower GrillBurger	1	1060	75	680	26	2	165	1980	41	2	54	3 carb, 6 med-fat meat, 9 fat

FAST FOOD

	Serving	Calories	Fat (g)	Cal. from Fat	Sat. Fat (g)	Trans Fat (g)	Chol. (mg)	Sod. (mg)	Carb. (g)	Fiber (g)	Prot. (g)	Servings/Exchanges
Hot Dogs												
All-Beef Hot Dog	1	250	14	130	5	0	25	770	21	1	9	1 1/2 carb, 1 med-fat meat, 2 fat
All-Beef Chili Cheese Dog	1	430	22	220	10	0	50	1010	39	2	18	2 1/2 carb, 2 med-fat meat, 2 fat
Sandwiches/Baskets												
Grilled Chicken Sandwich	1	370	16	150	2.5	0	55	780	32	1	24	2 carb, 3 med-fat meat
Crispy Chicken Sandwich	1	560	28	250	3.5	0	35	980	48	3	20	3 carb, 2 med-fat meat, 4 fat
Chicken Strip Basket with Gravy	4 pieces	1360	63	570	11	1	100	2910	103	8	39	7 carb, 3 med-fat meat, 10 fat
Side Items												
French Fries, Kid's	1	190	8	70	1	0	0	400	27	2	2	2 carb, 2 fat
French Fries Regular	1	310	13	120	2	0	0	640	43	3	4	3 carb, 3 fat

French Fries, Large	1	500	21	190	3.5	0	0	1040	70	5	6	4 1/2 carb, 4 fat
Onion Rings	1 order	360	16	140	2	0	0	840	47	2	6	3 carb, 3 fat
Side Salad	1	45	0	0	0	0	0	50	11	3	2	2 vegetable

Cones

Vanilla Cone, Kids	1	140	14	35	2.5	0	15	60	22	0	4	1 1/2 carb, 3 fat
Vanilla Cone, Small	1	230	7	60	4.5	0	25	100	31	0	6	2 carb, 1 fat
Vanilla Cone, Medium	1	330	10	90	6	0.5	30	140	53	0	9	3 1/2 carb, 2 fat
Vanilla Cone, Large	1	470	14	130	9	0.5	45	200	74	0	12	5 carb, 3 fat
Dipped Cone, Chocolate, Small	1	330	15	140	6	0	25	105	36	0	6	3 carb, 3 fat
Dipped Cone, Chocolate, Medium	1	470	22	200	9	0.5	30	150	60	1	9	4 carb, 4 fat
Dipped Cone, Chocolate, Large	1	660	30	270	13	0.5	45	220	84	1	13	5 1/2 carb, 6 fat

Malts, Shakes, and Arctic Rush

Chocolate Malt, Small	1	650	16	150	10	1	55	310	110	0	15	7 1/2 carb, 3 fat

FAST FOOD

	Serving	Calories	Fat (g)	Cal. from Fat	Sat. Fat (g)	Trans Fat (g)	Chol. (mg)	Sod. (mg)	Carb. (g)	Fiber (g)	Prot. (g)	Servings/Exchanges
Chocolate Malt, Medium	1	900	22	200	14	1	70	430	154	0	20	10 carb, 4 fat
Chocolate Malt, Large	1	1310	33	290	21	1.5	105	630	220	0	30	14 1/2 carb, 7 fat
Chocolate Shake, Small	1	570	15	140	10	0.5	50	250	92	0	13	6 carb, 3 fat
Chocolate Shake, Medium	1	790	21	190	13	1	70	350	130	0	18	8 1/2 carb, 4 fat
Chocolate Shake, Large	1	1130	31	280	20	1.5	100	510	184	0	26	12 carb, 6 fat
Arctic Rush, All Flavors, Small	1	240	0	0	0	0	0	0	48	0	0	3 carb
Arctic Rush, All Flavors, Medium	1	310	0	0	0	0	0	0	63	0	0	4 carb
MooLatte Frozen Blended Coffee												
Cappuccino MooLatte	16 oz	500	18	160	15	0.5	35	170	71	0	8	4 1/2 carb, 4 fat
Caramel MooLatte	16 oz	630	19	170	15	0.5	40	240	101	0	9	6 1/2 carb, 4 fat
French Vanilla MooLatte	16 oz	560	18	160	14	0.5	35	160	88	0	8	6 carb, 4 fat

Mocha MooLatte	16 oz	590	23	200	15	0.5	35	190	82	0	9	5 1/2 carb, 5 fat

Sundaes

Chocolate Sundae, Small	1	280	7	60	4.5	0	25	115	48	0	5	3 carb, 1 fat
Chocolate Sundae, Medium	1	400	10	90	6	0.5	30	170	70	0	8	4 1/2 carb, 2 fat
Chocolate Sundae, Large	1	570	14	120	9	0.5	45	240	98	0	11	6 1/2 carb, 3 fat

Treats

Banana Split	1	520	13	120	10	0.5	30	160	94	3	9	6 1/2 carb, 3 fat
Oreo Brownie Earthquake	1	760	27	240	16	0	60	400	117	2	11	8 carb, 5 fat
Peanut Buster Parfait	1	700	30	270	16	0.5	35	360	94	2	16	6 carb, 6 fat
Plain Waffle Cone with Soft Serve	1	420	13	110	7	0.5	40	140	67	0	10	4 1/2 carb, 3 fat
Turtle Waffle Bowl Sundae	1	810	34	310	18	0.5	40	320	116	2	12	7 1/2 carb, 7 fat

Novelties

Buster Bar Treat	1	480	31	280	15	0	20	220	45	2	11	3 carb, 6 fat

FAST FOOD

	Serving	Calories	Fat (g)	Cal. from Fat	Sat. Fat (g)	Trans Fat (g)	Chol. (mg)	Sod. (mg)	Carb. (g)	Fiber (g)	Prot. (g)	Servings/Exchanges
Cherry Starkiss Bar	1	80	0	0	0	0	0	10	21	0	0	1 1/2 carb
Chocolate Dilly Bar	1	240	15	140	9	0	15	70	24	1	4	1 1/2 carb, 3 fat
Dilly Bar, No Sugar Added	1	190	13	120	10	0	15	60	24	5	3	1 1/2 carb, 3 fat
DQ Fudge Bar, No Sugar Added	1	50	0	0	0	0	0	70	13	6	4	1 carb
DQ Sandwich	1	190	5	45	3	0	10	135	31	1	4	2 carb, 1 fat
DQ Vanilla Orange Bar, No Sugar Added	1	60	0	0	0	0	0	45	18	6	2	1 carb
Blizzard Treats												
Oreo Cookies Blizzard, Small	1	550	20	180	10	0.5	40	410	81	1	12	5 1/2 carb, 4 fat
Oreo Cookies Blizzard, Medium	1	820	35	320	19	1	105	610	108	1	16	7 carb, 7 fat

Oreo Cookies Blizzard, Large	1	1140	49	440	26	1	140	840	151	1	23	10 carb, 10 fat
Chocolate Chip Cookie Dough Blizzard, Small	1	710	27	250	14	3	55	350	103	1	13	7 carb, 6 fat
Chocolate Chip Cookie Dough Blizzard, Medium	1	1010	40	360	20	4.5	75	500	148	1	18	10 carb, 8 fat
Chocolate Chip Cookie Dough Blizzard, Large	1	1300	51	460	26	6	95	640	189	2	22	12 1/2 carb, 10 fat
DQ Cake (8" round cake)	1/8 cake	410	15	140	10	1	30	210	59	1	9	4 carb, 3 fat

DOMINO'S

Hand-Tossed, Large

Cheese	1/8 pizza	240	8	70	3	0	10	490	34	2	10	2 carb, 1 med-fat meat, 1 fat
Pepperoni	1/8 pizza	290	13	110	5	0	20	680	34	2	12	2 1/2 carb, 1 med-fat meat, 1 fat

FAST FOOD

	Serving	Calories	Fat (g)	Cal. from Fat	Sat. Fat (g)	Trans Fat (g)	Chol. (mg)	Sod. (mg)	Carb. (g)	Fiber (g)	Prot. (g)	Servings/Exchanges
Sausage	1/8 pizza	300	13	120	5	0	20	670	36	3	12	2 1/2 carb, 1 med-fat meat, 2 fat
Ham	1/8 pizza	255	9	75	3	0	15	625	34	2	12	2 carb, 1 med-fat meat, 1 fat
Beef	1/8 pizza	290	13	110	5	0	20	590	34	2	13	2 carb, 1 med-fat meat, 2 fat
Deep Dish, Large												
Cheese	1/8 pizza	330	14	130	5	0	15	760	40	5	12	2 1/2 carb, 1 med-fat meat, 2 fat
Pepperoni	1/8 pizza	380	15	170	7	0	25	950	40	5	12	2 1/2 carb, 1 med-fat meat, 2 fat
Sausage	1/8 pizza	390	19	180	7	0	25	940	42	6	14	3 carb, 1 med-fat meat, 4 fat
Ham	1/8 pizza	345	16	135	5	0	20	895	40	5	14	2 1/2 carb, 1 med-fat meat, 2 fat

	Serving	Calories	Fat (g)		Sat. Fat (g)		Chol. (mg)	Sodium (mg)	Carb. (g)	Fiber (g)	Prot. (g)	Exchanges/Choices
Beef	1/8 pizza	380	19	170	7	0	25	860	40	5	12	2 1/2 carb, 1 med-fat meat, 3 fat
Thin Crust, Large												
Cheese	1/8 pizza	180	10	90	4	0	15	340	19	1	7	1 carb, 1 med-fat meat, 1 fat
Pepperoni	1/8 pizza	230	15	130	5	0	25	530	19	1	9	1 carb, 1 med-fat meat, 2 fat
Sausage	1/8 pizza	240	15	140	6	0	25	520	19	2	9	1 carb, 1 med-fat meat, 2 fat
Ham	1/8 pizza	195	11	95	4	0	20	475	19	1	9	1 carb, 1 med-fat meat, 1 fat
Breadbowl Pasta												
Chicken Alfredo	1/2	700	25	230	11	0.5	50	1070	93	3	26	6 carb, 1 med-fat meat, 4 fat
Italian Sausage Marinara	1/2	730	26	240	11	0	35	1410	97	4	26	6 1/2 carb, 1 med-fat meat, 4 fat
Three Cheese Mac-N-Cheese	1/2	730	28	250	14	1	55	1420	95	3	27	6 1/2 carb, 1 med-fat meat, 5 fat

FAST FOOD

	Serving	Calories	Fat (g)	Cal. from Fat	Sat. Fat (g)	Trans Fat (g)	Chol. (mg)	Sod. (mg)	Carb. (g)	Fiber (g)	Prot. (g)	Servings/Exchanges
Oven Baked Sandwiches												
Chicken Bacon Ranch	1	890	45	400	16	1	115	2210	72	2	49	5 carb, 5 med-fat meat, 4 fat
Italian	1	880	45	410	22	1	120	2560	71	3	47	4 1/2 carb, 5 med-fat meat, 4 fat
Philly Cheese Steak	1	690	27	250	14	1	90	2080	72	3	41	5 carb, 4 med-fat meat, 1 fat
Salads (no dressing)												
Garden Fresh	1/2 salad	70	4	35	3	0	10	80	5	2	4	1 vegetable, 1 fat
Grilled Chicken Caesar	1/2 salad	100	5	40	2	0	20	310	6	2	10	1 vegetable, 1 med-fat meat
Side Items												
Barbeque Buffalo Wings	2 pieces	230	14	130	3.5	0	50	410	6	0	17	1/2 carb, 2 med-fat meat, 1 fat

Item	Serving											Exchanges
Blue Cheese Dipping Sauce	1 container	210	22	200	4	0	20	390	2	0	1	4 fat
Breadsticks	1	110	6	60	2	0	0	100	11	0	2	1 carb, 1 fat
Buffalo Chicken Kickers	2 pieces	100	5	40	0.5	0	20	280	7	1	9	1/2 carb, 1 med-fat meat
Cheesy Bread	1	120	6	60	2	0	5	150	11	0	4	1 carb, 1 fat
Cinna Stix	1	120	6	60	1	0	0	85	14	1	2	1 carb, 1 fat
Garlic Dipping Sauce	1 container	250	28	250	5	0	0	160	0	0	0	6 fat
Hot Buffalo Wings	2 pieces	200	14	120	3.5	0	50	690	2	0	16	2 med-fat meat, 1 fat
Hot Dipping Sauce	1 container	50	5	40	5	0	0	1480	3	0	0	1 fat
Marinara Dipping Sauce	1 container	25	0	0	0	0	0	270	5	1	1	free
Ranch Dipping Sauce	1 container	190	21	190	3	0	10	390	2	0	1	4 fat
Sweet Icing	1 container	250	3	25	1	0	0	0	57	0	0	4 carb, 1 fat

FAST FOOD

EINSTEIN BROS. BAGELS

Bagels

	Serving	Calories	Fat (g)	Cal. from Fat	Sat. Fat (g)	Trans Fat (g)	Chol. (mg)	Sod. (mg)	Carb. (g)	Fiber (g)	Prot. (g)	Servings/Exchanges
Asiago Cheese	1	330	5	50	3	0	15	660	59	2	15	4 starch, 1 fat
Blueberry	1	290	1.5	10	0	0	0	480	64	3	9	4 starch
Chocolate Chip	1	290	3	25	1	0	0	460	60	3	10	4 starch , 1 fat
Cinnamon Raisin Swirl	1	290	1	10	0	0	0	450	64	3	10	4 starch
Cinnamon Sugar Bagel, Chicago Style	1	310	2.5	20	0.5	0	0	510	66	3	10	4 1/2 starch, 1 fat
Cranberry	1	290	1	10	0	0	0	450	64	3	9	4 starch
Egg	1	300	6	50	1.5	0	150	480	52	2	12	3 1/2 starch, 1 fat
Everything	1	270	2	15	0	0	0	610	56	2	10	3 1/2 starch
Garlic Dip'd	1	290	2.5	20	0	0	0	490	60	2	10	4 starch, 1 fat
Good Grains	1	290	2.5	20	0	0	0	480	62	4	10	4 starch, 1 fat
Honey Whole Wheat	1	270	1	10	0	0	0	480	61	3	9	4 starch

Onion Dip'd	1	270	1	10	0	0	460	59	2	9	4 starch
Plain	1	260	1	10	0	0	460	56	2	9	3 1/2 starch
Poppy Dip'd	1	280	3	25	0	0	460	56	2	10	3 1/2 starch, 1 fat
Potato	1	260	1	10	0	0	540	58	2	9	4 starch
Power Bagel, Fruit & Nut	1	380	6	50	1	0	330	72	5	13	5 starch, 1 fat
Pumpernickel	1	250	1.5	10	0	0	710	55	3	9	3 1/2 starch
Sesame Dip'd	1	280	3	25	0	0	460	56	2	10	3 1/2 starch, 1 fat
Sun-Dried Tomato	1	270	1.5	15	0	0	570	58	3	10	4 starch
Gourmet Bagels											
Dutch Apple	1	340	7	60	1.5	0	540	66	2	8	4 1/2 starch, 1 fat
Green Chile	1	370	8	70	4.5	25	710	62	2	16	4 starch, 2 fat
Six Cheese	1	350	6	60	3.5	15	680	60	2	16	4 starch, 1 fat
Spinach Florentine	1	360	8	70	4	20	620	61	2	16	4 starch, 2 fat
Bagel Pretzels											
Asiago Cheese	1	300	7	70	2.5	5	710	52	2	11	3 1/2 starch, 1 fat

FAST FOOD

	Serving	Calories	Fat (g)	Cal. from Fat	Sat. Fat (g)	Trans Fat (g)	Chol. (mg)	Sod. (mg)	Carb. (g)	Fiber (g)	Prot. (g)	Servings/Exchanges
Cinnamon Sugar	1	320	5	50	1	0	0	630	66	3	8	4 1/2 starch, 1 fat
Plain	1	270	5	50	1	0	0	630	52	2	8	3 1/2 starch, 1 fat
Cream Cheese												
Whipped Plain	2 Tbsp	70	7	60	4.5	0	20	65	1	0	1	1 fat
Whipped Plain, Reduced Fat	2 Tbsp	60	5	45	3.5	0	15	100	2	0	1	1 fat
Whipped Blueberry, Reduced Fat	2 Tbsp	70	5	45	3.5	0	15	50	6	0	1	1/2 carb, 1 fat
Whipped Garlic Herb, Reduced Fat	2 Tbsp	60	5	45	3.5	0	15	100	3	0	1	1 fat
Whipped Garden Vegetable, Reduced Fat	2 Tbsp	60	5	45	3.5	0	15	100	3	0	1	1 fat
Whipped Honey Almond, Reduced Fat	2 Tbsp	70	5	45	3	0	15	45	6	0	1	1/2 carb, 1 fat

Whipped Jalapeño Salsa Reduced Fat	2 Tbsp	60	5	45	3.5	0	15	105	3	0	1	1 fat
Whipped Smoked Salmon	2 Tbsp	60	6	50	3.5	0	20	120	2	0	1	1 fat
Whipped Strawberry, Reduced Fat	2 Tbsp	70	5	45	3.5	0	15	50	5	0	1	1 fat
Whipped Sundried Tomato, Reduced Fat	2 Tbsp	60	5	45	3.5	0	15	100	2	0	1	1 fat
Wraps												
California Chicken Wrap	13.1 oz	630	28	250	8	0	110	1170	63	8	33	4 carb, 3 med-fat meat, 3 fat
Chipotle Turkey Wrap	13 oz	730	37	330	12	0	75	1990	70	9	34	4 1/2 carb, 3 med-fat meat, 4 fat
Salads (and Half Salads)												
Bros. Bistro House Salad	10.5 oz	820	68	610	11	0	25	320	38	7	14	2 1/2 carb, 1 med-fat meat, 13 fat

FAST FOOD

	Serving	Calories	Fat (g)	Cal. from Fat	Sat. Fat (g)	Trans Fat (g)	Chol. (mg)	Sod. (mg)	Carb. (g)	Fiber (g)	Prot. (g)	Servings/Exchanges
Bros. Bistro House Salad with Chicken	14 oz	940	71	630	12	0	105	810	39	7	36	2 1/2 carb, 4 med-fat meat, 10 fat
Caesar Salad	10 oz	690	63	570	15	0	55	1730	18	4	18	1 carb, 2 med-fat meat, 11 fat
Caesar Salad with Chicken	14 oz	820	66	600	16	0	145	2290	20	4	42	1 carb, 6 med-fat meat, 7 fat
Chicken Chipotle Salad	15.2 oz	710	41	370	9	0	95	1960	54	10	34	3 1/2 carb, 2 med-fat meat, 6 fat
Chipotle Salad	11.7 oz	590	38	340	8	0	20	1470	53	10	13	3 1/2 carb, 1 med-fat meat, 7 fat
Half Caesar Salad	4.5 oz	280	27	240	6	0	2	680	7	2	6	1/2 carb, 1 med-fat meat, 4 fat
Half Caesar Salad with Chicken	6.5 oz	350	28	260	6	0	65	960	8	2	18	1/2 carb, 2 med-fat meat, 4 fat

Half Chicken Chipotle Salad	7.8 oz	360	21	190	4.5	0	40	970	27	5	18	2 carb, 2 med-fat meat, 2 fat
Half Chipotle Salad	5.8 oz	290	18	170	4	0	10	730	26	5	6	2 carb, 4 fat
Sandwiches												
Deli Chicken Salad	9.7 oz	460	18	160	4	0.5	75	890	47	4	28	3 1/2 carb, 3 med-fat meat, 1 fat
Deli Ham	9.2 oz	520	26	230	5	0.5	45	1550	48	4	26	3 carb, 2 med-fat meat, 3 fat
Deli Pastrami	10.9 oz	630	33	300	9	1	80	1860	53	5	34	3 1/2 carb, 3 med-fat meat, 4 fat
Deli Tuna Salad	9.5 oz	440	15	130	2.5	0	35	920	50	4	29	3 carb, 3 med-fat meat
Deli Turkey	9.6 oz	510	15	130	8	0	75	1430	62	3	38	4 carb, 4 lean meat
Egg Way Original	8.7 oz	530	20	180	9	0	395	840	62	2	30	4 carb, 3 med-fat meat, 1 fat
Egg Way with Black Forest Ham	10.1 oz	570	21	190	9	0	410	1270	62	2	37	4 carb, 3 med-fat meat, 1 fat

FAST FOOD

	Serving	Calories	Fat (g)	Cal. from Fat	Sat. Fat (g)	Trans Fat (g)	Chol. (mg)	Sod. (mg)	Carb. (g)	Fiber (g)	Prot. (g)	Servings/Exchanges
Egg Way with Sausage	10.1 oz	600	24	210	10	0	425	1020	63	2	38	4 carb, 4 med-fat meat, 1 fat
Original Asiago Bagel Dog	6.8 oz	490	21	190	8	1	60	1230	56	2	22	3 1/2 carb, 2 med-fat meat, 2 fat
Original Bagel Dog	6.7 oz	470	20	180	7	1	55	1190	56	2	20	3 1/2 carb, 2 med-fat meat, 2 fat
Pepperoni Pizza Bagel	6.6 oz	470	16	140	8	0	45	1120	63	3	24	4 carb, 2 med-fat meat, 1 fat
Rachel, Regular Size	10.1 oz	910	64	580	16	1.5	130	2210	51	2	36	3 1/2 carb, 4 med-fat meat, 9 fat
Reuben, Regular Size	9.9 oz	650	38	340	12	1	105	2360	47	3	34	3 carb, 3 med-fat meat, 5 fat
Roasted Turkey & Swiss	10.9 oz	690	41	370	9	1	80	1460	49	4	35	5 carb, 2 lean meat
Sausage Ranchero Panini	12.2 oz	680	29	260	12	0	435	1360	64	4	32	4 1/2 carb, 3 med-fat meat, 3 fat

	Serving	Cal										Choices/Exchanges
Veg Out, on Sesame Seed Bagel	9.5 oz	440	14	120	7	0	30	760	66	4	17	4 1/2 carb, 1 med-fat meat, 2 fat
Paninis												
Italian Chicken	12.6 oz	800	40	360	12	0	120	2450	66	5	35	4 1/2 carb, 3 med-fat meat, 5 fat
Turkey Club	13.3 oz	790	41	370	11	1	100	2200	66	6	34	4 1/2 carb, 3 med-fat meat, 5 fat
Soups (Cup)												
Chicken Noodle	8.75 oz	120	3.5	35	1	0	30	770	14	1	5	1 carb, 1 fat
Corn Crab Chowder	8.75 oz	280	18	160	15	0	30	940	18	1	8	1 carb, 1 med-fat meat, 3 fat
Italian Wedding	8.75 oz	160	6	50	1.5	0	20	1060	15	2	11	1 carb, 1 med-fat meat
Seafood Minestrone	8.75 oz	130	4.5	40	1	0	40	1010	16	2	8	1 carb, 1 med-fat meat
Turkey Chili	8.75 oz	220	7	60	1.5	0	35	930	24	5	20	1 1/2 carb, 2 lean meat
Vegetarian Broccoli Cheese	8.75 oz	290	20	180	10	0	45	990	16	2	14	1 carb, 2 med-fat meat, 2 fat

FAST FOOD

	Serving	Calories	Fat (g)	Cal. from Fat	Sat. Fat (g)	Trans Fat (g)	Chol. (mg)	Sod. (mg)	Carb. (g)	Fiber (g)	Prot. (g)	Servings/Exchanges
HARDEE'S												
Breakfast												
Made from Scratch Biscuit	1	370	23	210	5	NA	0	890	35	0	5	2 carb, 5 fat
Bacon, Egg & Cheese Biscuit	1	530	36	320	11	NA	195	1390	36	0	15	2 1/2 carb, 1 med-fat meat, 6 fat
Biscuit 'N' Gravy	1	530	33	300	8	NA	10	1510	48	1	9	3 carb, 7 fat
Chicken Fillet Biscuit	1	600	34	310	7	NA	55	1680	50	1	24	3 carb, 2 med-fat meat, 5 fat
Country Ham Biscuit	1	440	26	240	6	NA	35	1710	36	0	14	2 1/2 carb, 1 med-fat meat, 4 fat
Country Steak Biscuit	1	630	43	390	11	NA	35	1330	45	0	16	3 carb, 1 med-fat meat, 8 fat
Frisco Breakfast Sandwich	1	400	18	160	7	NA	215	1350	27	2	23	2 carb, 2 med-fat meat, 2 fat

Loaded Biscuit 'N' Gravy Breakfast Bowl	1	740	52	460	14	NA	220	1920	49	1	20	3 carb, 2 med-fat meat, 8 fat
Loaded Breakfast Burrito	1	760	49	440	21	NA	445	1700	39	1	39	2 1/2 carb, 5 med-fat meat, 5 fat
Low Carb Breakfast Bowl	1	620	50	450	21	NA	325	1380	6	2	36	1/2 carb, 5 med-fat meat, 5 fat
Monster Biscuit	1	770	55	500	18	NA	250	2310	37	0	29	2 1/2 carb, 3 med-fat meat, 8 fat
Pancakes	3	300	5	45	1	NA	25	830	55	2	8	3 1/2 carb, 1 fat
Sausage & Egg Biscuit	1	590	42	380	11	NA	210	1300	36	0	16	2 1/2 carb, 2 med-fat meat, 6 fat
Sausage Biscuit	1	530	38	340	10	NA	30	1240	36	0	11	2 1/2 carb, 1 med-fat meat, 7 fat
Smoked Sausage Biscuit	1	620	46	420	15	NA	40	1680	37	0	14	2 1/2 carb, 1 med-fat meat, 8 fat
Sunrise Croissant with Ham	1	400	23	210	10	NA	225	1070	27	1	21	2 carb, 2 med-fat meat, 3 fat

FAST FOOD

Sandwiches

	Serving	Calories	Fat (g)	Cal. from Fat	Sat. Fat (g)	Trans Fat (g)	Chol. (mg)	Sod. (mg)	Carb. (g)	Fiber (g)	Prot. (g)	Servings/Exchanges
Small Hamburger	1	310	15	140	4	NA	35	500	32	1	14	2 carb, 1 med-fat meat, 2 fat
Small Cheeseburger	1	350	19	170	4	NA	45	730	32	1	16	2 carb, 1 med-fat meat, 3 fat
Little Thickburger	1	570	39	350	12	NA	80	1140	35	3	24	2 carb, 3 med-fat meat, 5 fat
1/3 lb Original Thickburger	1	770	48	430	16	NA	95	1560	53	4	35	3 1/2 carb, 3 med-fat meat, 8 fat
1/3 lb Low Carb Thickburger	1	420	32	280	12	NA	115	1010	5	2	30	4 med-fat meat, 2 fat
1/3 lb Cheeseburger	1	620	33	290	13	NA	80	1580	51	3	35	3 1/2 carb, 3 med-fat meat, 4 fat
1/3 lb Mushroom 'N Swiss Thickburger	1	650	36	320	14	NA	90	1620	47	3	39	3 carb, 4 med-fat meat, 3 fat

1/3 lb Bacon Cheese Thickburger	1	850	57	520	19	NA	105	1650	49	3	38	3 carb, 4 med-fat meat, 7 fat
2/3 lb Monster Thickburger	1	1320	95	860	36	NA	210	3020	46	2	70	3 carb, 9 med-fat meat, 10 fat
2/3 lb Bacon Cheese Thickburger	1	1200	84	750	30	NA	185	2450	50	3	65	3 carb, 8 med-fat meat, 9 fat
2/3 lb Double Thickburger	1	1150	78	700	28	NA	180	2410	53	4	62	3 1/2 carb, 7 med-fat meat, 9 fat
BBQ Chicken Sandwich	1	400	6	50	1	NA	45	1370	62	5	27	4 carb, 2 lean meat
Six Dollar Thickburger	1	930	59	530	21	NA	130	1960	57	4	46	4 carb, 5 med-fat meat, 7 fat
Charbroiled Chicken Club Sandwich	1	630	32	280	8	NA	80	1730	54	4	32	3 1/2 carb, 3 med-fat meat, 3 fat
Low Carb Charbroiled Chicken Club Sandwich	1	360	23	200	7	NA	75	1290	14	1	24	1 carb, 3 med-fat meat, 4 fat
Big Chicken Fillet Sandwich	1	710	38	350	7	NA	55	1610	62	5	33	4 carb, 3 med-fat meat, 5 fat

FAST FOOD

	Serving	Calories	Fat (g)	Cal. from Fat	Sat. Fat (g)	Trans Fat (g)	Chol. (mg)	Sod. (mg)	Carb. (g)	Fiber (g)	Prot. (g)	Servings/Exchanges
Spicy Chicken Sandwich	1	440	21	180	5	NA	50	1140	41	3	11	3 carb, 1 med-fat meat, 3 fat
Regular Roast Beef	1	310	15	130	5	NA	40	860	28	1	17	2 carb, 2 med-fat meat, 1 fat
Big Roast Beef	1	400	21	190	7	NA	60	1180	28	1	25	2 carb, 3 med-fat meat, 1 fat
Hot Ham 'N Cheese	1	280	12	100	4	NA	35	1090	29	1	18	2 carb, 2 med-fat meat
Big Hot Ham 'N Cheese	1	460	20	180	8	NA	75	2040	40	2	36	4 carb, 4 med-fat meat, 1 fat
Jumbo Hot Dog	1	400	26	240	9	NA	55	1170	25	1	16	2 carb, 2 med-fat meat, 3 fat
3 Piece Chicken Strips	1 order	370	26	230	6	NA	30	620	19	2	14	1 carb, 2 med-fat meat, 3 fat
5 Piece Chicken Strips	1 order	610	43	390	9	NA	50	1030	32	3	23	2 carb, 2 med-fat meat, 7 fat

Fried Chicken & Sides

Item	Serving											Exchanges/Choices
Fried Chicken Breast	1	370	15	130	4	NA	75	1190	29	0	29	2 carb, 3 med-fat meat
Fried Chicken Leg	1	170	7	60	2	NA	45	570	15	0	13	1 carb, 1 med-fat meat
Fried Chicken Thigh	1	330	15	130	4	NA	60	1000	30	0	19	2 carb, 2 med-fat meat, 1 fat
Fried Chicken Wing	1	200	8	70	2	NA	30	740	23	0	10	1 1/2 carb, 1 med-fat meat, 1 fat
Natural-Cut French Fries, Small	1 order	320	14	130	3	NA	0	710	45	3	4	3 carb, 3 fat
Natural-Cut French Fries, Medium	1 order	430	19	170	4	NA	5	960	60	4	5	4 carb, 4 fat
Natural-Cut French Fries, Large	1 order	470	21	190	4	NA	5	1640	65	5	5	4 1/2 carb, 4 fat
Crispy Curls, Small	1 order	340	17	150	4	NA	0	840	43	4	4	3 carb, 3 fat
Crispy Curls, Medium	1 order	410	20	180	5	NA	0	1020	52	4	5	3 1/2 carb, 4 fat
Crispy Curls, Large	1 order	480	23	210	6	NA	0	1190	60	5	6	4 carb, 5 fat
Coleslaw, Small	1 order	170	10	90	2	NA	10	140	20	2	1	1 carb, 2 fat

FAST FOOD

	Serving	Calories	Fat (g)	Cal. from Fat	Sat. Fat (g)	Trans Fat (g)	Chol. (mg)	Sod. (mg)	Carb. (g)	Fiber (g)	Prot. (g)	Servings/Exchanges
Mashed Potatoes, Small	1 order	90	2	15	0	NA	0	410	17	0	1	1 carb
Side Salad, No Dressing	1	120	7	70	5	NA	20	160	7	2	7	1 carb, 1 med-fat meat
IN-N-OUT BURGER												
Hamburger with Onion	1	390	19	170	5	0	40	650	39	3	16	2 1/2 carb, 2 med-fat meat, 2 fat
Hamburger, Protein Style	1	240	17	150	4	0	40	370	11	3	13	2 vegetable, 2 med-fat meat, 1 fat
Cheeseburger with Onion	1	480	27	240	10	0.5	60	1000	39	3	22	2 1/2 carb, 2 med-fat meat, 3 fat
Cheeseburger, Protein Style	1	330	25	220	9	0	60	720	11	3	18	2 vegetable, 2 med-fat meat, 3 fat
Double-Double with Onion	1	670	41	370	18	1	120	1440	39	3	37	2 1/2 carb, 4 med-fat meat, 4 fat
Double-Double, Protein Style	1	520	39	350	17	1	120	1160	11	3	33	2 vegetable, 4 med-fat meat, 4 fat

French Fries	1 order	400	18	160	5	0	0	245	54	2	7	3 1/2 carb, 4 fat
Chocolate Shake	15 oz	690	36	320	24	1	95	350	83	0	9	5 1/2 carb, 7 fat
Vanilla Shake	15 oz	680	37	330	25	1	90	390	78	0	9	5 carb, 7 fat
Strawberry Shake	15 oz	690	33	300	22	0.5	85	280	91	0	9	6 carb, 7 fat

JACK IN THE BOX

Healthy Dining

Chicken Fajita Pita	1	320	11	100	5	0.5	65	1110	33	4	24	2 carb, 2 med-fat meat
Chicken Teriyaki Bowl	1	580	5	50	1	0	35	1460	106	4	26	7 carb, 1 med-fat meat
Grilled Chicken Strip	1 order	180	2	20	0.5	0	125	700	3	0	37	5 lean meat
Hamburger Delue	1	340	18	170	6	1	40	550	31	2	14	2 carb, 1 med-fat meat, 3 fat
Steak Teriyaki Bowl	1	650	10	90	3	0	45	1740	106	4	30	7 carb, 1 med-fat meat, 1 fat

Burgers

Big Cheeseburger	1	650	40	360	15	1.5	70	1170	50	2	24	3 carb, 2 med-fat meat, 6 fat

FAST FOOD

	Serving	Calories	Fat (g)	Cal. from Fat	Sat. Fat (g)	Trans Fat (g)	Chol. (mg)	Sod. (mg)	Carb. (g)	Fiber (g)	Prot. (g)	Servings/Exchanges
Bacon Ultimate Cheeseburger	1	980	67	600	27	3	135	1880	52	2	43	3 1/2 carb, 5 med-fat meat, 8 fat
Hamburger	1	280	12	100	4.5	0.5	30	540	29	5	14	2 carb, 1 med-fat meat, 1 fat
Hamburger with Cheese	1	320	15	140	7	1	45	730	30	5	16	2 carb, 1 med-fat meat, 3 fat
Hamburger Deluxe	1	362	18	171	5	1	38	579	33	1	14	2 carb, 1 med-fat meat, 3 fat
Hamburger Deluxe with Cheese	1	430	25	230	10	1	65	920	33	7	19	2 carb, 2 med-fat meat, 3 fat
Jumbo Jack	1	580	33	300	11	1	50	920	51	10	20	3 1/2 carb, 1 med-fat meat, 6 fat
Junior Bacon Cheeseburger	1	400	23	210	8	1	55	800	30	1	18	2 carb, 2 med-fat meat, 3 fat

Sourdough Jack	1	680	46	410	17	1.5	75	1200	41	6	26	2 1/2 carb, 3 med-fat meat, 6 fat
Ultimate Cheeseburger	1	920	63	560	26	2.5	120	1530	52	11	38	3 1/2 carb, 4 med-fat meat, 9 fat
Sirloin Cheeseburger	1	950	60	540	19	2	145	1920	61	4	41	4 carb, 4 med-fat meat, 8 fat

Chicken & Fish

Chicken Breast Strips	4	500	25	220	6	6	80	1260	36	3	35	2 1/2 carb, 4 med-fat meat, 1 fat
Chicken Fajita Pita	1	326	10	95	6	0	64	987	35	3	23	2 carb, 2 med-fat meat
Chicken Sandwich	1	400	21	190	4.5	2.5	35	740	38	2	15	2 1/2 carb, 1 med-fat meat, 3 fat
Jack's Spicy Chicken	1	550	24	220	5	3	50	1050	59	8	24	4 carb, 2 med-fat meat, 3 fat
Sourdough Grilled Chicken Club	1	530	28	250	7	2	90	1440	34	3	36	2 carb, 4 med-fat meat, 2 fat

FAST FOOD

	Serving	Calories	Fat (g)	Cal. from Fat	Sat. Fat (g)	Trans Fat (g)	Chol. (mg)	Sod. (mg)	Carb. (g)	Fiber (g)	Prot. (g)	Servings/Exchanges
Fish & Chips	Small order	630	35	310	8	10	40	1290	61	5	19	4 carb, 1 med-fat meat, 6 fat
Snacks & Sides												
Bacon Cheddar Potato Wedges	1 order	760	52	470	16	13	45	960	53	4	21	3 1/2 carb, 2 med-fat meat, 8 fat
Egg Roll	1	130	6	60	2	1	5	310	15	1	5	1 carb, 1 fat
French Fries, Small	1	290	15	140	3.5	4.5	0	540	35	1	4	2 carb, 3 fat
French Fries, Medium	1	460	24	210	6	7	0	850	55	1	6	3 1/2 carb, 5 fat
French Fries, Large	1	620	32	290	7	9	0	1150	75	8	9	5 carb, 6 fat
Mozzarella Cheese Sticks	3	240	14	120	6	2	25	510	20	1	10	1 1/2 carb, 1 med-fat meat, 2 fat
Onion Rings	8	500	30	270	6	10	0	420	51	3	6	3 1/2 carb, 6 fat
Seasoned Curly Fries, Small	1	280	15	140	3	5	0	600	30	3	4	2 carb, 3 fat

Seasoned Curly Fries, Medium	1	420	24	210	5	7	0	920	46	5	6	3 carb, 5 fat
Seasoned Curly Fries, Large	1	570	32	290	7	10	0	1260	63	7	8	4 carb, 6 fat
Stuffed Jalapeños	3	230	13	110	6	2	20	690	22	2	7	1 1/2 carb, 3 fat
Jack's Ultimate Salads												
Asian Chicken Salad with Grilled Chicken	1	180	1.5	15	0	0	65	380	22	6	22	1 1/2 carb, 3 lean meat
Chicken Club Salad with Grilled Chicken	1	320	16	140	7	0	100	780	12	4	34	1 carb, 4 lean meat
Side Salad	1	50	3	25	1.5	0	10	60	5	2	3	1 vegetable, 1 fat
Southwest Chicken Salad	1	310	12	110	5	0	90	820	28	7	31	2 carb, 4 lean meat
Breakfast												
Bacon, Egg, & Cheese Biscuit	1	440	26	230	11	1	220	1030	37	2	16	2 1/2 carb, 1 med-fat meat, 4 fat
Breakfast Jack	1	290	12	110	4.5	0	220	760	29	1	17	2 carb, 2 med-fat meat

FAST FOOD

	Serving	Calories	Fat (g)	Cal. from Fat	Sat. Fat (g)	Trans Fat (g)	Chol. (mg)	Sod. (mg)	Carb. (g)	Fiber (g)	Prot. (g)	Servings/Exchanges
Extreme Sausage Sandwich	1	670	48	430	17	1.5	290	1300	31	2	29	2 carb, 3 med-fat meat, 7 fat
Sausage Breakfast Jack	1	450	28	250	10	1	245	840	29	1	20	2 carb, 2 med-fat meat, 4 fat
Sausage Croissant	1	580	39	350	13	4	255	770	37	2	21	2 1/2 carb, 2 med-fat meat, 6 fat
Sausage, Egg & Cheese Biscuit	1	590	40	360	16	1.5	245	1140	38	2	20	2 1/2 carb, 1 med-fat meat, 7 fat
Sourdough Breakfast Sandwich	1	420	24	220	8	2	230	980	31	2	20	2 carb, 2 med-fat meat, 3 fat
Supreme Croissant	1	450	25	230	9	3.5	235	860	36	1	20	2 1/2 carb, 2 med-fat meat, 3 fat
Ultimate Breakfast Sandwich	1	570	27	240	10	1	445	1700	49	2	34	3 carb, 4 med-fat meat, 1 fat

KFC

Salads

Crispy BLT Salad, with Chicken	1	340	19	170	5	0	70	840	14	3	30	1 carb, 4 med-fat meat
Crispy Caesar Salad, with Chicken	1	320	19	170	6	0	65	660	12	3	28	1 carb, 4 med-fat meat
House Side Salad	1	15	0	0	0	0	0	10	10	2	1	free
Roasted Caesar Salad	1	190	6	50	3	0	75	530	5	2	29	1 vegetable, 4 lean meat
Roasted Chicken BLT Salad	1	200	7	60	2	0	80	720	7	3	30	1/2 carb, 4 lean meat

Sandwiches & Wraps

Crispy Twister with Crispy Strip	1	580	30	270	7	0	60	1250	49	3	28	3 carb, 3 med-fat meat, 3 fat
Crispy Twister with Original Strip	1	540	26	230	7	0	65	1430	48	4	29	3 carb, 3 med-fat meat, 2 fat

FAST FOOD

	Serving	Calories	Fat (g)	Cal. from Fat	Sat. Fat (g)	Trans Fat (g)	Chol. (mg)	Sod. (mg)	Carb. (g)	Fiber (g)	Prot. (g)	Servings/Exchanges
Double Crunch, Original Strip	1	470	23	200	6	0	65	1020	35	2	27	2 carb, 3 med-fat meat, 2 fat
Honey BBQ Sandwich	1	310	4	35	1	0	70	810	42	1	23	3 carb, 2 lean meat
KFC Snacker with Crispy Strip	1	300	14	120	3	0	30	470	28	2	15	2 carb, 2 med-fat meat, 1 fat
KFC Snacker with Original Strip	1	270	12	100	3	0	30	560	28	2	15	2 carb, 1 med-fat meat, 1 fat
KFC Snacker, Fish	1	320	14	130	3	0	60	640	31	2	16	2 carb, 1 med-fat meat, 2 fat
KFC Snacker, Honey BBQ	1	210	3	30	1	0	35	470	32	2	13	2 carb, 1 med-fat meat
Oven Roast Filet Sandwich	1	480	23	210	4	0	85	1230	38	2	25	2 1/2 carb, 3 med-fat meat, 2 fat
Tender Roast	1	440	18	160	4	0	70	1120	42	2	29	3 carb, 3 med-fat meat, 1 fat

Item	Serving	Cal	Fat	Fat Cal	Sat Fat	Trans Fat	Chol	Sod	Carb	Fiber	Prot	Exchanges
Tender Roast Sandwich	1	400	15	130	3	0	90	810	29	1	34	2 carb, 4 lean meat
Toasted Wrap with Crispy Strip	1	360	20	180	6	0	40	730	27	2	17	2 carb, 2 med-fat meat, 2 fat
Toasted Wrap with Tender Roast Filet	1	310	14	130	5	0	60	740	24	1	22	1 1/2 carb, 2 med-fat meat, 1 fat

Chicken

Item	Serving	Cal	Fat	Fat Cal	Sat Fat	Trans Fat	Chol	Sod	Carb	Fiber	Prot	Exchanges
Original Chicken, Breast	1	370	21	190	5	0	120	1050	7	0	38	1/2 carb, 5 lean meat
Original Chicken, Breast without Skin or Breading	1	140	2	20	0	0	65	510	1	0	29	4 lean meat
Original Chicken, Drumstick	1	110	7	60	1.5	0	55	290	2	0	10	1 med-fat meat
Original Chicken, Thigh	1	260	19	170	5	0	85	670	6	0	16	1/2 carb, 3 med-fat meat, 2 fat
Original Chicken, Whole Wing	1	110	7	60	1.5	0	45	310	3	0	9	1 med-fat meat

FAST FOOD

	Serving	Calories	Fat (g)	Cal. from Fat	Sat. Fat (g)	Trans Fat (g)	Chol. (mg)	Sod. (mg)	Carb. (g)	Fiber (g)	Prot. (g)	Servings/Exchanges
Extra Crispy Chicken, Breast	1	490	31	280	7	0	120	1080	17	0	38	1 carb, 5 med-fat meat, 1 fat
Extra Crispy Chicken, Drumstick	1	150	9	80	2	0	50	360	6	0	11	1/2 carb, 1 med-fat meat, 1 fat
Extra Crispy Chicken, Thigh	1	370	27	250	6	0	85	840	12	0	18	1 carb, 2 med-fat meat, 3 fat
Extra Crispy Chicken, Whole Wing	1	150	10	90	2	0	50	320	6	1	11	1/2 carb, 1 med-fat meat, 1 fat
Grilled Chicken, Breast	1	180	4	35	1	0	110	440	0	0	35	5 lean meat
Grilled Chicken, Drumstick	1	70	4	35	1	0	50	200	0	0	10	1 med-fat meat
Grilled Chicken, Thigh	1	140	9	80	2.5	0	80	320	0	0	15	2 med-fat meat
Grilled Chicken, Wing	1	80	4	40	1	0	50	160	0	0	10	1 med-fat meat
Strips, Crispy strips	3	380	22	200	6	0	80	720	12	1	33	1 carb, 4 med-fat meat
Original Strips	3	310	15	140	5	0	80	990	11	2	32	1 carb, 4 lean meat

Popcorn Chicken

Individual	1 order	400	26	230	4.5	0	60	1160	22	3	21	1 1/2 carb, 3 med-fat meat, 2 fat
Large	1 order	550	35	320	6	0	80	1600	30	3	29	2 carb, 3 med-fat meat, 4 fat

Pot Pie & Bowls

Chicken Pot Pie	1	690	40	360	31	0	95	1760	57	3	27	4 carb, 2 med-fat meat, 6 fat
KFC Famous Bowls, Rice	1	790	28	250	7	1	55	2690	106	5	29	7 carb, 1 med-fat meat, 5 fat
KFC Famous Bowls, Mashed Potato	1	700	32	290	8	1	55	2260	77	6	26	5 carb, 2 med-fat meat, 4 fat

Wings

Honey BBQ Wings	1	80	5	45	1	0	20	170	5	1	4	1 med-fat meat
Honey BBQ Wings, Boneless	1	80	3.5	35	0.5	0	10	340	7	1	5	1/2 carb, 1 med-fat meat
Hot Wings	1	70	5	45	1	0	20	150	3	0	4	1 med-fat meat

FAST FOOD

	Serving	Calories	Fat (g)	Cal. from Fat	Sat. Fat (g)	Trans Fat (g)	Chol. (mg)	Sod. (mg)	Carb. (g)	Fiber (g)	Prot. (g)	Servings/Exchanges
Sides (Individual)												
Baked Beans	1	200	1.5	10	0	0	0	680	39	9	8	2 1/2 carb
Biscuit	1	180	8	70	6	0	0	530	23	1	4	1 1/2 carb, 2 fat
Coleslaw	1	180	10	90	1.5	0	5	270	22	3	1	1 1/2 carb, 2 fat
Corn on the Cob	3 inches	70	1.5	5	0.5	0	0	0	16	2	2	1 carb
Green Beans	1	25	0	0	0	0	0	380	5	2	1	1 vegetable
KFC Red Beans with Sausage & Rice	1	160	2.5	25	0.5	0	5	340	26	4	24	2 carb, 3 lean meat
Macaroni & Cheese	1	180	9	80	3	0	5	880	20	2	6	1 carb, 1 med-fat meat, 2 fat
Macaroni Salad	1	180	9	80	2	0	5	400	20	1	3	1 carb, 2 fat
Mashed Potatoes with Gravy	1	130	4.5	40	1	0	0	550	20	1	2	1 carb, 1 fat
Mashed Potatoes without Gravy	1	100	3	25	0.5	0	0	350	16	1	2	1 carb, 1 fat

Potato Salad	1	200	10	90	2	0	5	540	24	3	2	1 1/2 carb, 2 fat
Potato Wedges	1	260	13	110	2.5	0	0	740	33	3	4	2 carb, 3 fat
Seasoned Rice	1	140	0.5	5	0	0	0	560	31	1	3	2 carb

KRISPY KREME DONUTS

Apple Fritter	1	380	20	180	10	0	5	220	47	2	4	3 carb, 4 fat
Caramel Kreme Crunch	1	381	19	170	9	0	10	170	49	<1	4	3 carb, 4 fat
Chocolate Iced Custard Filled	1	300	17	150	8	0	5	150	35	<1	3	2 carb, 3 fat
Chocolate Iced Glazed	1	250	12	110	6	0	5	100	33	<1	3	2 carb, 2 fat
Chocolate Iced Kreme Filled	1	350	20	180	11	0	5	140	38	<1	3	2 1/2 carb, 4 fat
Cinnamon Bun	1	260	16	140	8	0	5	125	28	<1	3	2 carb, 3 fat
Cinnamon Twist	1	240	15	140	7	0	5	130	25	<1	3	1 1/2 carb, 3 fat
Glazed Chocolate Cake	1	300	15	130	7	0	20	250	42	2	3	3 carb, 3 fat
Glazed Cinnamon	1	210	12	110	6	0	5	100	24	<1	2	1 1/2 carb, 2 fat
Glazed Kreme Filled	1	340	20	180	10	0	5	140	39	<1	3	2 1/2 carb, 4 fat

FAST FOOD

	Serving	Calories	Fat (g)	Cal. from Fat	Sat. Fat (g)	Trans Fat (g)	Chol. (mg)	Sod. (mg)	Carb. (g)	Fiber (g)	Prot. (g)	Servings/Exchanges
Glazed Lemon Filled	1	290	16	140	8	0	5	135	35	<1	3	2 carb, 3 fat
Original Glazed	1	200	12	100	6	0	5	95	22	<1	2	1 1/2 carb, 2 fat
Powdered Cake	1	290	14	130	6	0	20	320	37	<1	3	2 1/2 carb, 3 fat
LONG JOHN SILVER'S												
Fish & Seafood												
Battered Fish	1 piece	260	16	140	4	4.5	35	790	17	0	12	1 carb, 1 med-fat meat, 2 fat
Baked Cod	1 piece	120	4.5	120	1	0	90	240	1	0	22	3 lean meat
Battered Shrimp	3 pieces	130	9	80	2.5	2.5	45	480	8	0	5	1/2 carb, 2 fat
Alaskan Flounder	1 piece	250	11	100	2.5	3	35	910	26	2	12	2 carb, 1 med-fat meat, 1 fat
Buttered Lobster Bites	1 snack box	230	9	80	3	3	60	520	24	2	13	1 1/2 carb, 2 med-fat meat
Grilled Pacific Salmon	2 filets	150	5	45	1	0	50	440	2	0	24	3 lean meat

Grilled Tilapia	1 filet	110	2.5	20	1	0	55	250	1	0	22	3 lean meat
Shrimp Scampi	8 pieces	110	5	45	1	0.5	150	610	1	0	16	2 lean meat
Lobster Stuffed Crab Cake	1 cake	170	9	80	2	0	30	390	16	1	6	1 carb, 1 med-fat meat, 1 fat
Breaded Clam Strips	1 snack box	320	19	170	4.5	7	35	1190	29	2	9	2 carb, 1 med-fat meat, 3 fat
Chicken												
Chicken Plank	1 piece	140	8	70	2	2.5	20	480	9	0	8	1/2 carb, 1 med-fat meat, 1 fat
Sandwiches												
Fish Sandwich	1	470	23	210	5	4.5	45	1210	48	3	18	3 carb, 1 med-fat meat, 4 fat
Ultimate Fish Sandwich	1	530	28	250	8	5	60	1400	49	3	21	3 carb, 2 med-fat meat, 4 fat
Chicken Sandwich	1	360	15	140	3.5	2.5	25	900	40	3	14	2 1/2 carb, 1 med-fat meat, 2 fat

FAST FOOD

	Serving	Calories	Fat (g)	Cal. from Fat	Sat. Fat (g)	Trans Fat (g)	Chol. (mg)	Sod. (mg)	Carb. (g)	Fiber (g)	Prot. (g)	Servings/Exchanges
Baja Fish Taco	1 taco	350	22	200	5	3.5	20	840	29	1	9	2 carb, 1 med-fat meat, 3 fat
Freshside Grille Smart Choice, Salmon	1 plate	280	7	60	2	0	50	1010	27	3	27	2 carb, 3 lean meat
Freshside Grille Smart Choice, Scampi	1 plate	250	7	60	2	0.5	155	1180	27	3	19	2 carb, 1 lean meat
Freshside Grille Smart Choice, Tilapia	1 plate	250	4.5	40	2	0	60	820	27	3	25	2 carb, 3 lean meat
Salmon Bowl with Sauce	1 bowl	460	8	70	2.5	0	50	1660	65	4	30	4 1/2 carb, 2 med-fat meat
Shrimp Bowl with Sauce	1 bowl	380	4.5	40	1.5	0	145	1580	64	4	21	4 carb, 1 med-fat meat
Sauces												
Cocktail Sauce	1 oz	25	0	0	0	0	0	250	6	0	0	1/2 carb

Tartar Sauce	1 oz	100	9	80	1.5	0	15	250	4	0	0	2 fat
Sides												
Breadsticks	1	170	3.5	30	1	1	0	290	29	1	6	2 carb, 1 fat
Broccoli Cheese Soup	1 bowl	220	18	160	8	0	30	650	8	1	5	1/2 carb, 1 med-fat meat, 3 fat
Coleslaw	4 oz	200	15	130	2.5	0	20	340	15	3	1	1 carb, 3 fat
Corn Cobbette with Butter Oil	1	150	10	90	2	0	0	30	14	3	3	1 carb, 2 fat
Crumblies	1 oz	170	12	110	2.5	4	0	410	14	1	1	1 carb, 2 fat
Fries, Basket Combo Portion	4 oz	310	14	120	3.5	3.5	0	460	45	4	3	3 carb, 3 fat
Fries, Platter Portion	3 oz	230	10	90	2.5	3	0	350	34	3	3	2 carb, 2 fat
Hushpuppy	1	60	2.5	20	0.5	1	0	200	9	1	1	1/2 carb, 1 fat
Rice	5 oz	180	1	10	0.5	0	0	470	37	2	4	2 1/2 carb
Desserts												
Chocolate Cream Pie	1 slice	310	22	200	14	2	15	170	24	1	5	1 1/2 carb, 4 fat

FAST FOOD

	Serving	Calories	Fat (g)	Cal. from Fat	Sat. Fat (g)	Trans Fat (g)	Chol. (mg)	Sod. (mg)	Carb. (g)	Fiber (g)	Prot. (g)	Servings/Exchanges
Pecan Pie	1 slice	370	15	140	3	2	40	190	55	2	4	3 1/2 carb, 3 fat
Pineapple Cream Pie	1 slice	290	13	110	7	2	15	210	39	1	4	2 1/2 carb, 3 fat
McDONALD'S												
Sandwiches												
Hamburger	1	250	9	80	3.5	0.5	25	520	31	2	12	2 carb, 1 med-fat meat, 1 fat
Cheeseburger	1	300	12	110	6	0.5	40	750	33	2	15	2 carb, 1 med-fat meat, 1 fat
McDouble	1	390	19	170	8	1	65	920	33	2	22	2 carb, 2 med-fat meat, 2 fat
Double Cheeseburger	1	440	23	210	11	1.5	80	1150	34	2	25	2 carb, 3 med-fat meat, 2 fat
Quarter Pounder	1	410	19	170	7	1	65	730	37	2	24	2 1/2 carb, 2 med-fat meat, 2 fat

Item												Exchanges
Quarter Pounder with Cheese	1	510	26	230	12	1.5	90	1190	40	3	29	2 1/2 carb, 3 med-fat meat, 2 fat
Double Quarter Pounder with Cheese	1	740	42	380	19	2.5	155	1380	40	3	48	2 1/2 carb, 6 med-fat meat, 2 fat
Big Mac	1	540	29	260	10	1.5	75	1040	45	3	25	3 carb, 2 med-fat meat, 4 fat
Big N' Tasty	1	460	24	220	8	1.5	70	720	37	3	24	2 1/2 carb, 2 med-fat meat, 3 fat
Angus Bacon & Cheese	1	790	39	350	17	2	145	2070	63	4	45	4 carb, 5 med-fat meat, 3 fat
Angus Deluxe	1	750	39	350	16	2	135	1700	61	4	40	4 carb, 5 med-fat meat, 3 fat
Angus Mushroom & Swiss	1	770	40	360	17	2	135	1170	59	4	44	4 carb, 5 med-fat meat, 3 fat
Filet-O-Fish	1	380	18	170	3.5	0	40	640	38	2	15	2 1/2 carb, 1 med-fat meat, 3 fat

FAST FOOD

	Serving	Calories	Fat (g)	Cal. from Fat	Sat. Fat (g)	Trans Fat (g)	Chol. (mg)	Sod. (mg)	Carb. (g)	Fiber (g)	Prot. (g)	Servings/Exchanges
McRib	1	500	26	240	10	0	70	980	44	3	22	3 carb, 2 med-fat meat, 3 fat
McChicken	1	360	16	150	3	0	35	830	40	2	15	2 1/2 carb, 1 med-fat meat, 2 fat
Premium Grilled Chicken Classic	1	420	10	90	2	0	70	1190	51	3	32	3 1/2 carb, 3 lean meat
Premium Crispy Chicken Classic	1	530	20	180	3.5	0	50	1150	59	3	28	4 carb, 2 med-fat meat, 2 fat
Premium Grilled Chicken Club	1	530	17	160	6	0	95	1410	52	4	39	3 1/2 carb, 4 lean meat
Premium Crispy Chicken Club	1	630	28	250	7	0	75	1360	60	4	35	4 carb, 2 med-fat meat, 4 fat
Premium Grilled Chicken Ranch BLT	1	470	12	110	3	0	80	1440	54	3	36	3 1/2 carb, 4 lean meat

	Amount	Cal										Exchanges
Premium Crispy Chicken Ranch BLT	1	580	23	200	4.5	0	65	1400	62	3	31	4 carb, 3 med-fat meat, 2 fat
Southern Style Crispy Chicken	1	400	17	150	3	0	45	1030	39	1	24	2 1/2 carb, 2 med-fat meat, 1 fat
Honey Mustard Snack Wrap, Grilled	1	260	9	80	3.5	0	45	800	27	1	18	2 carb, 2 med-fat meat
Honey Mustard Snack Wrap, Crispy	1	330	16	140	4.5	0	30	780	34	1	14	2 carb, 1 med-fat meat, 2 fat
Ranch Snack Wrap, Grilled	1	270	10	90	4	0	45	830	26	1	18	2 carb, 2 med-fat meat
Ranch Snack Wrap, Crispy	1	340	17	150	4.5	0	30	810	33	1	14	2 carb, 1 med-fat meat, 2 fat
French Fries												
French Fries, Small	1	230	11	100	1.5	0	0	160	29	3	3	2 carb, 2 fat
French Fries, Medium	1	380	19	170	2.5	0	0	270	48	5	4	3 carb, 4 fat
French Fries, Large	1	500	25	220	3.5	0	0	350	63	6	6	4 carb, 5 fat

FAST FOOD

Chicken McNuggets, Chicken Strips, Sauces

	Serving	Calories	Fat (g)	Cal. from Fat	Sat. Fat (g)	Trans Fat (g)	Chol. (mg)	Sod. (mg)	Carb. (g)	Fiber (g)	Prot. (g)	Servings/Exchanges
Chicken McNuggets	4 pieces	190	12	100	2	0	30	400	11	0	10	1 carb, 1 med-fat meat, 1 fat
Chicken McNuggets	10 pieces	460	29	260	5	0	70	1000	27	0	24	2 carb, 3 med-fat meat, 3 fat
Chicken Selects Premium Breast Strips	3 pieces	400	24	210	3.5	0	17	1010	23	0	23	1 1/2 carb, 3 med-fat meat, 2 fat
Chicken Selects Premium Breast Strips	5 pieces	660	40	360	6	0	85	1680	39	0	38	2 1/2 carb, 4 med-fat meat, 4 fat
BBQ Sauce	1 pkg	50	0	0	0	0	0	260	12	0	0	1 carb
Honey	1 pkg	50	0	0	0	0	0	12	0	0	0	1 carb
Sweet 'N Sour Sauce	1 pkg	50	0	0	0	0	0	150	12	0	0	1 carb
Creamy Ranch Sauce	1.5 oz	200	22	200	3.5	0	10	320	2	0	0	4 fat

Premium Bacon Ranch Salad with Grilled Chicken	1	260	9	90	4	0	90	1010	12	3	33	1 carb, 4 lean meat
Premium Bacon Ranch Salad with Crispy Chicken	1	370	20	180	6	0	75	970	20	3	29	1 carb, 4 med-fat meat
Premium Caesar Salad	1	90	4	35	2.5	0	10	180	9	3	7	1/2 carb, 1 med-fat meat
Premium Caesar Salad with Grilled Chicken	1	220	6	60	3	0	75	890	12	3	30	1 carb, 4 lean meat
Premium Caesar Salad with Crispy Chicken	1	330	17	150	4.5	0	60	840	20	3	26	1 carb, 3 med-fat meat
Premium Southwest Salad with Grilled Chicken	1	320	9	80	3	0	70	960	30	6	30	2 carb, 1 1/2 lean meat
Premium Southwest Salad with Crispy Chicken	1	430	20	180	4	0	55	920	38	6	26	2 1/2 carb, 3 med-fat meat, 1 fat

FAST FOOD

	Serving	Calories	Fat (g)	Cal. from Fat	Sat. Fat (g)	Trans Fat (g)	Chol. (mg)	Sod. (mg)	Carb. (g)	Fiber (g)	Prot. (g)	Servings/Exchanges
Side Salad	1	20	0	0	0	0	0	10	4	1	1	1 vegetable
Snack Size Fruit & Walnut Salad	1	210	8	70	1.5	0	5	60	31	2	4	2 carb, 2 fat
Salad Dressings												
Newman's Own Creamy Caesar	2 oz	190	18	170	3.5	0	20	500	4	0	2	4 fat
Newman's Own Creamy Southwest	1.5 oz	100	6	50	1	0	20	340	11	0	1	1 carb, 1 fat
Newman's Own Low Fat Balsamic	1.5 oz	40	3	25	0	0	0	730	4	0	0	1 fat
Newman's Own Low Fat Italian	1.5 oz	60	2.5	20	0	0	0	730	8	0	1	1/2 carb, 1 fat
Newman's Own Ranch	2 oz	170	15	130	2.5	0	20	530	9	0	1	1/2 carb, 3 fat
Breakfast												

	Serving	Calories	Fat (g)	Calories from Fat	Sat. Fat (g)	Trans Fat (g)	Cholesterol (mg)	Sodium (mg)	Carbs (g)	Fiber (g)	Protein (g)	Exchanges
Egg McMuffin	1	300	12	110	5	0	260	820	30	2	18	2 carb, 2 med-fat meat
Sausage McMuffin	1	370	22	200	8	0	45	850	29	2	14	2 carb, 1 med-fat meat, 3 fat
Sausage McMuffin with Egg	1	450	27	250	10	0	285	920	30	2	21	2 carb, 2 med-fat meat, 3 fat
English Muffin	1	160	3	30	0.5	0	0	280	27	2	5	2 carb
Biscuit	Regular size	260	12	110	7	0	0	740	33	2	5	2 carb, 2 fat
Bacon, Egg & Cheese Biscuit	Regular size	420	23	210	12	0	235	1160	37	2	15	2 1/2 carb, 1 med-fat meat, 4 fat
Sausage Biscuit with Egg	Regular size	510	33	290	14	0	250	1170	36	2	18	2 1/2 carb, 2 med-fat meat, 5 fat
Sausage Biscuit	Regular size	430	27	240	12	0	30	1080	34	2	11	2 carb, 1 med-fat meat, 4 fat
Southern Style Chicken Biscuit	Regular size	410	20	180	8	0	30	1180	41	2	17	3 carb, 1 med-fat meat, 1 fat

FAST FOOD

	Serving	Calories	Fat (g)	Cal. from Fat	Sat. Fat (g)	Trans Fat (g)	Chol. (mg)	Sod. (mg)	Carb. (g)	Fiber (g)	Prot. (g)	Servings/Exchanges
Bacon, Egg & Cheese McGriddle	1	420	18	160	8	0	240	1110	48	2	15	3 carb, 1 med-fat meat, 3 fat
Sausage McGriddle	1	420	22	200	8	0	35	1030	44	2	11	3 carb, 4 fat
Sausage, Egg & Cheese McGriddle	1	560	32	290	12	0	265	1360	48	2	20	3 carb, 2 med-fat meat, 4 fat
Big Breakfast	Regular size	740	48	430	17	0	555	1560	51	3	28	3 1/2 carb, 3 med-fat meat, 7 fat
Deluxe Breakfast	Regular size	1090	56	510	19	0	575	2150	111	6	36	7 1/2 carb, 2 med-fat meat, 9 fat
Hash Browns	2 oz	150	9	80	1.5	0	0	310	15	2	1	4 carb, 3 fat
Hotcakes & Sausage	1	520	24	210	7	0	50	930	61	3	15	4 carb, 5 fat
McSkillet Burrito with Sausage	1	610	36	320	14	0.5	410	1390	44	3	27	3 carb, 3 med-fat meat, 4 fat
Sausage Burrito	1	300	16	140	7	0.5	130	830	26	1	12	2 carb, 1 med-fat meat, 2 fat

Scrambled Eggs	3.3 oz	170	11	100	4	0	520	180	1	0	15	2 med-fat meat

Desserts/Shakes

Apple Dippers	1 pkg	35	0	0	0	0	0	0	8	0	0	1/2 fruit
Baked Hot Apple Pie	1	250	13	110	7	0	0	170	32	4	2	2 carb, 3 fat
Cinnamon Melts	4 oz	460	19	170	9	0	15	370	66	3	6	4 1/2 carb, 4 fat
Fruit 'n Yogurt Parfait	5.3 oz	160	2	20	1	0	5	85	31	1	4	2 carb
Hot Caramel Sundae	6.4 oz	340	8	70	5	0	30	160	60	1	7	4 carb, 2 fat
Hot Fudge Sundae	6.3 oz	330	10	90	7	0	25	180	54	2	8	3 1/2 carb, 2 fat
Kiddie Cone	1 oz	45	1	10	0.5	0	5	20	8	0	1	1/2 carb
Low Fat Caramel Dip	0.8 oz	70	0.5	5	0	0	5	35	15	0	0	1 carb
M&M'S McFlurry	12.3 oz	620	20	180	12	1	55	190	96	1	14	6 1/2 carb, 4 fat
OREO McFlurry	11.9 oz	550	17	150	9	1	50	250	88	0	13	6 carb, 3 fat
Vanilla Reduced Fat Ice Cream Cone	3.2 oz	150	3.5	35	2	0	15	60	24	0	4	1 1/2 carb, 1 fat
Chocolate Triple Thick Shake, Small	12 oz	440	10	90	6	0.5	40	190	76	1	10	5 carb, 2 fat

FAST FOOD

	Serving	Calories	Fat (g)	Cal. from Fat	Sat. Fat (g)	Trans Fat (g)	Chol. (mg)	Sod. (mg)	Carb. (g)	Fiber (g)	Prot. (g)	Servings/Exchanges
Chocolate Triple Thick Shake, Medium	16 oz	580	14	120	8	1	50	250	102	1	13	7 carb, 3 fat
Chocolate Triple Thick Shake, Large	21 oz	770	18	160	11	1	70	330	134	1	18	9 carb, 4 fat
Vanilla Triple Thick Shake, Small	12 oz	420	10	90	6	0.5	40	140	72	0	9	5 carb, 2 fat
Vanilla Triple Thick Shake, Medium	16 oz	550	13	120	8	1	50	190	96	0	13	6 1/2 carb, 3 fat
Vanilla Triple Thick Shake, Large	21 oz	740	18	160	11	1	70	250	128	0	17	8 1/2 carb, 4 fat
McDonaldland Cookies	2 oz	260	8	70	2.5	0	0	300	43	1	4	3 carb, 2 fat
Chocolate Chip Cookie	1	160	8	70	3.5	0	10	90	21	1	2	1 1/2 carb, 2 fat
McCafe Coffee, Nonfat Milk												
Nonfat Cappuccino, Small	12 oz	60	0	0	0	0	5	85	9	0	6	1 skim milk

Item	Size									Exchanges
Nonfat Cappuccino, Medium	16 oz	80	0	0	5	110	12	0	8	1 skim milk
Nonfat Cappuccino, Large	20 oz	90	0	0	5	130	13	0	9	1 skim milk
Nonfat Latte, Small	12 oz	90	0	0	5	115	13	0	9	1 skim milk
Nonfat Latte, Medium	16 oz	110	0	0	5	140	15	0	10	1 1/2 skim milk
Nonfat Latte, Large	20 oz	120	0	0	5	160	18	0	12	1 1/2 skim milk
Nonfat Caramel Cappuccino, Medium	16 oz	190	0	0	5	150	41	0	6	1 skim milk, 2 carb
Nonfat Caramel Latte, Medium	16 oz	220	0	0	5	180	45	0	9	1 skim milk, 2 carb
Nonfat Vanilla Cappuccino, Medium	16 oz	190	0	0	5	90	42	0	6	1 skim milk, 2 carb
Nonfat Vanilla Latte, Medium	16 oz	220	0	0	5	115	46	0	9	1 skim milk, 2 carb
Nonfat Cappuccino with Sugar Free Vanilla Syrup	16 oz	70	0	0	5	130	19	0	7	1 skim milk, 1/2 carb

FAST FOOD

	Serving	Calories	Fat (g)	Cal. from Fat	Sat. Fat (g)	Trans Fat (g)	Chol. (mg)	Sod. (mg)	Carb. (g)	Fiber (g)	Prot. (g)	Servings/Exchanges
Nonfat Latte with Sugar Free Vanilla Syrup	16 oz	90	0	0	0	0	5	160	22	0	9	1 skim milk, 1/2 carb
Iced Nonfat Latte, Medium	16 oz	60	0	0	0	0	5	90	9	0	6	1 skim milk
Iced Nonfat Caramel Latte, Medium	16 oz	150	0	0	0	0	5	120	32	0	5	1 skim milk, 1 carb
Iced Nonfat Vanilla Latte, Medium	16 oz	150	0	0	0	0	5	70	33	0	5	1 skim milk, 1 1/2 carb
Iced Nonfat Latte with Sugar Free Vanilla Syrup	16 oz	50	0	0	0	0	5	100	14	0	5	1 skim milk
McCafe Coffee, Whole Milk												
Cappuccino, Small	12 oz	120	7	60	4	0	20	85	9	0	6	1 whole milk
Cappuccino, Medium	16 oz	140	8	70	4.5	0	25	105	11	0	8	1 whole milk
Cappuccino, Large	20 oz	180	10	90	6	0	30	130	13	0	9	1 whole milk

Item												
Latte, Small	12 oz	150	8	70	4.5	0	25	105	11	0	8	1 whole milk
Latte, Medium	16 oz	180	10	90	6	0	30	130	13	0	10	1 whole milk
Latte, Large	20 oz	210	11	100	7	0	35	150	16	0	11	1 1/2 whole milk
Caramel Cappuccino, Medium	16 oz	240	6	50	3.5	0	20	150	41	0	6	1/2 whole milk, 2 carb
Caramel Latte, Medium	16 oz	280	8	70	4.5	0	25	170	43	0	8	1 whole milk, 2 carb
Vanilla Cappuccino, Medium	16 oz	240	6	50	3.5	0	20	85	42	0	6	1 whole milk, 2 carb
Vanilla Latte, Medium	16 oz	280	8	70	4.5	0	25	110	44	0	8	1 whole milk, 2 carb
Cappuccino with Sugar Free Vanilla Syrup, Medium	16 oz	120	6	60	3.5	0	20	130	18	0	6	1 whole milk
Latte with Sugar Free Vanilla Syrup, Medium	16 oz	160	8	70	5	0	25	150	21	0	8	1 whole milk, 1/2 carb
Iced Latte, Medium	16 oz	100	6	50	3.5	0	15	80	8	0	6	1/2 whole milk
Iced Caramel Latte, Medium	16 oz	180	4.5	40	2.5	0	15	120	31	0	4	1/2 whole milk, 1 1/2 carb

FAST FOOD

	Serving	Calories	Fat (g)	Cal. from Fat	Sat. Fat (g)	Trans Fat (g)	Chol. (mg)	Sod. (mg)	Carb. (g)	Fiber (g)	Prot. (g)	Servings/Exchanges
Iced Vanilla Latte, Medium	16 oz	190	4.5	40	2.5	0	15	70	33	0	5	1/2 whole milk, 2 carb
Iced Latte with Sugar Free Vanilla Syrup	16 oz	90	5	40	3	0	15	105	14	0	5	1/2 whole milk, 1/2 carb
PANDA EXPRESS												
Chicken												
Black Pepper Chicken	5.5 oz	200	11	100	2.5	0	90	740	11	2	14	1 carb, 2 med-fat meat
Broccoli Chicken	5.5 oz	180	9	80	2	0	65	630	11	3	13	1 carb, 1 med-fat meat, 1 fat
Kung Pao Chicken	6.1 oz	300	20	180	4	0	110	900	13	2	20	1 carb, 2 med-fat meat, 2 fat
Mandarin Chicken	5.8 oz	310	16	150	4	0	115	740	8	0	34	1/2 carb, 4 lean meat
Orange Chicken	5.4 oz	400	20	170	3.5	0	90	640	42	0	15	3 carb, 1 med-fat meat, 3 fat

	Size	Cal									Exchanges
Pineapple Chicken	6.5 oz	230	10	90	2	0	75	710	21	2	13	1 1/2 carb, 1 med-fat meat, 1 fat
Pineapple Chicken Breast	6.1 oz	230	12	110	2	0	30	560	19	1	11	1 carb, 1 med-fat meat, 1 fat
Potato Chicken	6 oz	190	9	80	2	0	70	660	13	3	12	1 carb, 1 med-fat meat, 1 fat
String Bean Chicken	6 oz	190	9	80	2	0	70	660	13	3	12	1 carb, 1 med-fat meat, 1 fat
String Bean Chicken Breast	6 oz	200	12	100	2	0	30	550	12	2	10	1 carb, 1 med-fat meat, 1 fat
Sweet & Sour Chicken	5.5 oz	400	17	150	3	0	40	370	46	1	15	3 carb, 1 med-fat meat, 2 fat
Thai Cashew Chicken Breast	6.3 oz	330	22	190	3.5	0	35	630	17	2	15	1 carb, 2 med-fat meat, 2 fat
Beef											
Beijing Beef	4.9 oz	660	41	360	7	0	60	860	52	4	24	3 1/2 carb, 2 med-fat meat, 6 fat

FAST FOOD

	Serving	Calories	Fat (g)	Cal. from Fat	Sat. Fat (g)	Trans Fat (g)	Chol. (mg)	Sod. (mg)	Carb. (g)	Fiber (g)	Prot. (g)	Servings/Exchanges
Broccoli Beef	5.4 oz	150	6	50	1.5	0	25	720	12	3	11	1 carb, 1 med-fat meat
Mongolian Beef	6.1 oz	200	9	80	2	0	40	830	16	3	15	1 carb, 2 med-fat meat
Pork												
BBQ Pork	4.6 oz	360	19	180	8	0	120	1310	12	1	34	1 carb, 4 med-fat meat
Sweet & Sour Pork	5.6 oz	400	23	210	4.5	0	30	360	36	2	13	2 1/2 carb, 1 med-fat meat, 4 fat
Shrimp												
Crispy Shrimp	3.5 oz	260	13	120	2.5	0	60	810	26	1	9	2 carb, 3 fat
Kung Pao Shrimp	6.4 oz	230	14	130	2.5	0	110	850	13	2	13	1 carb, 1 med-fat meat, 2 fat
Tangy Shrimp	5.3 oz	140	4.5	40	1	0	85	660	16	1	8	1 carb, 1 med-fat meat
Veggies												
Eggplant & Tofu	6.1 oz	310	24	220	3	0	0	680	19	3	7	1 carb, 1 med-fat meat, 4 fat

Mixed Veggies, Side	4.8 oz	100	6	60	1	0	0	220	7	3	3	1 vegetable. 1 fat
Mixed Veggies, Entrée	9.6 oz	190	13	120	2	0	0	440	14	5	5	3 vegetable, 3 fat
Rice & Noodles												
Chow Mein	8.3 oz	400	12	110	2	0	0	1060	61	8	12	4 carb, 2 fat
Fried Rice	10 oz	570	18	160	4	0	130	900	85	8	16	5 1/2 carb, 4 fat
Steamed Rice	8.7 oz	420	0	0	0	0	0	0	93	0	8	6 carb
Appetizers												
Chicken Egg Roll	3 oz, 1 roll	200	12	100	4	0	20	390	16	2	8	1 carb, 1 med-fat meat, 1 fat
Chicken Potsticker	3.3 oz, 3 pcs	220	11	100	2.5	0	20	280	23	1	7	1 1/2 carb, 1 med-fat meat, 1 fat
Cream Cheese Rangoon	2.4 oz, 3 pcs	190	8	70	5	0	35	180	24	2	5	1 1/2 carb, 2 fat
Veggie Spring Roll	3.4 oz, 2 rolls	160	7	60	1	0	0	540	22	4	4	1 1/2 carb, 1 fat
Soup												
Hot & Sour Soup	10.6 oz	90	3.5	30	0.5	0	65	970	12	1	4	1 carb, 1 fat

FAST FOOD

	Serving	Calories	Fat (g)	Cal. from Fat	Sat. Fat (g)	Trans Fat (g)	Chol. (mg)	Sod. (mg)	Carb. (g)	Fiber (g)	Prot. (g)	Servings/Exchanges
Sauces & Cookie												
Fortune Cookie	1	32	0	2	0	0	0	8	7	0	1	1/2 carb
Mandarin Sauce	1.8 oz	160	0	0	0	0	0	340	40	0	0	2 1/2 carb
Sweet & Sour Sauce	1.8 oz	80	0	0	0	0	0	180	21	0	0	1 1/2 carb
PAPA JOHN'S												
Original Crust, Large (14 inches)												
Cheese	1 slice	280	10	90	3	0	15	700	38	2	12	2 1/2 carb, 1 med-fat meat, 1 fat
Pepperoni	1 slice	310	13	120	4	0	20	810	38	2	13	2 1/2 carb, 1 med-fat meat, 2 fat
Sausage	1 slice	330	15	130	4.5	0	20	810	37	3	13	2 1/2 carb, 1 med-fat meat, 2 fat
The Meats	1 slice	350	16	140	5	0	30	930	38	2	15	2 1/2 carb, 2 med-fat meat, 1 fat

Garden Fresh	1 slice	280	9	80	2.5	0	15	680	39	2	11	2 1/2 carb, 1 med-fat meat, 1 fat
The Works	1 slice	330	11	100	6	0	25	890	39	3	14	2 1/2 carb, 1 med-fat meat, 1 fat
Spinach Alfredo	1 slice	280	11	100	4.5	0	20	630	36	2	11	2 1/2 carb, 1 med-fat meat, 1 fat
Tuscan Six Cheese	1 slice	320	13	110	4.5	0	25	780	38	2	15	2 1/2 carb, 1 med-fat meat, 2 fat
Spicy Italian	1 slice	370	11	100	10	0	30	960	38	4	15	2 1/2 carb, 1 med-fat meat, 1 fat
BBQ Chicken & Bacon	1 slice	340	11	100	3.5	0	30	960	44	2	15	3 carb, 1 med-fat meat, 1 fat
Hawaiian BBQ Chicken	1 slice	340	11	100	3.5	0	30	960	46	2	16	3 carb, 1 med-fat meat, 1 fat

Thin Crust, Large (14 inches)

| Cheese | 1 slice | 220 | 12 | 100 | 3 | 0 | 15 | 490 | 21 | 1 | 9 | 1 1/2 carb, 1 med-fat meat, 1 fat |

FAST FOOD

	Serving	Calories	Fat (g)	Cal. from Fat	Sat. Fat (g)	Trans Fat (g)	Chol. (mg)	Sod. (mg)	Carb. (g)	Fiber (g)	Prot. (g)	Servings/Exchanges
Sausage	1 slice	270	16	150	5	0	20	600	21	2	9	1 1/2 carb, 1 med-fat meat, 2 fat
The Meats	1 slice	280	17	160	5	0	30	720	21	1	12	1 1/2 carb, 1 med-fat meat, 2 fat
Garden Fresh	1 slice	210	11	90	2.5	0	15	470	23	2	8	1 1/2 carb, 1 med-fat meat, 1 fat
The Works	1 slice	260	13	110	6	0	25	680	22	2	11	1 1/2 carb, 1 med-fat meat, 2 fat
Spinach Alfredo	1 slice	220	13	110	4.5	0	20	420	19	1	8	1 carb, 1 med-fat meat, 2 fat
Tuscan Six Cheese	1 slice	250	14	130	5	0	25	580	21	1	12	1 1/2 carb, 1 med-fat meat, 2 fat
Spicy Italian	1 slice	310	13	110	11	0	30	760	22	3	12	1 1/2 carb, 1 med-fat meat, 2 fat
BBQ Chicken & Bacon	1 slice	270	13	110	3.5	0	30	750	27	<1	12	2 carb, 1 med-fat meat, 2 fat

	Serving											Exchanges
Hawaiian BBQ Chicken	1 slice	290	14	120	3.5	0	30	740	31	1	13	2 carb, 1 med-fat meat, 2 fat
Pan Crust, Large (14 inches)												
Cheese	1 slice	410	23	200	7	0	20	750	38	1	13	2 1/2 carb, 1 med-fat meat, 4 fat
Pepperoni	1 slice	410	24	210	8	0	20	820	37	1	13	2 1/2 carb, 1 med-fat meat, 4 fat
Sausage	1 slice	420	25	230	8	0	20	790	37	2	12	2 1/2 carb, 1 med-fat meat, 4 fat
The Meats	1 slice	440	28	230	8	0	30	890	37	1	15	2 1/2 carb, 1 med-fat meat, 1 fat
Garden Fresh	1 slice	370	19	170	6	0	15	660	39	2	11	2 1/2 carb, 1 med-fat meat, 3 fat
The Works	1 slice	420	21	190	9	0	25	860	38	2	14	2 1/2 carb, 1 med-fat meat, 3 fat
Spinach Alfredo	1 slice	380	22	200	8	0	20	610	35	1	11	2 carb, 1 med-fat meat, 3 fat

FAST FOOD

	Serving	Calories	Fat (g)	Cal. from Fat	Sat. Fat (g)	Trans Fat (g)	Chol. (mg)	Sod. (mg)	Carb. (g)	Fiber (g)	Prot. (g)	Servings/Exchanges
Tuscan Six Cheese	1 slice	410	23	200	8	0	25	760	37	1	15	2 1/2 carb, 1 med-fat meat, 4 fat
Spicy Italian	1 slice	470	21	190	14	0	30	950	38	3	15	2 1/2 carb, 1 med-fat meat, 3 fat
BBQ Chicken & Bacon	1 slice	430	22	200	7	0	30	940	43	1	15	3 carb, 1 med-fat meat, 3 fat
Hawaiian BBQ Chicken	1 slice	440	22	200	7	0	30	940	45	1	15	3 carb, 1 med-fat meat, 3 fat
Side Items												
BBQ Wings	2	160	10	90	3	0	85	560	4	0	14	2 med-fat meat
Bread Sticks	2	290	4.5	40	0.5	0	0	540	53	2	9	3 1/2 carb, 1 fat
Buffalo Wings	2	160	11	100	3.5	0	90	680	1	1	14	2 med-fat meat
Cheese Sticks	4	370	16	150	4.5	0	25	830	42	2	15	3 carb, 1 med-fat meat, 2 fat

Chicken Strips	2	160	8	70	2	0	25	350	10	0	10	1/2 carb, 1 med-fat meat, 1 fat
Cinnamon Sweetsticks	4 sticks	580	16	140	4.5	0	0	740	98	3	11	6 1/2 carb, 3 fat
Cinnaple	4 sticks	560	19	170	6	0	0	540	90	2	8	6 carb, 4 fat
Garlic Parmesan Bread Sticks	2	330	10	90	1.5	0	0	720	54	2	10	3 1/2 carb, 2 fat
Honey Chipotle Wings	2	190	12	110	3	0	50	730	8	0	12	1/2 carb, 1 med-fat meat, 1 fat
Cheese Sauce	1	40	3.5	30	1	0	0	160	2	0	1	1 fat
Garlic Sauce	1	150	17	150	3	0	0	310	0	0	0	3 fat
Pizza Sauce	1	20	1	10	0	0	0	230	3	0	0	free
Ranch	1	100	10	90	1.5	0	10	260	1	0	1	2 fat
Honey Mustard	1	150	15	140	2.5	0	10	120	5	0	0	3 fat

PIZZA HUT

P'Zone

All Natural Pepperoni	1/2 order	630	24	220	11	0.5	70	1580	76	2	28	5 carb, 2 med-fat meat, 3 fat

FAST FOOD

	Serving	Calories	Fat (g)	Cal. from Fat	Sat. Fat (g)	Trans Fat (g)	Chol. (mg)	Sod. (mg)	Carb. (g)	Fiber (g)	Prot. (g)	Servings/Exchanges
Classic	1/2 order	630	23	210	11	0.5	65	1480	77	3	28	5 carb, 2 med-fat meat, 3 fat
Meaty	1/2 order	740	33	300	15	1	95	1840	76	3	34	5 carb, 3 med-fat meat, 4 fat
Appetizers												
Baked Hot Wings	2	120	7	70	2	0	65	500	1	0	11	2 lean meat
Bread Sticks	1	140	6	60	1.5	0	0	240	18	1	4	1 carb, 1 fat
Cheese Breadsticks	1	180	7	70	3.5	0	15	370	20	1	7	1 carb, 1 fat
Wing Ranch Dipping Sauce	1.5 oz	220	23	210	4	0	25	400	3	0	1	5 fat
Marinara Dipping Sauce	3 oz	60	0	0	0	0	0	440	12	2	2	1 carb
Desserts												
Cinnamon Sticks	2 pieces	170	6	50	1.5	0	0	200	26	1	4	2 carb, 1 fat
White Icing Dipping Cup	2 oz	190	0	0	0	0	0	0	47	0	0	3 carb

14-Inch Large Pan Pizzas

Cheese	1 slice	350	14	140	6	0	35	740	37	2	15	2 1/2 carb, 1 med-fat meat, 2 fat
All Natural Pepperoni	1 slice	370	18	160	7	0	35	850	37	2	15	2 1/2 carb, 1 med-fat meat, 3 fat
Ham & Pineapple	1 slice	320	13	110	5	0	25	740	38	2	14	2 1/2 carb, 1 med-fat meat, 2 fat
Supreme	1 slice	400	20	180	8	0	40	890	38	2	17	2 1/2 carb, 1 med-fat meat, 4 fat
Dan's Original	1 slice	400	20	180	8	0	40	890	37	2	17	2 1/2 carb, 1 med-fat meat, 3 fat
Meat Lover's	1 slice	470	27	240	10	0	60	1170	37	2	21	2 1/2 carb, 2 med-fat meat, 3 fat
Veggie Lover's	1 slice	320	13	120	4.5	0	20	690	38	2	13	2 1/2 carb, 1 med-fat meat, 2 fat
All Natural Pepperoni & Mushroom	1 slice	340	15	140	6	0	30	740	37	2	14	2 1/2 carb, 1 med-fat meat, 2 fat

FAST FOOD

	Serving	Calories	Fat (g)	Cal. from Fat	Sat. Fat (g)	Trans Fat (g)	Chol. (mg)	Sod. (mg)	Carb. (g)	Fiber (g)	Prot. (g)	Servings/Exchanges
Triple Meat Italiano	1 slice	410	21	190	8	0	45	1010	37	2	18	2 1/2 carb, 2 med-fat meat, 2 fat
14-Inch Large Thin 'N Crispy Pizzas												
Cheese	1 slice	260	11	100	6	0	35	740	29	1	12	2 carb, 1 med-fat meat, 1 fat
All Natural Pepperoni	1 slice	290	14	120	6	0	35	860	28	1	12	2 carb, 1 med-fat meat, 2 fat
Ham & Pineapple	1 slice	240	9	80	4	0	25	750	31	1	11	2 carb, 1 med-fat meat, 1 fat
Supreme	1 slice	320	16	150	7	0	40	900	30	2	14	2 carb, 1 med-fat meat, 2 fat
Dan's Original	1 slice	320	16	150	7	0	40	900	29	2	15	2 carb, 1 med-fat meat, 2 fat
Meat Lover's	1 slice	400	23	210	9	0	60	1190	29	1	19	2 carb, 2 med-fat meat, 3 fat

Veggie Lover's	1 slice	240	9	80	4	0	20	710	30	2	10	2 carb, 1 med-fat meat, 1 fat
All Natural Pepperoni & Mushroom	1 slice	260	11	100	5	0	30	740	29	1	12	2 carb, 1 med-fat meat, 1 fat
Triple Meat Italiano	1 slice	320	17	150	7	0	45	1010	28	1	15	2 carb, 1 med-fat meat, 2 fat
14-Inch Large Hand-Tossed Style Pizzas												
Cheese	1 slice	320	12	110	6	0	35	820	38	2	15	2 1/2 carb, 1 med-fat meat, 1 fat
All Natural Pepperoni	1 slice	340	15	130	7	0	35	930	37	2	14	2 1/2 carb, 1 med-fat meat, 2 fat
Ham & Pineapple	1 slice	300	10	90	5	0	25	820	39	2	13	2 1/2 carb, 1 med-fat meat, 1 fat
Supreme	1 slice	380	17	160	8	0	40	970	39	3	16	2 1/2 carb, 1 med-fat meat, 2 fat
Dan's Original	1 slice	370	17	160	8	0	40	970	38	2	17	2 1/2 carb, 1 med-fat meat, 2 fat

FAST FOOD

	Serving	Calories	Fat (g)	Cal. from Fat	Sat. Fat (g)	Trans Fat (g)	Chol. (mg)	Sod. (mg)	Carb. (g)	Fiber (g)	Prot. (g)	Servings/Exchanges
Meat Lover's	1 slice	450	24	210	10	0	60	1250	38	2	20	2 1/2 carb, 2 med-fat meat, 3 fat
Veggie Lover's	1 slice	290	10	90	4.5	0	20	770	39	3	12	2 1/2 carb, 1 med-fat meat, 1 fat
Triple Meat Italiano	1 slice	380	18	160	8	0	45	1090	38	2	17	2 1/2 carb, 2 med-fat meat, 3 fat
All Natural Pepperoni & Mushroom	1 slice	310	12	110	6	0	30	820	38	2	14	2 1/2 carb, 1 med-fat meat, 1 fat
14-Inch Large Stuffed Crust Pizzas												
Cheese	1 slice	340	14	130	8	0	40	910	39	2	15	2 1/2 carb, 1 med-fat meat, 2 fat
All Natural Pepperoni	1 slice	380	18	160	8	0	45	1060	39	2	16	2 1/2 carb, 1 med-fat meat, 3 fat
Ham & Pineapple	1 slice	330	13	110	7	0	35	940	41	2	15	2 1/2 carb, 1 med-fat meat, 2 fat

	Amount	Calories	Fat (g)	Cal. from Fat	Sat. Fat (g)	Trans Fat (g)	Chol. (mg)	Sod. (mg)	Carb. (g)	Fiber (g)	Pro. (g)	Exchanges
Supreme	1 slice	410	20	180	9	0	50	1090	40	3	18	2 1/2 carb, 2 med-fat meat, 2 fat
Meat Lover's	1 slice	480	26	240	12	0.5	70	1370	39	2	22	2 1/2 carb, 2 med-fat meat, 3 fat
Veggie Lover's	1 slice	330	13	110	6	0	30	890	40	3	14	2 1/2 carb, 1 med-fat meat, 2 fat
Triple Meat Italiano	1 slice	440	23	200	11	0	65	1290	40	2	21	2 1/2 carb, 2 med-fat meat, 3 fat
All Natural Pepperoni & Mushroom	1 slice	350	15	130	7	0	40	940	39	2	15	2 1/2 carb, 1 med-fat meat, 2 fat

12 Large Fit 'N Delicious Pizzas

	Amount	Calories	Fat (g)	Cal. from Fat	Sat. Fat (g)	Trans Fat (g)	Chol. (mg)	Sod. (mg)	Carb. (g)	Fiber (g)	Pro. (g)	Exchanges
All Natural Chicken, Mushroom & Jalapeño	1 slice	180	4.5	40	1.5	0	25	710	22	1	12	1 1/2 carb, 1 med-fat meat
All Natural Chicken, Red Onion & Green Pepper	1 slice	180	4.5	40	1.5	0	25	500	24	1	11	1 1/2 carb, 1 med-fat meat
Green Pepper, Red Onion & Diced Tomato	1 slice	150	4	35	1.5	0	10	400	24	2	6	1 1/2 carb, 1 fat

FAST FOOD

	Serving	Calories	Fat (g)	Cal. from Fat	Sat. Fat (g)	Trans Fat (g)	Chol. (mg)	Sod. (mg)	Carb. (g)	Fiber (g)	Prot. (g)	Servings/Exchanges
Ham, Pineapple & Diced Red Tomato	1 slice	160	4.5	40	1.5	0	15	560	24	1	7	1 1/2 carb, 1 fat
Ham, Red Onion & Mushroom	1 slice	160	4.5	40	1.5	0	15	550	23	1	8	1 1/2 carb, 1 med-fat meat
Tomato, Mushroom & Jalapeño	1 slice	150	4	35	1.5	0	10	640	23	2	6	1 1/2 carb, 1 fat
Tuscani Pastas (1/4 Full Pan or 1/2 Half Pan)												
All Natural Chicken Alfredo	1 piece	640	33	300	11	0.5	70	1190	56	4	28	3 1/2 carb, 3 med-fat meat, 4 fat
Bacon Mac 'N Cheese	1 piece	520	22	200	12	0.5	60	1170	54	4	24	3 1/2 carb, 2 med-fat meat, 2 fat
Lasagna	1 piece	570	30	270	13	1	105	1670	45	5	29	3 carb, 3 med-fat meat, 3 fat
Meaty Marinara	1 piece	510	24	220	10	1	80	1310	48	5	25	3 carb, 2 med-fat meat, 3 fat

RUBIOS

Burritos

	Amount											
Baja Grill, Chicken	1	620	26	230	9	NA	125	1890	53	4	46	3 1/2 carb, 5 med-fat meat
Baja Grill, Steak	1	670	34	310	14	NA	100	2320	53	4	38	3 1/2 carb, 4 med-fat meat, 3 fat
Bean & Cheese	1	700	33	290	17	NA	85	1750	75	12	29	5 carb, 2 med-fat meat, 5 fat
Big Burrito Especial Chicken	1	830	32	290	7	NA	80	2030	99	7	38	6 1/2 carb, 3 med-fat meat, 3 fat
Big Burrito Especial Steak	1	870	38	350	11	NA	65	2360	99	7	32	6 1/2 carb, 2 med-fat meat, 6 fat
Carnitas Rajas	1	740	39	360	13	NA	85	1970	75	4	34	5 carb, 3 med-fat meat, 5 fat
Fish	1	710	40	360	8	NA	80	1520	71	6	25	4 1/2 carb, 2 med-fat meat, 6 fat
Grilled Shrimp	1	710	34	300	11	NA	220	2100	72	5	30	5 carb, 2 med-fat meat, 5 fat

FAST FOOD

	Serving	Calories	Fat (g)	Cal. from Fat	Sat. Fat (g)	Trans Fat (g)	Chol. (mg)	Sod. (mg)	Carb. (g)	Fiber (g)	Prot. (g)	Servings/Exchanges
Grilled Veggie	1	630	29	260	9	NA	35	1290	73	4	19	5 carb, 6 fat
HealthMe, Chicken	1	500	10	90	2.5	NA	70	1700	70	6	34	4 1/2 carb, 3 lean meat
HealthMe, Mahi Mahi	1	510	15	130	3	NA	25	1190	68	6	29	4 1/2 carb, 2 med-fat meat, 1 fat
Mahi Mahi	1	700	42	380	12	NA	65	1150	49	4	34	3 carb, 3 med-fat meat, 5 fat
Tacos												
Carnitas Rajas	1	210	11	100	2	NA	20	420	23	3	9	1 1/2 carb, 1 med-fat meat, 1 fat
Especial Fish	1	330	20	180	4.5	NA	50	510	30	4	13	2 carb, 1 med-fat meat, 3 fat
Garlic Herb Shrimp	1	360	22	200	7	NA	80	580	23	3	19	1 1/2 carb, 2 med-fat meat, 2 fat
Grilled Chicken	1	280	15	130	4	NA	40	450	22	3	15	1 1/2 carb, 2 med-fat meat, 1 fat

Grilled Chicken, Gourmet	1	360	21	190	7	NA	65	670	23	3	22	1 1/2 carb, 3 med-fat meat, 1 fat
Grilled Mahi Mahi	1	300	17	160	4	NA	25	250	22	4	15	1 1/2 carb, 2 med-fat meat, 1 fat
Grilled Portobello & Poblano	1	310	19	170	6	NA	25	340	25	4	12	1 1/2 carb, 1 med-fat meat, 3 fat
Grilled Shrimp	1	230	12	110	2	NA	90	540	22	3	9	1 1/2 carb, 1 med-fat meat, 1 fat
Grilled Steak	1	220	10	90	4	NA	30	520	22	3	13	1 1/2 carb, 1 med-fat meat, 1 fat
Grilled Steak, Gourmet	1	370	23	210	8	NA	55	800	23	3	20	1 1/2 carb, 3 med-fat meat, 2
HealthMe, Chicken	1	150	1.5	15	0	NA	30	400	21	3	12	1 1/2 carb, 1 lean meat
HealthMe, Mahi Mahi	1	160	4	35	0.5	NA	10	200	21	3	12	1 1/2 carb, 1 med-fat meat
Street Taco, Carnitas	1	100	5	45	1.5	NA	20	250	9	2	7	1/2 carb, 1 med-fat meat
Street Taco, Chicken	1	100	4	30	0.5	NA	25	240	9	2	10	1/2 carb, 1 med-fat meat

FAST FOOD

	Serving	Calories	Fat (g)	Cal. from Fat	Sat. Fat (g)	Trans Fat (g)	Chol. (mg)	Sod. (mg)	Carb. (g)	Fiber (g)	Prot. (g)	Servings/Exchanges
Street Taco, Steak	1	120	6	50	2	NA	20	380	9	2	8	1/2 carb, 1 med-fat meat
World Famous	1	270	14	130	2	NA	35	420	29	3	10	2 carb, 1 med-fat meat, 2 fat
Kid's Meals												
Bean & Cheese Burrito	1	530	23	200	11	NA	50	1200	63	8	20	4 carb, 1 med-fat meat, 4 fat
Cheese Quesadilla	1	500	27	240	14	NA	70	1030	44	1	23	3 carb, 2 med-fat meat, 3 fat
Taquitos	2	230	10	90	4.5	NA	50	270	21	2	15	1 1/2 carb, 1 med-fat meat, 1 fat
Rubio's Favorites												
Cheese Quesadilla	1	1070	67	600	28	NA	125	1820	85	8	38	5 1/2 carb, 3 med-fat meat, 10 fat
Chicken Quesadilla	1	1190	69	620	29	NA	195	2370	87	8	61	6 carb, 7 med-fat meat, 7 fat

Chicken Taquitos	3	270	8	70	2	NA	45	360	33	4	16	2 carb, 1 med-fat meat, 1 fat
Nachos Grande	1	1270	78	710	27	NA	120	1850	112	20	37	7 carb, 2 med-fat meat, 14 fat
Nachos Grande Chicken	1	1390	80	720	28	NA	190	2400	114	20	60	7 1/2 carb, 5 med-fat meat, 11 fat
Nachos Grande Steak	1	1430	87	780	31	NA	175	2730	114	20	54	7 1/2 carb, 4 med-fat meat, 13 fat
Steak Quesadilla	1	1230	75	680	32	NA	175	2710	87	8	55	6 carb, 5 med-fat meat, 10 fat
Sides												
Black Beans, Regular	1	100	1	5	1	NA	0	340	17	2	6	1 carb
Black Beans, Large	1	280	0.5	5	0	NA	0	950	50	7	17	3 carb, 1 lean meat
Chips, Regular	1	260	13	120	1	NA	0	290	33	4	3	2 carb, 3 fat
Chips, Large	1	570	29	260	2.5	NA	0	650	74	9	7	5 carb, 6 fat
Churro	1	170	8	70	2	NA	20	140	22	0	2	1 1/2 carb, 2 fat
Guacamole & Chips	1	790	49	440	6	NA	0	920	85	16	10	5 1/2 carb, 5 fat

FAST FOOD

	Serving	Calories	Fat (g)	Cal. from Fat	Sat. Fat (g)	Trans Fat (g)	Chol. (mg)	Sod. (mg)	Carb. (g)	Fiber (g)	Prot. (g)	Servings/Exchanges
Pinto Beans, Regular	1	110	2	10	0.5	NA	0	340	22	8	2	1 1/2 carb
Pinto Beans, Large	1	300	2.5	25	1	NA	0	940	65	24	5	4 1/2 carb, 1 fat
Rice, Regular	1	120	1	10	0	NA	0	220	25	1	2	1 1/2 carb
Rice, Large	1	310	3	25	0	NA	0	580	67	2	5	4 1/2 carb, 1 fat
Salads, Wrapsalada, Bowls (dressing/sauce included)												
Chicken Chipotle Ranch Salad	1	520	35	310	6	NA	80	1460	24	6	30	1 1/2 carb, 4 med-fat meat, 3 fat
Chicken Chipotle Ranch Wrapsalada	1	770	42	380	8	NA	80	2070	65	9	36	4 carb, 3 med-fat meat, 5 fat
Chicken Chopped Salad	1	570	33	300	9	NA	100	1480	34	7	36	2 carb, 4 med-fat meat, 3 fat
Chicken Chopped Wrapsalada	1	800	40	360	10	NA	100	2070	72	9	41	5 carb, 4 med-fat meat, 4 fat
Chicken Fiesta Salad	1	590	46	410	11	NA	105	1130	13	4	32	1 carb, 4 med-fat meat, 5 fat

	Serving	Cal	Fat (g)	Fat Cal	Sat Fat (g)	Trans Fat	Chol (mg)	Sod (mg)	Carb (g)	Fiber (g)	Prot (g)	Exchanges/Choices
Chicken Fiesta Wrapsalada	1	830	53	480	12	NA	105	1740	53	8	38	3 1/2 carb, 4 med-fat meat, 7 fat
Chicken Tropical Salad	1	410	23	200	3.5	NA	75	720	25	5	27	1 1/2 carb, 3 med-fat meat, 2 fat
Chicken Tropical Wrapsalada	1	650	30	270	5	NA	75	1320	64	8	32	4 carb, 3 med-fat meat, 3 fat
STARBUCKS												
Brewed Coffees												
Caffè Misto/Caffè AuLait, 2% Milk	12 oz	80	3	30	2	0	15	70	7	0	5	1/2 low-fat milk
Iced Brewed Coffee	12 oz	60	0	0	0	0	0	0	15	0	0	1 carb
Iced Coffee, 2% Milk	12 oz	90	1	10	0.5	0	5	25	18	0	2	1 carb
Espresso, Hot												
Caffè Americano	12 oz	10	0	0	0	0	0	0	5	2	1	free
Caffè Latte, 2% Milk	12 oz	150	6	50	3.5	0	25	115	14	0	10	1 low-fat milk
Caffè Mocha, 2% Milk with Whipped Cream	12 oz	270	12	110	7	0	40	105	33	1	10	1 low-fat milk, 1 1/2 carb, 1 fat

FAST FOOD

	Serving	Calories	Fat (g)	Cal. from Fat	Sat. Fat (g)	Trans Fat (g)	Chol. (mg)	Sod. (mg)	Carb. (g)	Fiber (g)	Prot. (g)	Servings/Exchanges
Cappuccino, 2% Milk	12 oz	90	3.5	30	2	0	15	70	9	0	6	1 low-fat milk
Caramel Macchiato, 2% Milk	12 oz	180	5	45	3.5	0	20	100	25	0	8	1 low-fat milk, 1 carb
Espresso Solo	1 oz	5	0	0	0	0	0	0	1	0	0	free
Espresso Truffle with Whipped Cream	12 oz	360	15	130	9	0	35	115	45	5	15	1 low-fat milk, 2 carb, 2 fat
Peppermint Mocha with Whipped Cream	12 oz	320	13	120	7	0	40	100	46	2	10	1 low-fat meat, 2 carb, 2 fat
Skinny Caramel Latte, Nonfat Milk	12 oz	130	0	0	0	0	5	170	19	0	12	1 skim milk, 1/2 carb
Skinny Latte, Nonfat Milk	12 oz	100	0	0	0	0	5	120	15	0	10	1 skim milk
Skinny Vanilla Latte, Nonfat Milk	12 oz	90	0	0	0	0	5	125	14	0	9	1 skim milk
Vanilla Latte, 2% Milk	12 oz	190	5	45	3.5	0	20	110	27	0	9	1 low-fat milk, 1 carb

White Chocolate Mocha, 2% Milk with Whipped Cream	12 oz	370	15	130	10	0	45	190	48	0	12	1 low-fat milk, 2 1/2 carb, 2 fat

Espresso, Iced

Iced Caffè Americano	12 oz	10	0	0	0	0	0	5	2	0	1	free
Iced Caffè Latte, 2% Milk	12 oz	100	3.5	30	2.5	0	15	80	10	0	6	1 low-fat milk
Iced Caffè Mocha, 2% Milk with Whipped Cream	12 oz	230	12	110	7	0	40	70	29	1	7	1 low-fat milk, 1 carb, 1 fat
Iced Caramel Macchiato, 2% Milk	12 oz	170	5	45	3	0	20	95	24	0	7	1 low-fat milk, 1 carb
Iced Espresso Truffle with Whipped Cream	12 oz	270	13	120	8	0	40	75	29	3	8	1 low-fat milk, 1 carb, 2 fat
Iced Sugar Free Syrup Latte, 2% Milk	12 oz	90	3	30	2	0	15	85	9	0	6	1 low-fat milk

FAST FOOD

	Serving	Calories	Fat (g)	Cal. from Fat	Sat. Fat (g)	Trans Fat (g)	Chol. (mg)	Sod. (mg)	Carb. (g)	Fiber (g)	Prot. (g)	Servings/Exchanges
Iced Vanilla Latte, 2% Milk	12 oz	140	3	30	2	0	15	70	23	0	6	1 low-fat milk, 1 carb
Frappuccino Blended Coffee												
Caffè Vanilla with Whipped Cream	12 oz	320	10	90	6	0	40	190	52	0	4	3 carb, 2 fat
Caramel with Whipped Cream	12 oz	300	11	100	7	0	40	190	46	0	4	3 carb, 2 fat
Coffee	12 oz	180	2.5	20	1.5	0	10	170	37	0	4	2 1/2 carb, 1 fat
Mocha with Whipped Cream	12 oz	280	11	100	6	0	40	180	43	0	5	3 carb, 2 fat
Pumpkin Spice with Whipped Cream	12 oz	310	11	100	7	0	40	210	49	0	5	3 carb, 2 fat
Frappuccino Light Blended Coffee												
Caffè Vanilla	12 oz	140	0.5	5	0	0	0	180	30	2	4	2 carb

Caramel	12 oz	130	1	10	0	0	5	180	25	2	4	1 1/2 carb
Coffee	12 oz	90	0.5	5	0	0	0	160	18	2	4	1 carb
Mocha	12 oz	110	1	10	0	0	0	170	23	2	4	1 1/2 carb
Pumpkin	12 oz	120	0.5	5	0	0	0	190	25	2	5	1 1/2 carb
Frappuccino Blended Crème												
Double Chocolaty Chip with Whipped Cream	12 oz	380	14	120	8	0	35	240	59	2	11	4 carb, 3 fat
Pumpkin Spice with Whipped Cream	12 oz	360	10	90	5	0	35	280	58	0	10	4 carb, 2 fat
Strawberries & Crème with Whipped Cream	12 oz	360	10	90	6	0	30	310	58	1	9	4 carb, 2 fat
Vanilla Bean with Whipped Cream	12 oz	470	14	120	7	0	50	320	75	0	12	5 carb, 3 fat
Brownies, Cookies, Bars												
Chocolate Chunk Cookie	1	360	17	150	10	0	65	170	50	2	4	3 carb, 3 fat

FAST FOOD

	Serving	Calories	Fat (g)	Cal. from Fat	Sat. Fat (g)	Trans Fat (g)	Chol. (mg)	Sod. (mg)	Carb. (g)	Fiber (g)	Prot. (g)	Servings/Exchanges
Double Chocolate Brownie	1	410	24	220	7	0	95	75	46	3	6	3 carb, 5 fat
Marshmallow Dream Bar	1	210	4	35	2.5	0	10	250	43	0	1	3 carb, 1 fat
Outrageous Oatmeal Cookie	1	370	14	120	8	0	65	170	56	3	5	3 1/2 carb, 3 fat
Starbuck's Indulgent Cookie	1	320	19	170	11	0	60	85	40	3	4	2 1/2 carb, 4 fat
Rich Toffee Pecan Bar	1	380	22	200	8	0	85	120	42	<1	4	3 carb, 4 fat
Cakes, Pies, Tarts												
Cherry Cherry Pie	1 piece	370	19	170	11	0	40	410	46	2	4	3 carb, 4 fat
Luscious Lemon Tart	1	410	25	220	14	0.5	145	25	42	<1	5	3 carb, 5 fat
Croissants, Bagels												
Butter Croissant	1	310	18	160	11	1	45	290	32	<1	5	2 carb, 4 fat

Item	Serving											Exchanges
Chonga Bagel	1	310	5	50	2	0	0	10	540	52	3	12	3 1/2 carb, 1 fat
Doughnuts, Sweet Rolls, Danish												
Apple Fritter	1	420	20	180	9	0	0		360	59	1	5	4 carb, 4 fat
Cheese Danish	1	420	25	230	16	0	115		370	39	<1	7	2 1/2 carb, 5 fat
Chocolate Old Fashioned Doughnut	1	420	21	190	9	0	20		340	57	2	5	4 carb, 4 fat
Classic Glazed	1	420	21	190	10	0	15		260	57	<1	4	4 carb, 4 fat
Double Iced Cinnamon Roll	1	490	20	180	12	1	65		480	70	3	7	4 1/2 carb, 4 fat
Morning Bun	1	350	16	140	9	0	75		330	45	2	6	3 carb, 3 fat
Loaves, Coffee Cakes												
Banana Nut Bread	1 slice	480	19	170	2.5	0	25		210	73	4	7	5 carb, 4 fat
Classic Coffee Cake	1 slice	420	19	170	10	0	90		530	59	1	6	4 carb, 4 fat
Pumpkin Loaf	1 slice	320	12	110	2	0	45		400	50	1	5	3 carb, 2 fat
Reduced-Fat Cinnamon Swirl Coffee Cake	1 slice	290	7	60	3.5	0	10		390	55	2	4	3 1/2 carb, 1 fat

FAST FOOD

	Serving	Calories	Fat (g)	Cal. from Fat	Sat. Fat (g)	Trans Fat (g)	Chol. (mg)	Sod. (mg)	Carb. (g)	Fiber (g)	Prot. (g)	Servings/Exchanges
Reduced-Fat Very Berry Coffee Cake	1 slice	320	9	90	3.5	0	55	470	54	4	6	3 1/2 carb, 2 fat
Muffins, Scones												
Apple Bran Muffin	1	350	9	80	2.5	0	65	520	64	7	6	4 carb, 2 fat
Blueberry Scone	1	460	22	190	12	0.5	75	420	61	2	7	4 carb, 4 fat
Blueberry Streusel Muffin	1	360	11	100	6	0	80	390	59	2	7	4 carb, 2 fat
Petite Vanilla Bean Scone	1	140	5	45	2.5	0	15	90	21	0	0	1 1/2 carb, 1 fat
SUBWAY												
6-Inch Low Fat Sandwiches												
Black Forest Ham	1	290	4.5	40	1	0	25	1200	47	5	18	3 carb, 1 med-fat meat
Oven Roasted Chicken Breast	1	320	4.5	40	1	0	25	750	49	5	23	3 carb, 2 lean meat

												Exchanges/Choices
Roast Beef	1	310	4.5	40	1.5	0	25	840	46	5	26	3 carb, 2 lean meat
Subway Club	1	320	5	45	1.5	0	35	1160	47	5	26	3 carb, 2 lean meat
Sweet Onion Chicken Teriyaki	1	380	4.5	40	1	0	50	1010	60	5	26	4 carb, 2 lean meat
Turkey Breast	1	280	3.5	30	1	0	20	920	47	5	18	3 carb, 1 med-fat meat
Veggie Delite	1	230	2.5	20	0.5	0	0	410	45	5	8	3 carb, 1 fat
6-Inch Sandwiches												
Big Philly Cheesesteak	1	520	18	160	9	0.5	90	1570	53	6	39	3 1/2 carb, 4 med-fat meat
BLT	1	360	13	120	6	0	30	990	45	5	17	3 carb, 1 med-fat meat, 2 fat
Chicken & Bacon Ranch	1	570	28	250	10	0.5	95	1190	49	6	35	3 carb, 4 med-fat meat, 2 fat
Cold Cut Combo	1	410	16	150	6	0.5	60	1450	48	5	21	3 carb, 2 med-fat meat, 1 fat
Italian BMT	1	450	20	180	8	0.5	55	1730	48	5	22	3 carb, 2 med-fat meat, 2 fat

FAST FOOD

	Serving	Calories	Fat (g)	Cal. from Fat	Sat. Fat (g)	Trans Fat (g)	Chol. (mg)	Sod. (mg)	Carb. (g)	Fiber (g)	Prot. (g)	Servings/Exchanges
Meatball Marinara	1	580	23	200	9	1	45	1530	70	9	24	4 1/2 carb, 2 med-fat meat, 3 fat
Spicy Italian	1	520	28	250	11	0.5	65	1830	47	5	22	3 carb, 2 med-fat meat, 4 fat
Subway Melt	1	380	11	100	5	0	45	1530	49	5	25	3 carb, 2 med-fat meat
The Feast	1	540	22	200	9	0.5	85	2470	50	5	39	3 carb, 4 med-fat meat
Tuna	1	530	30	270	6	0.5	45	930	46	5	21	3 carb, 2 med-fat meat, 4 fat
Flatbread Sandwiches												
Black Forest Ham	1	320	7	60	1.5	0	25	1270	47	3	18	3 carb, 1 med-fat meat
Oven Roasted Chicken Breast	1	350	7	70	1.5	0	25	820	48	3	24	3 carb, 2 lean meat
Roast Beef	1	340	8	70	2	0	25	920	45	3	27	3 carb, 3 lean meat
Subway Club	1	350	8	70	1.5	0	35	1230	47	3	26	3 carb, 2 med-fat meat

Sweet Onion Teriyaki	1	410	7	70	1.5	0	50	1080	59	3	26	4 carb, 2 lean meat
Turkey Breast	1	310	6	60	1	0	20	990	47	3	18	3 carb, 1 med-fat meat
Veggie Delite	1	260	5	45	1	0	0	490	44	3	9	3 carb, 1 fat

Salads (dressing & croutons not included)

Ham	1	110	3	25	1	0	25	850	12	4	12	2 vegetable, 1 lean meat
Oven Roasted Chicken Breast	1	130	2.5	25	0.5	0	50	280	10	4	20	2 vegetable, 2 lean meat
Roast Beef	1	140	3.5	30	1	0	25	500	10	4	21	2 vegetable, 2 lean meat
Subway Club	1	140	3.5	30	1	0	35	810	12	4	20	2 vegetable, 2 lean meat
Sweet Onion Chicken Teriyaki	1	200	3	30	1	0	50	660	25	4	20	1 1/2 carb, 2 lean meat
Turkey Breast	1	110	2	20	0.5	0	20	570	12	4	12	2 vegetable, 1 lean meat

FAST FOOD

	Serving	Calories	Fat (g)	Cal. from Fat	Sat. Fat (g)	Trans Fat (g)	Chol. (mg)	Sod. (mg)	Carb. (g)	Fiber (g)	Prot. (g)	Servings/Exchanges
Veggie Delite	1	50	1	10	0	0	0	65	10	4	3	2 vegetable
Salad Dressing												
Fat Free Italian	1 pkg	35	0	0	0	0	0	720	7	0	1	1/2 carb
Ranch	1 pkg	290	30	270	4.5	0.5	15	540	3	0	1	6 fat
Breakfast Sandwiches, 6-Inch Bread												
Black Forest Ham & Cheese	1	450	19	170	7	0	200	1450	47	5	27	3 carb, 3 med-fat meat, 1 fat
Cheese	1	420	18	160	7	0	190	1060	46	5	22	3 carb, 2 med-fat meat, 2 fat
Double Bacon & Cheese	1	520	25	220	11	0	210	1440	47	5	29	3 carb, 3 med-fat meat, 2 fat
Mega	1	720	45	400	18	0	235	1580	47	5	33	3 carb, 3 med-fat meat, 6 fat
Sausage & Cheese	1	670	41	370	16	0	225	1390	46	5	30	3 carb, 3 med-fat meat, 5 fat

Item	Serving	Cal.	Fat (g)	Fat Cal.	Sat. Fat (g)	Trans Fat (g)	Chol. (mg)	Sod. (mg)	Carb. (g)	Fiber (g)	Pro. (g)	Exchanges/Choices
Western Egg with Cheese	1	450	19	170	7	0	200	1460	48	5	27	3 carb, 3 med-fat meat, 1 fat
Cookies & Desserts												
Apple Pie	1	250	10	90	2	0	NA	290	37	1	0	2 1/2 carb, 2 fat
Apple Slices	1 pkg	35	0	0	0	0	0	0	9	2	0	1/2 fruit
Chocolate Chip Cookie	1	210	10	90	6	0	15	150	30	1	2	2 carb, 2 fat
Chocolate Chunk Cookie	1	220	10	90	5	0	10	100	30	<1	2	2 carb, 2 fat
M&M Cookie	1	210	10	90	5	0	10	100	32	<1	2	2 carb, 2 fat
Oatmeal Raisin Cookie	1	200	8	70	4	0	15	170	30	1	3	2 carb, 2 fat
Peanut Butter Cookie	1	220	12	110	5	0	15	190	26	1	4	2 carb, 2 fat
Sugar Cookie	1	220	12	110	6	0	15	140	28	<1	2	2 carb, 2 fat
White Chip Macadamia Nut Cookie	1	220	11	100	5	0	15	160	29	<1	2	2 carb, 2 fat
Soup												
Chicken & Dumpling	10 oz	170	6	45	2	0	35	810	23	2	8	1 1/2 carb, 1 med-fat meat

FAST FOOD

	Serving	Calories	Fat (g)	Cal. from Fat	Sat. Fat (g)	Trans Fat (g)	Chol. (mg)	Sod. (mg)	Carb. (g)	Fiber (g)	Prot. (g)	Servings/Exchanges
Chicken Tortilla	10 oz	110	1.5	20	0.5	0	10	440	11	3	6	1 carb
Chili Con Carne	10 oz	340	11	100	5	0	60	650	35	10	20	2 carb, 2 med-fat meat
Chipotle Chicken Corn Chowder	10 oz	140	3	30	1.5	0	15	900	22	2	6	1 1/2 carb, 1 fat
Cream of Potato with Bacon	10 oz	240	13	120	5	0	15	870	26	3	5	2 carb, 3 fat
Golden Broccoli & Cheese	10 oz	180	11	100	5	0	25	990	16	4	5	1 carb, 2 fat
Minestrone	10 oz	90	1	10	0	0	<5	910	17	3	4	1 carb
New England Style Clam Chowder	10 oz	150	5	45	1	0	10	990	20	4	6	1 carb, 1 fat
Roasted Chicken Noodle	10 oz	80	2	20	0.5	0	15	950	12	1	6	1 carb
Vegetable Beef	10 oz	100	2	20	0.5	0	10	960	17	3	5	1 carb

TACO BELL

Fresco Menu

Crunchy Taco	1	150	7	70	2.5	0	20	350	12	3	7	1 carb, 1 med-fat meat
Soft Taco, Beef	1	180	7	60	3	0	20	640	22	3	8	1 1/2 carb, 1 med-fat meat
Ranchero Chicken Soft Taco	1	170	4	35	1.5	0	25	740	22	2	12	1 1/2 carb, 1 med-fat meat
Grilled Steak Soft Taco	1	160	4.5	40	1.5	0	15	600	21	2	9	1 1/2 carb, 1 med-fat meat
Burrito Supreme, Chicken	1	340	8	70	2.5	0	25	1390	49	6	18	3 carb, 1 med-fat meat, 1 fat
Burrito Supreme, Steak	1	330	8	70	2.5	0	15	1310	49	6	15	3 carb, 1 med-fat meat, 1 fat

Value Menu

Bean Burrito	1	350	9	80	3.5	0.5	5	1220	54	9	13	3 1/2 carb, 1 med-fat meat, 1 fat

FAST FOOD

	Serving	Calories	Fat (g)	Cal. from Fat	Sat. Fat (g)	Trans Fat (g)	Chol. (mg)	Sod. (mg)	Carb. (g)	Fiber (g)	Prot. (g)	Servings/Exchanges
Caramel Apple Empanada	1	310	15	140	2.5	0	0	310	39	2	3	2 1/2 carb, 3 fat
Cheese Roll-Up	1	200	10	90	5	0	20	530	19	2	9	1 carb, 1 med-fat meat, 1 fat
Cinnamon Twists	1 order	170	7	60	0	0	0	200	26	1	1	2 carb, 1 fat
Crispy Potato Soft Taco	1	260	13	120	3	0	10	690	31	3	6	2 carb, 3 fat
Crunchy Taco	1	170	10	90	3.5	0	30	330	12	3	8	1 carb, 1 med-fat meat, 1 fat
Grilled Chicken Soft Taco	1	440	20	180	5	0	40	1260	48	3	16	3 carb, 1 med-fat meat, 3 fat
Grilled Chicken Soft Taco	1	200	8	70	3	0	35	640	19	1	12	1 carb, 1 med-fat meat, 1 fat
Soft Taco	1	210	9	80	4	0	30	620	21	3	10	1 1/2 carb, 1 med-fat meat, 1 fat
Triple Layer Nachos	1	340	18	160	1.5	0	0	720	38	6	7	2 1/2 carb, 4 fat

Tacos

Crunchy Taco Supreme	1	200	12	100	5	0	35	350	15	3	9	1 carb, 1 med-fat meat, 1 fat
Double Decker Taco	1	320	13	120	4.5	0.5	30	800	38	7	14	2 1/2 carb, 1 med-fat meat, 2 fat
Double Decker Taco Supreme	1	350	15	140	6	1	35	820	40	7	14	2 1/2 carb, 1 med-fat meat, 2 fat
Grilled Steak Soft Taco	1	250	14	130	4	0	30	710	20	2	11	1 carb, 1 med-fat meat, 2 fat
Ranchero Chicken Soft Taco	1	270	14	120	4	0	40	840	21	2	14	1 1/2 carb, 1 med-fat meat, 2 fat
Soft Taco Supreme, Beef	1	240	11	100	5	0	35	650	24	3	11	1 1/2 carb, 1 med-fat meat, 1 fat

Gorditas

Gordita Baja, Beef	1	360	21	190	5	0	35	800	30	5	13	2 carb, 1 med-fat meat, 3 fat

FAST FOOD

	Serving	Calories	Fat (g)	Cal. from Fat	Sat. Fat (g)	Trans Fat (g)	Chol. (mg)	Sod. (mg)	Carb. (g)	Fiber (g)	Prot. (g)	Servings/Exchanges
Gordita Baja, Chicken	1	340	18	160	3.5	0	40	840	29	3	17	2 carb, 2 med-fat meat, 2 fat
Gordita Baja, Steak	1	330	18	160	4	0	30	760	28	3	14	2 carb, 1 med-fat meat, 2 fat
Gordita Nacho Cheese, Beef	1	320	16	150	3.5	0	20	780	31	4	12	2 carb, 1 med-fat meat, 2 fat
Gordita Nacho Cheese, Chicken	1	300	13	120	2	0	25	820	30	2	15	2 carb, 1 med-fat meat, 2 fat
Gordita Nacho Cheese, Steak	1	290	13	120	2	0	15	740	29	2	13	2 carb, 1 med-fat meat, 2 fat
Gordita Supreme, Beef	1	320	16	150	5	0	35	640	30	4	13	2 carb, 1 med-fat meat, 2 fat
Gordita Supreme, Chicken	1	300	13	120	3.5	0	35	680	29	3	17	2 carb, 2 med-fat meat, 1 fat
Gordita Supreme, Steak	1	290	13	120	4	0	30	610	29	3	14	2 carb, 1 med-fat meat, 2 fat

Chalupas

Chalupa Baja, Beef	1	410	26	230	5	0	35	770	31	4	13	2 carb, 1 med-fat meat, 4 fat
Chalupa Baja, Chicken	1	390	23	200	4	0	40	800	29	2	17	2 carb, 2 med-fat meat, 3 fat
Chalupa Nacho Cheese, Beef	1	370	21	190	3.5	0	25	750	32	3	12	2 carb, 1 med-fat meat, 4 fat
Chalupa Nacho Cheese, Chicken	1	350	18	160	2	0	25	780	30	2	16	2 carb, 1 med-fat meat, 3 fat
Chalupa Supreme, Beef	1	370	21	190	6	0.5	35	310	31	3	14	2 carb, 1 med-fat meat, 3 fat
Chalupa Supreme, Chicken	1	350	18	160	4	0	40	650	30	2	17	2 carb, 2 med-fat meat, 2 fat
Chalupa Supreme, Steak	1	340	18	160	4	0	30	580	29	2	15	2 carb, 1 med-fat meat, 3 fat

Burritos

1/2 lb Combo Burrito	1	450	17	160	7	1	50	1610	51	9	21	3 1/2 carb, 2 med-fat meat, 1 fat

FAST FOOD

	Serving	Calories	Fat (g)	Cal. from Fat	Sat. Fat (g)	Trans Fat (g)	Chol. (mg)	Sod. (mg)	Carb. (g)	Fiber (g)	Prot. (g)	Servings/Exchanges
1/2 lb Nacho Crunch Burrito	1	520	25	230	8	0.5	50	1400	54	6	19	3 1/2 carb, 1 med-fat meat, 4 fat
7-Layer Burrito	1	490	17	160	6	1	20	1360	67	10	17	4 1/2 carb, 1 med-fat meat, 2 fat
Bean Burrito	1	350	9	80	3.5	0.5	5	1220	54	9	13	3 1/2 carb, 1 med-fat meat, 1 fat
Burrito Supreme, Chicken	1	390	12	110	5	0	40	1390	51	6	20	3 1/2 carb, 2 med-fat meat
Burrito Supreme, Steak	1	380	12	110	5	0.5	30	1320	50	6	17	3 carb, 1 med-fat meat, 1 fat
Cheesy Bean & Rice Burrito	1	470	21	180	5	0	15	1420	60	6	12	4 carb, 4 fat
Cheesy Double Beef Burrito	1	470	20	180	6	0.5	40	1580	54	6	18	3 1/2 carb, 1 med-fat meat, 3 fat

Food	Amount										Exchanges/Choices
Grilled Stuft Burrito, Beef	1	690	30	270	10	1	60	2110	79	10	26	5 carb, 2 med-fat meat, 4 fat
Grilled Stuft Burrito, Chicken	1	650	23	210	7	0.5	70	2180	76	7	33	5 carb, 3 med-fat meat, 2 fat
Grilled Stuft Burrito, Steak	1	630	24	220	8	1	50	2040	75	7	28	5 carb, 2 med-fat meat, 3 fat
Volcano Menu											
Volcano Nachos	1 order	990	61	550	9	1.5	45	1880	88	14	20	6 carb, 12 fat
Volcano Taco	1	240	17	150	5	0	35	470	14	3	8	1 carb, 1 med-fat meat, 2 fat
Volcano Burrito	1	800	42	380	12	1	70	2010	81	8	24	5 1/2 carb, 1 med-fat meat, 7 fat
Taco Salads											
Chicken Ranch Taco Salad	1	960	57	510	10	1	70	1710	78	8	36	5 carb, 3 med-fat meat, 8 fat
Chipotle Steak Taco Salad	1	950	59	530	11	1	65	1760	76	8	29	5 carb, 2 med-fat meat, 10 fat

FAST FOOD

	Serving	Calories	Fat (g)	Cal. from Fat	Sat. Fat (g)	Trans Fat (g)	Chol. (mg)	Sod. (mg)	Carb. (g)	Fiber (g)	Prot. (g)	Servings/Exchanges
Fiesta Taco Salad	1	820	43	380	10	1.5	60	1740	81	15	30	5 1/2 carb, 2 med-fat meat, 7 fat
Fiesta Taco Salad without Shell	1	460	22	200	8	1.5	60	1470	41	13	24	2 1/2 carb, 2 med-fat meat, 2 fat
Specialties												
Chicken Grilled Taquito	1	320	11	100	4.5	0	40	1000	37	2	18	2 1/2 carb, 2 med-fat meat
Steak Grilled Taquito	1	310	11	100	5	0	30	930	37	2	15	2 1/2 carb, 1 med-fat meat, 1 fat
Chicken Quesadilla	1	520	27	240	12	0.5	80	1490	41	4	28	2 1/2 carb, 3 med-fat meat, 2 fat
Steak Quesadilla	1	510	28	250	12	1	65	1340	40	4	25	2 1/2 carb, 2 med-fat meat, 4 fat
Crunchwrap Supreme	1	540	21	190	7	0	30	1400	71	6	16	4 1/2 carb, 1 med-fat meat, 3 fat

	Amount	Calories						Sodium				Exchanges
Enchirito, Beef	1	360	17	150	8	1	45	1410	35	7	18	2 carb, 2 med-fat meat, 1 fat
Enchirito, Chicken	1	340	13	120	7	0.5	50	1450	33	6	22	2 carb, 2 med-fat meat, 1 fat
Enchirito, Steak	1	330	14	120	7	0.5	45	1370	33	6	19	2 carb, 2 med-fat meat, 1 fat
Express Taco Salad	1	600	30	270	9	1.5	60	1380	57	15	25	4 carb, 2 med-fat meat, 4 fat
Mexican Pizza	1	530	30	270	8	1	45	990	46	7	20	3 carb, 2 med-fat meat, 4 fat
MexiMelt	1	280	14	130	7	0.5	45	870	23	4	15	1 1/2 carb, 2 med-fat meat, 1 fat

Nacho, Sides

	Amount	Calories						Sodium				Exchanges
Cheesy Fiesta Potatoes	1 order	270	16	140	2.5	0	5	840	28	3	4	2 carb, 3 fat
Mexican Rice	1 order	130	3.5	35	0	0	0	410	21	1	2	1 1/2 carb, 1 fat
Nachos	1 order	330	21	190	2	0	0	520	31	2	4	2 carb, 4 fat

FAST FOOD

	Serving	Calories	Fat (g)	Cal. from Fat	Sat. Fat (g)	Trans Fat (g)	Chol. (mg)	Sod. (mg)	Carb. (g)	Fiber (g)	Prot. (g)	Servings/Exchanges
Nachos Supreme	1 order	430	24	220	4.5	0.5	30	780	41	7	13	2 1/2 carb, 1 med-fat meat, 4 fat
Nachos BellGrande	1 order	760	42	380	6	1	30	1250	77	12	19	5 carb, 1 med-fat meat, 7 fat
Pintos 'n Cheese	1 order	170	6	60	3	0.5	15	670	18	7	9	1 carb, 1 med-fat meat
TACO JOHN'S												
Burritos												
Bean Burrito	1	380	9	80	3	0	15	830	58	9	15	4 carb, 2 fat
Beefy Burrito	1	440	20	180	7	1	50	860	45	7	22	3 carb, 2 med-fat meat, 2 fat
Beef Grilled Burrito	1	600	32	280	13	1	75	1230	52	8	27	3 1/2 carb, 2 med-fat meat, 4 fat
Chicken & Potato Burrito	1	470	19	170	4.5	0	30	1220	54	7	17	3 1/2 carb, 1 med-fat meat, 3 fat

Item	Serving											Exchanges
Chicken Grilled Burrito	1	590	29	260	11	0.5	90	1510	50	6	32	3 carb, 3 med-fat meat, 3 fat
Combination Burrito	1	400	14	130	5	0.5	35	830	50	8	18	3 carb, 1 med-fat meat, 2 fat
Meat & Potato Burrito	1	500	23	210	6	0.5	30	1100	58	8	15	4 carb, 5 fat
Super Burrito	1	450	18	160	7	0.5	40	920	54	9	19	3 1/2 carb, 1 med-fat meat, 3 fat
Desserts												
Apple Grande	1	270	12	110	3	0	5	420	38	2	5	2 1/2 carb, 2 fat
Choco Taco	1	390	20	180	15	0	15	160	48	1	5	3 carb, 4 fat
Churros	1	190	7	60	1.5	0	20	170	15	4	2	1 carb, 1 fat
Local Favorites												
Chili Cheese Potato Oles	1	590	36	320	8	0.5	25	2130	55	8	13	3 1/2 carb, 1 med-fat meat, 6 fat
Chili Enchilada	1	310	16	140	7	1	50	1000	24	4	18	1 1/2 carb, 2 med-fat meat, 1 fat

FAST FOOD

	Serving	Calories	Fat (g)	Cal. from Fat	Sat. Fat (g)	Trans Fat (g)	Chol. (mg)	Sod. (mg)	Carb. (g)	Fiber (g)	Prot. (g)	Servings/Exchanges
Chillito	1	510	20	180	8	1	45	1330	60	10	23	4 carb, 2 med-fat meat, 2 fat
Mexi Rolls with Nacho Cheese	4 pieces	260	10	90	4	0.5	20	370	28	4	13	2 carb, 1 med-fat meat, 1 fat
Ranch Burrito, Beef	1	440	22	220	6	0	45	850	45	6	17	3 carb, 1 med-fat meat, 3 fat
Ranch Burrito, Chicken	1	400	17	160	4.5	0	45	970	44	5	19	3 carb, 1 med-fat meat, 2 fat
Smothered Burrito	1	510	20	180	8	1	45	1330	60	10	23	4 carb, 2 med-fat meat, 2 fat
Sides												
Chili without Crackers	1 order	220	11	100	5	0	35	1240	17	4	14	1 carb, 2 med-fat meat
Mexican Rice	1 order	250	6	50	0	0	0	1080	45	0	5	3 carb, 1 fat
Nachos	1 order	380	23	210	6	0	10	750	38	1	6	2 1/2 carb, 5 fat
Potato Oles, Small	1 order	430	26	230	3.5	0	0	1220	45	6	4	3 carb, 5 fat

Potato Oles, Medium	1 order	600	36	330	5	0.5	0	1710	62	8	6	4 carb, 7 fat
Potato Oles, Large	1 order	770	46	420	6	1	0	2200	80	11	7	5 carb, 9 fat
Refried Beans	1 order	320	6	60	3.5	1	15	1020	47	11	18	3 carb, 1 med-fat meat
Specialties												
Taco Salad, No Dressing	1	520	33	290	11	1	60	860	37	7	21	2 1/2 carb, 2 med-fat meat, 5 fat
Chicken Taco Salad, No Dressing	1	480	27	240	9	0.5	65	24	35	6	24	2 carb, 3 med-fat meat, 2 fat
Quesadilla Melt, Cheesy	1	440	22	220	10	0.5	55	1050	43	5	19	3 carb, 1 med-fat meat, 3 fat
Quesadilla Melt, Fajita Chicken	1	510	23	210	11	0.5	75	1360	47	6	28	3 carb, 3 med-fat meat, 2 fat
Quesadilla Melt, Fajita Beef	1	540	28	250	12	1	70	1240	49	7	26	3 1/2 carb, 2 med-fat meat, 4 fat
Super Nachos	Regular order	810	48	430	16	1	55	1450	74	5	22	5 carb, 1 med-fat meat, 9 fat
Super Potato Oles	Regular order	1030	65	580	19	1.5	55	2850	87	13	24	5 1/2 carb, 1 med-fat meat, 12 fat

FAST FOOD

	Serving	Calories	Fat (g)	Cal. from Fat	Sat. Fat (g)	Trans Fat (g)	Chol. (mg)	Sod. (mg)	Carb. (g)	Fiber (g)	Prot. (g)	Servings/Exchanges
Tacos												
Chicken Softshell Taco	1	190	6	50	3	0	30	700	19	1	13	1 carb, 1 med-fat meat
Crispy Taco	1	180	10	90	3.5	0	25	270	13	2	9	1 carb, 1 med-fat meat, 1 fat
Softshell Taco	1	220	11	90	4.5	0.5	25	580	21	2	11	1 1/2 carb, 1 med-fat meat, 1 fat
Taco Bravo	1	340	13	120	4.5	0.5	25	750	40	5	15	2 1/2 carb, 1 med-fat meat, 2 fat
Taco Burger	1	270	12	110	4	0.5	30	600	28	3	14	2 carb, 1 med-fat meat, 1 fat
WENDY'S												
Sandwiches												
Hamburger Kid's Meal	1	220	8	70	3	0	30	490	25	1	12	1 1/2 carb, 1 med-fat meat, 1 fat

Cheeseburger, Kid's Meal	1	260	11	100	5	0.5	40	700	26	1	15	2 carb, 1 med-fat meat, 1 fat
Jr. Hamburger	1	230	8	70	3	0	30	490	26	1	13	2 carb, 1 med-fat meat, 1 fat
Jr. Cheeseburger	1	270	11	100	5	0.5	40	700	26	1	15	2 carb, 1 med-fat meat, 2 fat
Jr. Cheeseburger Deluxe	1	300	14	130	6	0.5	45	730	28	2	15	2 carb, 1 med-fat meat, 2 fat
Jr. Bacon Cheeseburger	1	310	16	140	6	0.5	50	670	25	1	17	1 1/2 carb, 2 med-fat meat, 1 fat
Single with Everything	1	430	20	180	7	1	75	870	38	2	25	2 1/2 carb, 3 med-fat meat, 1 fat
Double with Everything & Cheese	1	700	40	360	17	2	160	1440	38	2	47	2 1/2 carb, 6 med-fat meat, 2 fat
Triple with Everything & Cheese	1	970	60	540	27	3.5	245	2010	39	2	69	2 1/2 carb, 9 med-fat meat, 3 fat

FAST FOOD

	Serving	Calories	Fat (g)	Cal. from Fat	Sat. Fat (g)	Trans Fat (g)	Chol. (mg)	Sod. (mg)	Carb. (g)	Fiber (g)	Prot. (g)	Servings/Exchanges
Double Stack	1	360	18	160	8	1	70	810	26	1	23	2 carb, 2 med-fat meat, 2 fat
Baconator	1	830	51	460	23	2.5	195	1880	35	1	56	2 carb, 7 med-fat meat, 3 fat
Crispy Chicken Sandwich	1	360	18	160	3.5	0	30	710	36	2	15	2 1/2 carb, 1 med-fat meat, 3 fat
Grilled Chicken Go Wrap	1	250	10	90	3	0	45	730	24	1	17	1 1/2 carb, 2 med-fat meat
Homestyle Chicken Fillet Sandwich	1	440	16	140	3	0	50	1050	47	2	25	3 carb, 2 med-fat meat, 1 fat
Spicy Chicken Fillet Sandwich	1	440	16	140	3	0	55	1200	49	2	26	3 carb, 2 med-fat meat, 1 fat
Ultimate Chicken Grill Sandwich	1	320	7	60	1.5	0	70	950	36	2	28	2 1/2 carb, 3 lean meat

Item	Serving											Exchanges
Chicken Club Sandwich	1	550	26	230	8	0	75	1290	48	2	34	3 carb, 4 med-fat meat, 1 fat

Chicken

Item	Serving											Exchanges
4-Piece Kid's Chicken Nuggets Meal	4 pieces	190	13	120	3	0	25	380	9	0	9	1/2 carb, 1 med-fat meat, 2 fat
5-Piece Chicken Nuggets	5 pieces	230	16	50	3.5	0	30	480	11	0	12	1 carb, 1 med-fat meat, 2 fat
Bold Buffalo Boneless Wings	1 order	520	18	160	3.5	0	75	2630	58	2	31	4 carb, 3 med-fat meat, 1 fat
Honey BBQ Boneless Wings	1 order	580	18	160	3.5	0	75	1990	75	2	32	5 carb, 2 med-fat meat, 2 fat
BBQ Nugget Sauce	1 pkt	45	0	0	0	0	0	160	11	0	1	1 carb
Honey Mustard Nugget Sauce	1 pkt	130	12	110	2	0	10	220	6	0	0	1/2 carb, 2 fat
Sweet & Sour Sauce	1 pkt	50	0	0	0	0	0	120	12	0	0	1 carb

Salads

Item	Serving											Exchanges
Chicken Caesar	1	370	20	170	4	0	85	1015	18	3	31	1 carb, 4 med-fat meat

FAST FOOD

	Serving	Calories	Fat (g)	Cal. from Fat	Sat. Fat (g)	Trans Fat (g)	Chol. (mg)	Sod. (mg)	Carb. (g)	Fiber (g)	Prot. (g)	Servings/Exchanges
Mandarin Chicken	1	550	26	230	3	0	65	1250	49	4	31	3 carb, 3 med-fat meat, 2 fat
Southwest Taco	1	645	39	350	16	1	105	1565	44	8	31	3 carb, 3 med-fat meat, 5 fat
Sides												
Baked Potato, Plain	1	270	0	0	0	0	0	25	61	7	7	4 carb
Baked Potato, Sour Cream & Chives	1	320	3.5	30	0	0	10	50	63	7	8	4 carb, 1 fat
Caesar Side Salad	1	70	4	40	0	0	10	170	4	2	6	1 vegetable, 1 fat
Chili, Small	1	190	6	50	2.5	0	40	830	19	5	14	1 carb, 2 lean meat
Chili, Large	1	280	9	80	3.5	0.5	60	1240	29	7	21	2 carb, 2 med-fat meat
Fries, Small	1 order	330	16	140	0	0	0	300	44	4	4	3 carb, 3 fat
Fries, Medium	1 order	420	20	180	4	0	0	380	55	5	5	3 1/2 carb, 4 fat
Fries, Large	1 order	540	26	230	5	0	0	500	71	7	7	4 1/2 carb, 5 fat

Mandarin Orange Cup	1	80	0	0	0	0	0	15	19	1	1	1 fruit
Side Salad	1	35	0	0	0	0	0	25	8	2	1	1 vegetable
Frosty, Vanilla, Small	1	310	8	70	5	0	35	180	52	0	8	3 1/2 carb, 2 fat
Frosty, Vanilla, Large	1	500	12	110	8	0.5	45	220	88	0	9	5 1/2 carb, 2 fat

FROZEN MEALS, MEAT, CHICKEN, FISH

FROZEN MEALS, ENTRÉES

Aunt Jemima Entrees

	Serving	Calories	Fat (g)	Cal. from Fat	Sat. Fat (g)	Trans Fat (g)	Chol. (mg)	Sod. (mg)	Carb (g)	Fiber (g)	Prot. (g)	Servings/Exchanges
Eggs & Bacon	1	300	20	180	6	0	340	910	14	1	15	1 carb, 2 med-fat meat, 2 fat
Ham & Cheese Omelet	1	260	13	120	3.5	0	195	920	21	2	16	1 1/2 carb, 2 med-fat meat, 1 fat
Pancakes & Bacon	1	450	17	150	4.5	0	65	1100	61	3	14	4 carb, 3 fat
Sausage & Egg Scramble	1	300	18	160	5	0	200	890	21	2	15	1 1/2 carb, 2 med-fat meat, 2 fat

Banquet Meals

	Serving	Calories	Fat (g)	Cal. from Fat	Sat. Fat (g)	Trans Fat (g)	Chol. (mg)	Sod. (mg)	Carb (g)	Fiber (g)	Prot. (g)	Servings/Exchanges
Beef Pot Pie	1	450	27	250	11	0.5	30	730	36	2	14	2 1/2 carb, 1 med-fat meat, 4 fat
Chicken Fingers	1	460	15	130	3.5	0.5	20	730	69	11	13	4 1/2 carb, 1 med-fat meat, 2 fat

Food											
Chicken Pot Pie	1	370	21	190	9	0	35	850	34	2	10	2 carb, 1 med-fat meat, 3 fat
Corn Dog	1	470	18	160	4	4	35	730	68	8	11	4 1/2 carb, 4 fat
Country Fried Beefsteak	1	390	19	170	6	0.5	35	1040	41	3	14	2 1/2 carb, 1 med-fat meat, 3 fat
Country Fried Pork	1	420	23	210	7	0	20	1140	40	5	13	2 1/2 carb, 1 med-fat meat, 4 fat
Macaroni & Cheese	1	260	6	60	3	0	15	770	40	4	11	2 1/2 carb, 1 med-fat meat
Meatloaf	1	280	13	120	5	0	40	1000	28	4	12	2 carb, med-fat meat, 2 fat
Meatloaf	1	300	15	140	6	1	35	820	28	5	14	2 carb, 1 med-fat meat, 3 fat
Original Fried Chicken	1	380	20	210	5	0	30	930	35	5	14	2 carb, 1 med-fat meat, 3 fat
Salisbury Steak	1	300	16	150	6	1	25	1090	25	5	14	1 1/2 carb, 2 med-fat meat, 2 fat

FROZEN MEALS, MEAT, CHICKEN, FISH

	Serving	Calories	Fat (g)	Cal. from Fat	Sat. Fat (g)	Trans Fat (g)	Chol. (mg)	Sod. (mg)	Carb. (g)	Fiber (g)	Prot. (g)	Servings/Exchanges
Spaghetti & Meatballs	1	380	16	150	6	0	25	650	42	5	17	3 carb, 1 med-fat meat, 2 fat
Swedish Meatballs	1	430	23	210	10	0.5	90	950	35	4	20	2 carb, 2 med-fat meat, 3 fat
Turkey	1	200	8	80	2	0	30	980	27	5	14	2 carb, 1 med-fat meat, 1 fat
Boston Market												
Beef Sirloin & Noodles	14 oz	460	12	110	5	1	105	960	58	4	29	4 carb, 2 med-fat meat
Chicken Parmesan	16.1 oz	620	24	220	8	1	50	1580	69	7	33	4 1/2 carb, 3 med-fat meat, 2 fat
Chicken Pot Pie	8 oz	560	36	330	13	55	0	930	43	2	16	3 carb, 1 med-fat meat, 6 fat
Lasagna with Meat Sauce	12.6 oz	500	23	210	11	1	85	1290	49	4	22	3 carb, 2 med-fat meat, 3 fat

Meatloaf	16.1 oz	710	42	380	15	3	95	1590	53	5	30	3 1/2 carb, 3 med-fat meat, 5 fat
Salisbury Steak	16 oz	710	40	360	17	3	95	1760	53	5	34	3 1/2 carb, 3 med-fat meat, 5 fat
Turkey Breast Medallions	15.1 oz	360	14	130	3	1	55	1570	35	5	24	2 carb, 3 med-fat meat
Eating Right												
Beef Portabello	9 oz	260	7	60	2	0	30	680	42	4	16	3 carb, 1 med-fat meat
Cashew Chicken	9.7 oz	290	4	35	1	0	30	460	44	3	18	3 carb, 1 med-fat meat
Cheese Ravioli	8.5 oz	280	8	70	4.5	0	55	610	38	3	12	2 1/2 carb, 1 med-fat meat, 1 fat
Chicken Poblano	9 oz	310	8	70	3	0	40	490	37	2	22	2 1/2 carb, 2 med-fat meat
Chicken Teriyaki	8.2 oz	270	4	35	1	0	20	580	44	3	15	3 carb, 1 med-fat meat
Five Grain Beef & Vegetables	8.75 oz	280	5	45	1	0	25	500	43	4	13	3 carb, 1 med-fat meat

FROZEN MEALS, MEAT, CHICKEN, FISH

	Serving	Calories	Fat (g)	Cal. from Fat	Sat. Fat (g)	Trans Fat (g)	Chol. (mg)	Sod. (mg)	Carb. (g)	Fiber (g)	Prot. (g)	Servings/Exchanges
Lasagna with Meat Sauce	10.7 oz	370	8	70	3.5	0	25	630	55	3	15	3 1/2 carb, 1 med-fat meat, 1 fat
Lemongrass Chicken	9.25 oz	230	7	60	3	0	40	500	26	3	16	2 carb, 1 med-fat meat
Macaroni & Cheese	10 oz	330	8	70	4.5	0	25	770	46	2	18	3 carb, 1 med-fat meat, 1 fat
Roasted Turkey	9.75 oz	320	7	80	2	0	55	790	40	3	21	2 1/2 carb, 2 lean meat
Sesame Chicken	9 oz	370	5	45	0.5	0	25	450	67	3	16	4 1/2 carb, 1 med-fat meat
Spaghetti with Meat Sauce	11.5 oz	330	9	80	3	0	15	800	47	4	14	3 carb, 1 med-fat meat, 1 fat
Turkey Lasagna	11.25 oz	370	9	90	3	0	60	640	48	5	21	3 carb, 2 med-fat meat
Green Giant Complete Skillet Meal												
Cheesy Macaroni & Beef	1 cup	370	14	120	6	0	35	1170	48	2	15	3 carb, 1 med-fat meat, 2 fat

	Amount	Cal.	Fat (g)	Cal. Fat	Sat. Fat (g)	Trans Fat (g)	Chol. (mg)	Sod. (mg)	Carb. (g)	Fiber (g)	Pro. (g)	Exchanges
Chicken Alfredo	1 1/4 cup	260	5	45	2.5	0	30	660	39	3	17	2 1/2 carb, 2 lean meat
Mexican Style Rice & Beef	1 cup	280	7	70	3.5	0	20	810	42	4	11	3 carb, 1 fat
Pasta Primavera	1 1/2 cup	300	6	50	3	0	30	730	45	4	19	3 carb, 1 med-fat meat
Healthy Choice Café Steamers												
Cajun Style Chicken & Shrimp	10.4 oz	260	4	40	1	0	50	570	40	3	15	2 1/2 carb, 1 med-fat meat
Chicken Margherita	10 oz	320	7	70	1.5	0	35	580	45	5	18	3 carb, 1 med-fat meat
Chicken Red Pepper Alfredo	10.3 oz	250	5	45	2	0	35	520	30	4	20	2 carb, 2 lean meat
Grilled Chicken Marinara	10 oz	270	4.5	45	1.5	0	30	550	35	5	21	2 carb, 2 lean meat
Grilled Whiskey Steak	9.5 oz	250	4	40	1.5	0	35	560	37	6	15	2 1/2 carb, 1 med-fat meat
Roasted Beef Merlot	10 oz	230	8	80	2	0	35	600	21	5	17	1 1/2 carb, 2 med-fat meat

FROZEN MEALS, MEAT, CHICKEN, FISH

	Serving	Calories	Fat (g)	Cal. from Fat	Sat. Fat (g)	Trans Fat (g)	Chol. (mg)	Sod. (mg)	Carb. (g)	Fiber (g)	Prot. (g)	Servings/Exchanges
Sweet Sesame Chicken	10.3 oz	340	6	50	1	0	30	330	53	3	17	3 1/2 carb, 1 med-fat meat
Healthy Choice Meals												
Beef Pot Roast	11.1 oz	310	7	45	3	0	45	500	45	5	15	3 carb, 1 med-fat meat
Beef Tips Portabella	11.4 oz	300	8	80	2.5	0	35	600	33	7	20	2 carb, 2 med-fat meat
Chicken Alfredo Florentine	8.5 oz	230	3.5	35	1.5	0	25	560	31	4	17	2 carb, 2 lean meat
Chicken Parmigiana	11.1 oz	370	9	90	2	0	15	500	56	6	16	3 1/2 carb, 1 med-fat meat, 1 fat
Classic Meatloaf	10 oz	300	7	70	2.5	0	35	530	44	7	15	3 carb, 1 med-fat meat
Classic Meatloaf	12 oz	300	7	70	2.5	0	35	530	44	7	15	3 carb, 1 med-fat meat
Country Breaded Chicken	10.8 oz	370	9	90	2	0	25	560	53	6	15	3 1/2 carb, 1 med-fat meat, 1 fat
Country Herb Chicken	11.5 oz	240	5	45	1.5	0	30	600	34	5	15	2 carb, 1 med-fat meat
Fajita Steak	12.5 oz	360	6	60	6	2	40	590	56	7	20	3 1/2 carb, 2 lean meat

	Serving	Cal	Fat (g)	Cal from Fat	Sat Fat (g)	Trans Fat (g)	Chol (mg)	Sod (mg)	Carb (g)	Fiber (g)	Pro (g)	Exchanges/Choices
Golden Roast Turkey Breast	8.6 oz	300	4	40	1	0	25	550	42	6	21	3 carb, 2 lean meat
Grilled Chicken Teriyaki	11.1 oz	300	5	45	1	0	30	590	49	5	14	3 carb, 1 med-fat meat
Homestyle Salisbury Steak	12.8 oz	360	9	80	3.5	0	40	600	46	7	20	3 carb, 2 med-fat meat
Honey Ginger Chicken	8.5 oz	310	4.5	45	1	0	25	310	53	3	14	3 1/2 carb, 1 med-fat meat
Lemon Pepper Fish	10.8 oz	310	4.5	45	1	0	20	440	53	5	13	3 1/2 carb, 1 med-fat meat
Marina Manicotti Formaggio	11.1 oz	380	6	60	3	0	25	600	63	8	16	4 carb, 1 med-fat meat
Sesame Chicken	9.1 oz	230	4.5	40	1	0	15	600	34	5	12	2 carb, 1 med-fat meat
Sweet & Sour Chicken	11.1 oz	430	9	90	1	0	20	600	69	5	16	4 1/2 carb, 1 med-fat meat, 1 fat
Jimmy Dean												
Bacon, Egg, Cheese Biscuit	1	320	18	160	7	3	100	800	27	1	12	2 carb, 1 med-fat meat, 3 fat

FROZEN MEALS, MEAT, CHICKEN, FISH

	Serving	Calories	Fat (g)	Cal. from Fat	Sat. Fat (g)	Trans Fat (g)	Chol. (mg)	Sod. (mg)	Carb. (g)	Fiber (g)	Prot. (g)	Servings/Exchanges
Eggs, Potato, Ham Breakfast Bowl	1	390	23	210	9	0	360	1170	23	3	24	1 1/2 carb, 3 med-fat meat, 2 fat
Eggs, Potato, Sausage, Breakfast Bowl	1	490	34	310	13	0	370	1210	20	3	23	1 carb, 3 med-fat meat, 4 fat
Pancakes & Sausage Links	1	710	31	280	11	0	45	890	93	3	13	6 carb, 6 fat
Sausage Biscuit	1	360	24	220	8	3	30	600	26	1	8	2 carb, 5 fat
Lean Cuisine Café Classics												
Beef & Broccoli	9 oz	260	5	45	1.5	0	20	580	39	2	14	2 1/2 carb, 1 med-fat meat
Beef Portabello	9 oz	220	6	50	2.5	0	30	640	25	3	16	1 1/2 carb, 2 lean meat
Chicken & Almonds	8.5 oz	250	4	35	0.5	0	30	490	38	4	16	2 1/2 carb, 1 med-fat meat
Chicken Carbonara	9 oz	310	8	70	2	0	30	680	36	4	23	2 1/2 carb, 2 med-fat meat

Glazed Chicken	8.5 oz	220	3.5	30	1	0	40	500	25	1	21	1 1/2 carb, 2 lean meat
Grilled Chicken Caesar	8.5 oz	260	6	50	2	0	35	590	33	3	18	2 carb, 2 lean meat
Honey Dijon Grilled Chicken	8 oz	220	7	60	2.5	0	50	640	22	2	17	1 1/2 carb, 2 lean meat
Lemon Pepper Fish	9 oz	330	8	70	2.5	0	40	590	50	2	15	3 carb, 1 med-fat meat, 1 fat
Orange Chicken	9 oz	300	7	60	1.5	0	25	580	46	2	14	3 carb, 1 med-fat meat
Roasted Garlic Chicken	8.9 oz	180	7	60	2.5	0	40	650	9	1	20	1/2 carb, 3 lean meat
Sesame Chicken	9 oz	330	9	80	1.5	0	25	650	47	2	16	3 carb, 1 med-fat meat, 1 fat
Shrimp & Angel Hair Pasta	10 oz	220	4	35	1	0	50	590	32	2	14	2 carb, 1 med-fat meat
Shrimp Alfredo	9 oz	260	5	45	2	0	60	590	36	3	18	2 1/2 carb, 2 lean meat
Steak Tips Portabello	7.5 oz	160	7	60	2.5	0	40	450	10	3	15	1/2 carb, 2 lean meat
Sun Dried Tomato Pesto Chicken	8.6 oz	290	9	80	2	0	30	570	34	4	18	2 carb, 2 med-fat meat

FROZEN MEALS, MEAT, CHICKEN, FISH

	Serving	Calories	Fat (g)	Cal. from Fat	Sat. Fat (g)	Trans Fat (g)	Chol. (mg)	Sod. (mg)	Carb. (g)	Fiber (g)	Prot. (g)	Servings/Exchanges
Sweet & Sour Chicken	10 oz	300	3	25	0.5	0	30	560	51	2	18	3 1/2 carb, 1 lean meat
Thai-Style Chicken	9 oz	290	7	60	2	0	30	560	39	2	18	2 1/2 carb, 2 lean meat
Three Cheese Chicken	8 oz	210	9	90	3	0	40	500	10	3	21	1/2 carb, 3 lean meat
Lean Cuisine One Dish Favorites												
Angel Hair Pomodoro	10 oz	250	5	45	2	0	5	620	42	4	8	3 carb, 1 fat
BBQ Chicken Quesadilla	5 oz	260	7	60	2.5	0	15	630	35	2	16	2 carb, 1 med-fat meat
Cheddar Potatoes with Broccoli	10.25 oz	230	5	45	3	0	15	640	35	4	12	2 carb, 1 med-fat meat
Cheese Ravioli	8.5 oz	220	5	45	3	0	35	620	33	3	11	2 carb, 1 med-fat meat
Chicken Chow Mein with Rice	9 oz	260	4	25	1	0	25	550	41	3	14	2 1/2 carb, 1 med-fat meat
Chicken Enchilada Suiza	9 oz	270	4	35	1.5	0	20	550	47	3	12	3 carb, 1 med-fat meat
Chicken Fettucini	9.3 oz	270	6	50	3	0	40	690	32	0	22	2 carb, 2 lean meat

Classic Five Cheese Lasagna	11.5 oz	360	8	70	3.5	0	20	600	51	3.5	21	3 1/2 carb, 2 med-fat meat
Fettucini Alfredo	9.3 oz	330	7	60	3	0	15	600	54	3	12	3 1/2 carb, 1 fat
Lasagna with Meat Sauce	10.5 oz	320	8	70	4	0	30	630	45	4	17	3 carb, 1 med-fat meat, 2 fat
Linguine Cabrera	9.25 oz	300	8	70	2	0	15	590	43	2	14	3 carb, 1 med-fat meat, 1 fat
Macaroni & Cheese	10 oz	290	7	60	4	0	20	630	41	1	15	2 1/2 carb, 1 med-fat meat
Pasta Romano with Bacon	10 oz	280	7	60	2	0	10	650	43	4	12	3 carb, 1 med-fat meat
Roasted Chicken with Lemon Pepper Fettuccini	8.1 oz	260	6	50	1.5	0	30	650	36	3	16	2 1/2 carb, 1 med-fat meat
Sante Fe-Style Rice & Beans	10.4 oz	300	5	45	2.5	0	15	590	52	5	11	3 1/2 carb, 1 fat
Spaghetti	9.5 oz	270	5	45	2	0	25	560	38	2	18	2 1/2 carb, 2 lean meat

FROZEN MEALS, MEAT, CHICKEN, FISH

	Serving	Calories	Fat (g)	Cal. from Fat	Sat. Fat (g)	Trans Fat (g)	Chol. (mg)	Sod. (mg)	Carb. (g)	Fiber (g)	Prot. (g)	Servings/Exchanges
Stuffed Cabbage with Whipped Potatoes	9.5 oz	210	6	50	1.5	0	15	670	28	3	10	2 carb, 1 med-fat meat
Swedish Meatballs	9.125 oz	300	8	70	3	0	45	620	34	3	22	2 carb, 2 med-fat meat
Lean Cuisine Dinnertime Selects												
Balsamic Glazed Chicken	12 oz	330	7	60	2.5	0	40	660	41	4	25	2 1/2 carb, 3 lean meat
Chicken Fettuccini	12 oz	400	8	70	4	0	50	850	48	6	33	3 carb, 3 lean meat
Chicken Florentine	13.3 oz	410	9	80	3.5	0	45	840	54	6	28	3 1/2 carb, 2 med-fat meat
Grilled Chicken & Penne Pasta	12 oz	330	4.5	40	1.5	0	40	580	52	6	20	3 1/2 carb, 2 lean meat
Jumbo Rigatoni with Meatballs	15.4 oz	390	8	70	2.5	0	35	830	56	7	23	3 1/2 carb, 2 med-fat meat
Roasted Turkey Breast	12 oz	290	7	60	1	0	30	890	38	5	19	2 1/2 carb, 2 lean meat
Salisbury Steak	12.5 oz	270	8	70	4	0	45	650	27	10	22	2 carb, 2 med-fat meat

Steak Tips Dijon	12 oz	280	7	60	2.5	0	30	650	33	5	21	2 carb, 2 lean meat
Lean Cuisine Spa Cuisine												
Chicken in Peanut Sauce	9 oz	280	8	70	1.5	0	25	560	30	5	22	2 carb, 2 med-fat meat
Chicken Mediterranean	10.5 oz	240	4	35	1	0	40	590	32	6	19	2 carb, 2 lean meat
Chicken Pecan	9 oz	250	6	50	1	0	30	490	33	3	17	2 carb, 2 lean meat
Lemon Chicken	9 oz	300	9	80	2	0	25	550	41	3	13	2 1/2 carb, 1 med-fat meat, 1 fat
Lemongrass Chicken	9.4 oz	250	6	50	3.5	0	30	610	30	4	18	2 carb, 2 lean meat
Salmon with Basil	9.6 oz	220	6	50	2	0	20	660	23	4	19	1 1/2 carb, 2 lean meat
Marie Callender's Meals												
Beef Pot Pie	1 cup	540	32	290	12	2	25	700	46	4	16	3 carb, 1 med-fat meat, 5 fat
Beef Tips	1 meal	360	12	110	4.5	0	70	1450	35	6	26	2 carb, 2 med-fat meat
Cheesy Chicken Breast & Rice	1 meal	480	18	170	13	0.5	80	1500	47	5	31	3 carb, 3 med-fat meat, 1 fat

FROZEN MEALS, MEAT, CHICKEN, FISH

	Serving	Calories	Fat (g)	Cal. from Fat	Sat. Fat (g)	Trans Fat (g)	Chol. (mg)	Sod. (mg)	Carb. (g)	Fiber (g)	Prot. (g)	Servings/Exchanges
Chicken & Noodles	1 meal	610	34	310	14	0.5	100	1500	52	5	24	3 1/2 carb, 2 med-fat meat, 5 fat
Chicken Parmesan	1 meal	650	29	270	8	0	35	1000	66	5	31	4 1/2 carb, 3 med-fat meat, 3 fat
Chicken Pot Pie	1 cup	600	37	340	15	2	30	850	46	3	17	3 carb, 1 med-fat meat, 6 fat
Chicken Teriyaki	1 meal	430	4	40	1	0	45	1230	78	5	19	5 carb, 1 med-fat meat
Country Fried Beef	1 meal	540	28	260	11	1	45	1510	51	6	19	3 1/2 carb, 1 med-fat meat, 5 fat
Country Fried Chicken & Gravy	1 meal	500	21	190	7	0	30	1590	52	7	24	3 1/2 carb, 2 med-fat meat, 2 fat
Country Fried Pork Chop	1 meal	510	23	210	7	0	45	1560	53	11	21	3 1/2 carb, 2 med-fat meat, 3 fat
Creamy Mushroom Chicken Pot Pie	1 cup	560	35	320	13	2	30	700	45	3	15	3 carb, 1 med-fat meat, 6 fat

Creamy Parmesan Chicken Pot Pie	1 cup	530	32	290	12	2	30	720	43	2	17	3 carb, 1 med-fat meat, 5 fat
Fettuccini with Chicken & Broccoli	1 meal	630	37	340	15	0.5	90	900	43	6	30	3 carb, 3 med-fat meat, 4 fat
Fried Chicken Tenders	1 meal	470	19	180	8	0	40	1450	52	5	21	3 1/2 carb, 2 med-fat meat, 2 fat
Golden Battered Fish Fillet	1 meal	450	16	150	4.5	0	35	1170	53	4	22	3 1/2 carb, 2 med-fat meat, 1 fat
Grilled Chicken Bake	1 meal	610	35	320	14	0.5	75	990	43	5	30	3 carb, 3 med-fat meat, 4 fat
Herb Roasted Chicken	1 meal	460	25	230	7	0	65	1030	26	5	30	2 carb, 3 med-fat meat, 2 fat
Honey Roasted Chicken Pot Pie	1	530	30	270	12	2	25	880	47	7	16	3 carb, 1 med-fat meat, 1 fat
Lasagna Bake with Meat Sauce	1 cup	240	8	70	4	0	20	870	28	4	13	2 carb, 1 med-fat meat, 1 fat
Meat Lasagna	1 cup	240	9	80	5	0	45	950	24	2	14	1 1/2 carb, 1 med-fat meat, 1 fat

FROZEN MEALS, MEAT, CHICKEN, FISH

	Serving	Calories	Carb. (g)	Fat (g)	Cal from Fat.	Sat. Fat (g)	Trans Fat (g)	Chol. (mg)	Sod. (mg)	Fiber (g)	Prot. (g)	Servings/Exchanges
Meatloaf & Gravy	1 meal	480	22	200	9	0.5	60	1080	39	3	31	2 1/2 carb, 3 med-fat meat, 1 fat
Old Fashioned Beef Pot Roast	1 meal	330	10	90	4	0	45	970	32	9	27	2 carb, 3 lean meat
Salisbury Steak	1 meal	400	16	150	6	0	50	820	38	7	27	2 1/2 carb, 3 med-fat meat
Sweet & Sour Chicken	1 meal	600	18	160	20	0	25	860	88	10	22	6 carb, 1 med-fat meat, 3 fat
Turkey Pot Pie	1	670	41	370	16	2.5	25	1000	56	4	19	3 1/2 carb, 1 med-fat meat, 7 fat
Turkey with Stuffing	1 meal	400	9	90	2.5	0	65	1230	45	4	32	3 carb, 3 lean meat
Michael Angelo's												
Chicken Alfredo	1 cup	310	10	90	8	0	55	690	34	1	19	2 carb, 2 med-fat meat
Eggplant Parmesan	6 oz	250	15	140	7	0	60	540	16	3	13	1 carb, 1 med-fat meat, 2 fat

Lasagna with Meat Sauce	1 cup	300	11	100	6	0	55	560	30	3	20	2 carb, 2 med-fat meat
Vegetable Lasagna	1 cup	230	7	60	3	0	15	720	23	3	20	1 1/2 carb, 2 lean meat
Michelina's Authentico												
Chicken Fried Rice	8.1 oz	410	11	100	2	0	40	1100	64	2	12	4 carb, 2 fat
Chicken Primavera with Spirals	8.1 oz	320	7	60	3	0	25	630	48	3	14	3 carb, 1 med-fat meat
Chicken Primavira with Spirals	8.1 oz	320	7	60	3	0	25	630	48	3	14	3 carb, 1 med-fat meat
Fettucine Alfredo	9.1 oz	390	16	150	8	0.5	40	650	45	2	14	3 carb, 1 med-fat meat, 2 fat
Four Cheese Lasagna	8.1 oz	280	6	60	3	0	15	500	43	3	12	3 carb, 1 med-fat meat
Lasagana Mozarella	8.1 oz	260	7	60	3.5	0	20	540	39	3	9	2 1/2 carb, 1 med-fat meat
Lasagna with Meat Sauce	9.1 oz	320	10	90	4	0	35	740	40	3	14	2 1/2 carb, 1 med-fat meat, 1 fat

FROZEN MEALS, MEAT, CHICKEN, FISH

	Serving	Calories	Carb. (g)	Fat (g)	Cal from Fat.	Sat. Fat (g)	Trans Fat (g)	Chol. (mg)	Sod. (mg)	Fiber (g)	Prot. (g)	Servings/Exchanges
Macaroni & Cheese Bake	8.1 oz	240	4	35	2	0	10	540	41	2	9	2 1/2 carb, 1 fat
Pasta with Chicken	8.1 oz	290	10	90	4	0	35	800	38	2	12	2 1/2 carb, 1 med-fat meat, 1 fat
Penne with Chicken	8.6 oz	330	9	80	4	0	35	610	48	2	14	3 carb, 1 med-fat meat, 1 fat
Risotto Parmigiano	8.1 oz	420	18	160	9	0.5	45	770	49	1	16	3 carb, 1 med-fat meat, 2 fat
Stroganoff	8.1 oz	400	18	160	7	0	35	740	38	2	13	2 1/2 carb, 1 med-fat meat, 3 fat
Sweet & Sour Chicken	8.6 oz	370	2.5	25	0.5	0	15	970	68	1	10	4 1/2 carb, 1 fat
Wheels & Cheese	8.1 oz	350	11	90	4.5	0	20	780	48	2	13	3 carb, 1 med-fat meat, 1 fat
Michelina's Budget Gourmet												
Angel Hair Pasta	8 oz	290	5	50	2	0	10	410	48	4	11	3 carb, 1 fat

Chinese-Style Vegetables & White Chicken	8 oz	310	5	45	0.5	0	5	670	57	2	8	4 carb, 1 fat
Fettuccine Alfredo	8 oz	300	9	90	4.5	0	25	640	42	2	11	3 carb, 2 fat
Italian-Style Vegetables & White Chicken	8 oz	270	5	45	1	0	10	540	44	4	11	3 carb, 1 fat
Lasagna Alfredo with Broccoli	8 oz	300	12	110	6	0	30	560	36	2	10	2 1/2 carb, 1 med-fat meat, 1 fat
Lasagna with Meat Sauce	8 oz	260	8	70	2.5	0	15	680	34	3	10	2 carb, 1 med-fat meat, 1 fat
Macaroni & Cheese	8 oz	310	10	90	4	0	20	730	42	2	12	3 carb, 1 med-fat meat, 1 fat
Rigatoni in Sauce	8 oz	290	9	70	3.5	0	25	570	43	3	11	3 carb, 2 fat
Spaghetti Marinara	8 oz	270	3.5	30	1	0	0	620	49	3	9	3 carb, 1 fat
Stir Fry Rice & Vegetables	8 oz	450	20	180	4	0	10	700	60	2	7	4 carb, 4 fat

FROZEN MEALS, MEAT, CHICKEN, FISH

	Serving	Calories	Fat (g)	Cal. from Fat	Sat. Fat (g)	Trans Fat (g)	Chol. (mg)	Sod. (mg)	Carb. (g)	Fiber (g)	Prot. (g)	Servings/Exchanges
Szechwan-Style Vegetables & White Chicken	8 oz	280	2.5	20	0	0	5	880	51	2	10	3 1/2 carb, 1 fat
Wild Rice Pilaf with Vegetables	8 oz	320	6	50	2.5	0	10	630	59	2	7	4 carb, 1 fat
Ziti Parmesano	8 oz	250	7	60	3	0	10	500	37	3	10	2 1/2 carb, 1 fat
Michelina's Lean Gourmet												
Beef Pepper Steak & Rice	8.1 oz	270	4	30	1	0	10	700	47	2	11	3 carb, 1 fat
Cheese Stuffed Rigatoni	8.1 oz	220	6	50	3	0	30	510	33	3	8	2 carb, 1 fat
Chicken Alfredo Florentine	8.1 oz	250	7	60	3.5	0	40	690	34	2	12	2 carb, 1 med-fat meat
Creamy Parmesan Chicken	8.1 oz	250	4.5	40	2	0	30	580	37	2	13	2 1/2 carb, 1 med-fat meat
Enchilada Bake	8.6 oz	300	8	70	2.5	0	15	750	47	6	11	3 carb, 2 fat

	Serving	Calories									Exchanges/Choices
Five Cheese Lasagna	8.1 oz	290	5	50	2	0	10	560	50	8	13	3 carb, 1 med-fat meat
Glazed Chicken	8.1 oz	250	3	25	0.5	0	20	470	46	1	10	3 carb, 1 fat
Macaroni & Cheese	9.1 oz	270	3.5	35	1.5	0	10	520	47	2	10	3 carb, 1 fat
Meatloaf	8.1 oz	180	6	60	3	0	35	860	21	2	11	1 1/2 carb, 1 med-fat meat
Penne Primavera	8.1 oz	280	6	60	3	0	15	480	43	3	11	3 carb, 1 fat
Roasted Sirloin Supreme	8.1 oz	230	5	45	1.5	0	15	950	34	2	13	2 carb, 1 med-fat meat
Salisbury Steak	8.1 oz	190	6	60	3	0	35	760	23	2	11	1 1/2 carb, 1 med-fat meat
Sante Fe Style Rice & Beans	8.6 oz	330	9	80	4	0	15	710	55	4	8	3 1/2 carb, 2 fat
Shrimp with Pasta & Vegetables	8.1 oz	260	6	60	3	0	45	620	39	2	11	2 1/2 carb, 1 med-fat meat
Spaghetti & Meat Sauce	8.6 oz	330	5	45	1.5	0	10	400	55	4	12	3 1/2 carb, 1 fat
Swedish Meatballs	8.6 oz	310	9	80	4	0	25	620	42	2	14	3 carb, 1 med-fat meat, 1 fat

FROZEN MEALS, MEAT, CHICKEN, FISH

	Serving	Calories	Fat (g)	Cal. from Fat	Sat. Fat (g)	Trans Fat (g)	Chol. (mg)	Sod. (mg)	Carb. (g)	Fiber (g)	Prot. (g)	Servings/Exchanges
Red Baron												
Biscuit-Style Scrambles, Bacon	1	410	21	190	10	0.5	65	960	36	2	17	2 1/2carb, 2 med-fat meat, 2 fat
Biscuit-Style Scrambles, Western	1	350	16	140	7	0	60	760	36	2	15	2 1/2 carb, 1 med-fat meat, 2 fat
Stouffer's												
Baked Chicken Breast	8.9 oz	250	10	90	3	0	60	730	20	1	20	1 carb, 2 med-fat meat
Beef Pot Roast	16 oz	320	8	70	3	0	30	1570	41	8	20	2 1/2 carb, 2 med-fat meat
Beef Stroganoff	9.8 oz	380	17	150	5	0	70	990	34	2	22	2 carb, 2 med-fat meat, 1 fat
Chicken à la King	11.5 oz	360	12	110	4	0	35	800	44	0	18	3 carb, 1 med-fat meat, 1 fat
Corn Souffle	6 oz	150	5	45	1	0	65	490	22	2	5	1 1/2 carb, 1 fat

	Serving	Cal.	Fat	Cal. Fat	Sat. Fat		Chol.	Sod.	Carb.	Fiber	Prot.	Exchanges
Creamed Chipped Beef	5.5 oz	140	7	60	4	0	35	590	9	0	9	1/2 carb, 1 med-fat meat
Escalloped Chicken & Noodles	8 oz	330	18	160	4	0	35	910	28	2	14	2 carb, 1 med-fat meat, 3 fat
Fish Filet	9 oz	400	16	140	4.5	0.5	55	1050	36	4	27	2 1/2 carb, 3 med-fat meat
Five Cheese Lasagna	10.8 oz	370	14	130	7	0	35	960	39	4	21	2 1/2 carb, 2 med-fat meat, 1 fat
Fried Chicken Breast	8.9 oz	360	18	160	4.5	0	45	880	30	2	20	2 carb, 2 med-fat meat, 2 fat
Grilled Chicken Teriyaki	9.4 oz	300	3.5	30	1	0	40	880	45	3	21	3 carb, 2 lean meat
Grilled Herb Chicken	9 oz	250	6	50	1	0	35	740	29	3	19	2 carb, 2 lean meat
Grilled Lemon Pepper Chicken	9 oz	240	8	70	2	0	40	670	24	4	19	1 1/2 carb, 2 med-fat meat
Lasagna with Meat Sauce	10.5 oz	350	11	100	6	0.5	40	930	38	3	24	2 1/2 carb, 2 med-fat meat

FROZEN MEALS, MEAT, CHICKEN, FISH

	Serving	Calories	Fat (g)	Cal. from Fat	Sat. Fat (g)	Trans Fat (g)	Chol. (mg)	Sod. (mg)	Carb. (g)	Fiber (g)	Prot. (g)	Servings/Exchanges
Macaroni & Beef	12.8 oz	410	16	140	7	0	40	990	45	4	22	3 carb, 2 med-fat meat, 1 fat
Macaroni & Cheese	6 oz	340	16	140	7	0	25	820	33	3	15	2 carb, 1 med-fat meat, 2 fat
Meatloaf	16 oz	600	31	280	12	1.5	90	1310	45	5	35	3 carb, 3 med-fat meat, 3 fat
Roast Turkey	9.6 oz	290	12	110	3.5	0	45	970	30	2	16	2 carb, 1 med-fat meat, 1 fat
Roasted Chicken	9.6 oz	460	24	220	6	0	80	990	34	5	26	2 carb, 3 med-fat meat, 2 fat
Salisbury Steak	16 oz	710	39	350	16	1.5	100	1820	48	3	41	3 carb, 4 med-fat meat, 4 fat
Spaghetti with Meat Sauce	12 oz	350	12	110	4	0	30	660	44	5	17	3 carb, 1 med-fat meat, 1 fat

Spaghetti with Meatballs	12.6 oz	360	12	110	3.5	0	35	850	45	6	19	3 carb, 1 med-fat meat, 1 fat
Spinach Souffle	4 oz	150	10	90	2	0	110	390	9	1	6	1/2 carb, 1 med-fat meat, 1 fat
Swedish Meatballs	11.5 oz	560	27	240	12	1	100	1250	47	3	32	3 carb, 3 med-fat meat, 2 fat
Tuna Noodle Casserole	12 oz	450	20	180	6	0	70	990	45	3	22	3 carb, 2 med-fat meat, 2 fat
White Meat Chicken Pot Pie	10 oz	660	37	330	14	0.5	50	1060	62	2	19	4 carb, 1 med-fat meat, 6 fat
Stouffer's Easy Express Skillets												
Chicken Alfredo	12.5 oz	410	10	90	4	0	50	980	48	6	31	3 carb, 3 lean meat
Garlic Chicken	11.5 oz	320	6	50	2.5	0	40	1440	42	6	24	3 carb, 2 lean meat
Steak Teriyaki	11.8 oz	310	5	45	2	0	25	1390	49	6	17	3 carb, 1 med-fat meat
Swanson Hungry-Man												
Beer Battered Chicken	16 oz	900	46	410	10	0	100	2090	78	7	37	5 carb, 3 med-fat meat, 6 fat

FROZEN MEALS, MEAT, CHICKEN, FISH

	Serving	Calories	Fat (g)	Cal. from Fat	Sat. Fat (g)	Trans Fat (g)	Chol. (mg)	Sod. (mg)	Carb. (g)	Fiber (g)	Prot. (g)	Servings/Exchanges
Boneless Fried Chicken	16 oz	860	39	350	9	0	130	1340	85	6	39	5 1/2 carb, 3 med-fat meat, 5 fat
Classic Fried Chicken	16 oz	1040	59	530	13	0	180	1610	64	4	60	4 carb, 7 med-fat meat, 5 fat
Country Fried Beef Patties	16 oz	810	50	450	16	0	75	1850	72	5	23	5 carb, 1 med-fat meat, 9 fat
Grilled Bourbon Steak Strips	16 oz	620	15	140	4	0	55	1990	94	4	26	6 carb, 1 med-fat meat, 2 fat
Meatloaf	16 oz	690	29	260	9	0	95	1510	74	5	34	5 carb, 2 med-fat meat, 4 fat
Mexican Style Fiesta	18.1 oz	600	23	210	8	0	20	1570	87	10	18	6 carb, 5 fat
Roasted Carved Turkey	17 oz	560	18	160	6	0	55	1620	78	5	19	5 carb, 1 med-fat meat, 3 fat
Salisbury Steak	16 oz	580	31	280	11	0	85	1380	50	5	27	3 carb, 3 med-fat meat, 3 fat

Southwest Style Fried Chicken	16 oz	630	19	170	5	0	60	1630	85	3	29	5 1/2 carb, 2 med-fat meat, 2 fat
Weight Watchers Smart Ones												
Chicken Enchiladas Suiza	9.1 oz	290	5	50	2	0	25	640	49	3	11	3 carb, 1 fat
Chicken Marsala	9 oz	180	7	60	1	0	50	530	10	2	20	1/2 carb, 3 lean meat
Chicken Parmesan	11.1 oz	290	5	50	1.5	0	40	630	35	4	26	2 carb, 2 lean meat
Chicken Sante Fe	9 oz	140	2.5	20	0	0	30	800	11	4	20	1 carb, 2 lean meat
Creamy Parmesan Chicken	9 oz	250	8	70	3.5	0	45	570	24	3	21	1 1/2 carb, 2 med-fat meat
Fettucini Alfredo	9.3 oz	240	3.5	30	1.5	0	5	570	41	4	12	2 1/2 carb, 1 med-fat meat
Ravioli Florentine	8.5 oz	250	5	45	2	0	30	720	40	4	11	2 1/2 carb, 1 med-fat meat
Slow-Roasted Turkey Breast	10 oz	210	7	60	2	0	45	770	18	2	18	1 carb, 2 lean meat
Sweet & Sour Chicken	9 oz	210	2	20	0	0	20	510	31	2	16	2 carb, 2 lean meat

FROZEN MEALS, MEAT, CHICKEN, FISH

	Serving	Calories	Fat (g)	Cal. from Fat	Sat. Fat (g)	Trans Fat (g)	Chol. (mg)	Sod. (mg)	Carb. (g)	Fiber (g)	Prot. (g)	Servings/Exchanges
Thai Style Chicken & Rice Noodles	10.2 oz	260	4	35	0.5	0	25	570	43	2	14	3 carb, 1 med-fat meat
Traditional Lasagna with Meat Sauce	10.6 oz	300	6	50	3	0	25	780	43	5	17	3 carb, 1 med-fat meat
Tuna Noodle Gratin	9.6 oz	240	4.5	40	2	0	30	720	37	3	15	2 1/2 carb, 1 med-fat meat

FROZEN CHICKEN

Banquet

	Serving	Calories	Fat (g)	Cal. from Fat	Sat. Fat (g)	Trans Fat (g)	Chol. (mg)	Sod. (mg)	Carb. (g)	Fiber (g)	Prot. (g)	Servings/Exchanges
Chicken Breast Nuggets	6 pieces	240	16	140	2.5	0	20	540	12	1	12	1 carb, 1 med-fat meat, 2 fat
Chicken Breast Patty	1	200	13	120	2.5	0	15	340	11	1	9	1 carb, 1 med-fat meat, 2 fat
Chicken Breast Strips	2	190	10	90	1.5	0	15	500	14	2	12	1 carb, 1 med-fat meat, 1 fat

Chicken Breast Tenders	5 pieces	220	14	130	2	0	15	470	12	<1	11	1 carb, 1 med-fat meat, 2 fat
Chicken Nuggets	6 pieces	220	13	120	2.5	0	25	530	15	2	11	1 carb, 1 med-fat meat, 2 fat
Chicken Wings, Honey BBQ	3 oz	270	17	160	4.5	1	65	520	12	5	17	1 carb, 2 med-fat meat, 1 fat
Chicken, Crispy Fried	1 piece	330	21	190	5	1.5	75	890	12	<1	24	1 carb, 3 med-fat meat, 1 fat
Chicken, Popcorn	11 pieces	180	9	80	2.5	0	20	510	18	<1	8	1 carb, 1 med-fat meat, 1 fat
Foster Farms												
Breast Nuggets	4	160	9	80	2	0	25	360	9	1	13	1/2 carb, 2 med-fat meat
Buffalo Style Strips	3 oz	190	8	70	2	0	30	1100	15	0	14	1 carb, 2 med-fat meat
Crispy Strips	3 oz	200	8	70	1.5	0	35	790	14	0	18	1 carb, 2 med-fat meat
Honey BBQ Wings	4	170	10	90	3	0	50	390	5	0	13	2 med-fat meat
Hot & Spicy Wings	4	170	13	120	4	0	55	460	1	0	14	2 med-fat meat, 1 fat

FROZEN MEALS, MEAT, CHICKEN, FISH

	Serving	Calories	Fat (g)	Cal. from Fat	Sat. Fat (g)	Trans Fat (g)	Chol. (mg)	Sod. (mg)	Carb. (g)	Fiber (g)	Prot. (g)	Servings/Exchanges
Tyson												
Breaded Chicken Breast Fillets	1 piece	240	9	80	1.5	0	45	680	20	0	19	1 carb, 2 med-fat meat
Buffalo Style Hot Wings	3 pieces	230	15	130	4	0	115	580	1	0	21	3 med-fat meat
Chicken Breast Nuggets	5 pieces	270	17	160	4	0	50	470	15	0	14	1 carb, 2 med-fat meat, 1 fat
Chicken Breast Patties	1 patty	180	11	90	2.5	0	25	390	12	1	10	1 carb, 1 med-fat meat, 1 fat
Chicken Breast Strips	2 pieces	200	10	90	2	0	30	520	13	1	16	1 carb, 2 med-fat meat
Chicken Breast Tenderloins	1 piece	150	7	60	1.5	0	20	370	12	1	10	1 carb, 1 med-fat meat
Diced Roasted Chicken Strips	3 oz	110	2.5	20	1	0	65	330	2	0	20	3 lean meat
Fajita Chicken Breast Strips	3 oz	110	4	35	1	0	55	540	1	0	17	2 lean meat

Fun Shaped Chicken Nuggets	5 pieces	280	18	160	4	0	45	490	16	0	14	1 carb, 2 med-fat meat, 2 fat
Honey BBQ Wings	3 pieces	230	14	130	3.5	0	100	470	9	0	15	2 med-fat meat
Popcorn Chicken Bites	7 pieces	180	9	80	1.5	0	30	560	11	0	13	1 carb, 1 med-fat meat, 1 fat

FROZEN FISH

Fisher Boy

Crispy Battered Fish Portions	1 piece	170	10	90	2	0	20	320	15	0	7	1 carb, 1 med-fat meat, 1 fat
Crunchy Breaded Fish Tenders	4 pieces	230	11	100	1.5	0	30	450	22	0	11	1 1/2 carb, 1 med-fat meat, 1 fat
Fish Sticks	3 oz	210	9	80	1.5	0	10	520	24	0	10	1 1/2 carb, 1 med-fat meat, 1 fat

Gorton's

Classic Breaded Fish Sticks	3.7 oz	250	16	140	4	0	25	340	19	1	10	1 carb, 1 med-fat meat, 2 fat

FROZEN MEALS, MEAT, CHICKEN, FISH

	Serving	Calories	Fat (g)	Cal. from Fat	Sat. Fat (g)	Trans Fat (g)	Chol. (mg)	Sod. (mg)	Carb. (g)	Fiber (g)	Prot. (g)	Servings/Exchanges
Classic Crispy Battered Fillets	3.8 oz	230	12	110	3	0	25	650	22	3	8	1 1/2 carb, 1 med-fat meat, 1 fat
Classic Crunchy Golden Fish Fillets	1 fillet	170	9	80	1.5	0	20	260	16	0	7	1 carb, 1 med-fat meat, 1 fat
Crunchy Fish Portions	1 piece	200	10	90	1.5	0	15	460	19	2	9	1 carb, 1 med-fat meat, 1 fat
Crunchy Golden Popcorn Shrimp	3.2 oz	240	12	110	3	0	55	630	24	0	8	1 1/2 carb, 1 med-fat meat, 1 fat
Garlic Butter Grilled Fillets	3.8 oz	100	3	25	0	0	70	290	1	0	17	2 lean meat
Grilled Shrimp Classic	4 oz	110	1	15	0	0	50	960	5	0	18	3 lean meat
Lemon Pepper Grilled Fillets	3.8 oz	100	3	25	0	0	70	290	1	0	17	2 lean meat
Original Batter Fish Tenders	3.6 oz	230	12	110	3	0	20	660	23	2	8	1 1/2 carb, 1 med-fat meat, 1 fat

	Serving	Cal.	Fat (g)	Cal. Fat	Sat. Fat	Trans Fat	Chol.	Sod.	Carb.	Fiber	Prot.	Exchanges
Salmon Classic Grilled Fillets	3.1 oz	100	3	25	0	0	35	270	2	0	15	2 lean meat
Mrs. Paul's												
Battered Fish Tenders	4 pieces	210	10	90	3.5	0	20	700	22	1	9	1 1/2 carb, 1 med-fat meat, 1 fat
Breaded Fish Sticks	6	250	12	110	4.5	0	25	390	25	1	10	1 1/2 carb, 1 med-fat meat, 1 fat
Lightly Breaded Cod Fillets	1 fillet	220	11	100	5	0	40	430	17	1	12	1 carb, 1 med-fat meat, 1 fat
Lightly Breaded Flounder Fillets	1 fillet	150	7	60	3.5	0	25	290	12	1	8	1 carb, 1 med-fat meat
Van de Kamp's												
Breaded Popcorn Fish	8 pieces	220	12	110	5	0	30	480	18	2	11	1 carb, 1 med-fat meat, 1 fat
Breaded Popcorn Shrimp	4 oz	260	11	100	4.5	0	80	750	30	2	11	2 carb, 1 med-fat meat, 1 fat

FROZEN MEALS, MEAT, CHICKEN, FISH

	Serving	Calories	Fat (g)	Cal. from Fat	Sat. Fat (g)	Trans Fat (g)	Chol. (mg)	Sod. (mg)	Carb. (g)	Fiber (g)	Prot. (g)	Servings/Exchanges
Crisp & Healthy Breaded Fish Fillets	2 fillets	150	1.5	15	1	0	20	470	25	1	8	1 1/2 carb, 1 lean meat
Crisp & Healthy Breaded Fish Sticks	6 sticks	140	1	10	0.5	0	25	380	24	1	9	1 1/2 carb, 1 lean meat
Crunchy Breaded Fish Fillets	2 fillets	230	13	120	4.5	0	20	440	21	<1	8	1 1/2 carb, 1 med-fat meat, 2 fat
Crunchy Breaded Fish Shaped Nuggets	4 pieces	260	12	110	1.5	0	15	790	29	1	9	2 carb, 1 med-fat meat, 1 fat
Crunchy Golden Breaded Fish Sticks	6 sticks	230	11	100	4	0	25	370	23	1	10	1 1/2 carb, 1 med-fat meat, 1 fat

FROZEN PIZZA, SNACKS

FROZEN PIZZA

California Pizza Kitchen

	Serving	Calories	Fat (g)	Cal. from Fat	Sat. Fat (g)	Trans Fat (g)	Chol. (mg)	Sod. (mg)	Carb. (g)	Fiber (g)	Prot. (g)	Servings/Exchanges
Crispy Thin Crust, Margherita	1/3 pizza	300	13	120	5	1	20	520	33	2	14	2 carb, 1 med-fat meat, 2 fat
Crispy Thin Crust, Sicilian	1/3 pizza	310	13	120	5	0.5	35	810	32	2	17	2 carb, 2 med-fat meat, 1 fat
Crispy Thin Crust, White Pizza	1/3 pizza	300	12	100	6	1	25	540	32	2	16	2 carb, 1 med-fat meat, 1 fat
Five Cheese & Tomato	1/3 pizza	320	15	140	8	0.5	40	700	29	1	18	2 carb, 2 med-fat meat, 1 fat
Hawaiian	1/3 pizza	260	9	80	4	0	20	730	31	2	14	2 carb, 2 med-fat meat
Rising Crust BBQ Chicken	1/5 pizza	320	10	90	4	0	25	750	43	2	16	3 carb, 1 med-fat meat, 1 fat

FROZEN PIZZA, SNACKS

	Serving	Calories	Fat (g)	Cal. from Fat	Sat. Fat (g)	Trans Fat (g)	Chol. (mg)	Sod. (mg)	Carb. (g)	Fiber (g)	Prot. (g)	Servings/Exchanges
DiGiorno												
Cheese Stuffed Crust Pepperoni	1/5 pizza	380	16	150	8	0	40	720	40	3	15	2 1/2 carb, 2 med-fat meat, 1 fat
Cheese Stuffed Crust Supreme	1/6 pizza	350	16	150	7	0	40	950	35	3	17	2 carb, 2 med-fat meat, 1 fat
Cheese Stuffed Crust Three Meat	1/6 pizza	350	16	150	7	0.5	40	950	34	2	17	2 carb, 2 med-fat meat, 1 fat
Rising Crust Four Cheese	1/2 pizza	310	11	100	5	0	25	850	40	2	15	2 1/2 carb, 1 med-fat meat, 1 fat
Rising Crust Pepperoni	1/2 pizza	330	13	110	5	0	30	940	40	2	14	2 1/2 carb, 1 med-fat meat, 2 fat
Rising Crust Supreme	1/2 pizza	360	15	130	6	0	30	990	41	3	16	2 1/2 carb, 1 med-fat meat, 2 fat
Thin Crispy Crust Four Cheese	1/5 pizza	310	13	120	7	1	35	660	32	3	18	2 carb, 2 med-fat meat, 1 fat

Food	Serving											Exchanges/Choices
Thin Crispy Crust Four Meat	1/5 pizza	320	14	130	6	0.5	35	850	32	2	18	2 carb, 2 med-fat meat, 1 fat
Thin Crispy Crust Pepperoni	1/5 pizza	320	15	140	7	0.5	35	790	31	2	16	2 carb, 1 med-fat meat, 2 fat
Thin Crispy Crust Supreme	1/5 pizza	320	15	130	6	0.5	30	720	33	3	16	2 carb, 1 med-fat meat, 1 fat
Freschetta												
Brick Oven, 5 Italian Cheese	1/4 pizza	340	15	130	6	0	25	780	37	3	15	2 1/2 carb, 1 med-fat meat, 2 fat
Brick Oven, Italian Pepperoni	1/4 pizza	410	20	180	20	0.5	40	1120	38	2	19	2 1/2 carb, 2 med-fat meat, 2 fat
Brick Oven, Spinach and Mushroom	1/4 pizza	310	11	100	3.5	0	15	710	40	3	13	2 1/2 carb, 1 med-fat meat, 1 fat
Jenos Crisp 'n Tasty												
Cheese	6.9 oz	450	21	190	3.5	6	0	1020	51	2	14	3 1/2 carb, 1 med-fat meat, 3 fat

FROZEN PIZZA, SNACKS

	Serving	Calories	Fat (g)	Cal. from Fat	Sat. Fat (g)	Trans Fat (g)	Chol. (mg)	Sod. (mg)	Carb. (g)	Fiber (g)	Prot. (g)	Servings/Exchanges
Combination	7 oz	480	25	220	6	4.5	15	1140	50	2	15	3 carb, 1 med-fat meat, 4 fat
Hamburger	7.3 oz	500	25	230	6	25	0	1040	51	2	18	3 1/2 carb, 1 med-fat meat, 4 fat
Pepperoni	6.8 oz	490	26	230	7	2.5	15	1060	50	2	15	3 carb, 1 med-fat meat, 4 fat
Sausage	7 oz	480	25	220	6	4.5	10	1110	50	2	15	3 carb, 1 med-fat meat, 4 fat
Supreme	7.2 oz	480	24	220	6	4.5	15	1130	49	1	15	3 carb, 1 med-fat meat, 4 fat
Red Baron												
Classic 4-Cheese	1/4 pizza	380	16	150	9	0.5	30	690	40	2	18	2 1/2 carb, 1 med-fat meat, 2 fat
Classic 4-Meat	1/4 pizza	380	16	150	8	0	30	770	41	2	17	2 1/2 carb, 1 med-fat meat, 2 fat

Classic Hamburger	1/4 pizza	360	15	130	7	0.5	30	770	40	2	17	2 1/2 carb, 1 med-fat meat, 1 fat
Classic Mexican Style Supreme	1/5 pizza	370	16	150	8	0	25	670	42	3	15	3 carb, 1 med-fat meat, 1 fat
Classic Pepperoni	1/5 pizza	370	16	150	8	0	30	740	40	2	16	2 1/2 carb, 1 med-fat meat, 1 fat
Classic Supreme	1/5 pizza	310	14	130	7	0	25	590	34	2	13	2 carb, 1 med-fat meat, 2 fat
Deep Dish Mini Pizza, Cheese	4 pieces	420	20	180	11	0	25	770	44	2	16	3 carb, 1 med-fat meat, 3 fat
Deep Dish Mini Pizza, Pepperoni	4 pieces	460	25	220	12	0	40	990	44	2	16	3 carb, 1 med-fat meat, 4 fat
Deep Dish Singles, Pepperoni	1	420	19	170	9	0	25	870	45	2	17	3 carb, 1 med-fat meat, 3 fat
Deep Dish Singles, Supreme	1	420	19	170	9	0	30	770	45	2	17	3 carb, 1 med-fat meat, 3 fat

FROZEN PIZZA, SNACKS

	Serving	Calories	Fat (g)	Cal. from Fat	Sat. Fat (g)	Trans Fat (g)	Chol. (mg)	Sod. (mg)	Carb. (g)	Fiber (g)	Prot. (g)	Servings/Exchanges
Fire Baked Pepperoni	1/4 pizza	370	17	150	7	0	30	910	40	3	16	2 1/2 carb, 1 med-fat meat, 2 fat
French Bread 5 Cheese & Garlic	1	410	22	200	8	0	25	880	39	2	14	2 1/2 carb, 1 med-fat meat, 3 fat
French Bread Pepperoni	1	360	15	130	7	0	30	1070	42	2	16	3 carb, 1 med-fat meat, 2 fat
Thin & Crispy 5-Cheese	1/3 pizza	360	16	140	8	0	25	780	39	2	16	2 1/2 carb, 1 med-fat meat, 2 fat
Thin & Crispy Pepperoni	1/3 pizza	410	20	180	9	0.5	35	970	40	2	17	2 1/2 carb, 1 med-fat meat, 3 fat
Tombstone												
Original Deluxe Cheese	1/5 pizza	290	12	110	5	0	30	580	31	3	14	2 carb, 1 med-fat meat, 1 fat
Original Hamburger	1/4 pizza	350	15	140	7	0.5	35	720	37	4	18	2 1/2 carb, 2 med-fat meat, 1 fat

Original Pepperoni	1/3 pizza	280	14	120	6	0	30	620	28	3	13	2 carb, 1 med-fat meat, 2 fat
Original Pepperoni & Sausage	1/3 pizza	290	14	130	6	0	30	650	28	3	14	2 carb, 1 med-fat meat, 2 fat
Original Supreme	1/5 pizza	300	14	120	6	0	30	640	31	3	14	2 carb, 1 med-fat meat, 2 fat
Original Xtra Cheese	1/2 pizza	360	14	130	7	0.5	30	680	42	4	17	3 carb, 1 med-fat meat, 2 fat

Tony's

Original Cheese	1/3 pizza	290	12	100	5	0	15	570	37	2	11	2 1/2 carb, 1 med-fat meat, 1 fat
Original Four Cheese	1/3 pizza	300	13	110	6	0	20	570	36	2	12	3 1/2 carb, 1 med-fat meat, 2 fat
Original Meat Trio	1/3 pizza	340	16	140	7	0	15	680	37	2	13	2 1/2 carb, 1 med-fat meat, 2 fat
Original Pepperoni	1/3 pizza	310	14	120	7	0	10	620	36	2	11	2 1/2 carb, 1 med-fat meat, 2 fat

FROZEN PIZZA, SNACKS

	Serving	Calories	Fat (g)	Cal. from Fat	Sat. Fat (g)	Trans Fat (g)	Chol. (mg)	Sod. (mg)	Carb. (g)	Fiber (g)	Prot. (g)	Servings/Exchanges
Original Sausage & Pepperoni	1/3 pizza	340	17	150	8	0	15	660	37	2	12	2 1/2 carb, 1 med-fat meat, 2 fat
Original Supreme	1/3 pizza	330	16	140	7	0	10	630	37	2	12	2 1/2 carb, 1 med-fat meat, 2 fat
Thin Crust Supreme	1/3 pizza	360	19	170	5	0	15	930	34	2	14	2 carb, 1 med-fat meat, 3 fat
Totino's Party Pizza												
Crisp Crust Canadian Style Bacon	1/2 pizza	320	15	130	2.5	4	10	890	34	1	13	2 carb, 1 med-fat meat, 2 fat
Crisp Crust Combination	1/2 pizza	370	20	180	4.5	4	10	910	35	1	12	2 carb, 1 med-fat meat, 3 fat
Crisp Crust Mexican Style	1/2 pizza	370	19	180	4.5	4	15	890	36	2	14	2 1/2 carb, 1 med-fat meat, 3 fat
Crisp Crust Pepperoni	1/2 pizza	360	20	180	4.5	4	10	920	34	1	12	2 carb, 1 med-fat meat, 3 fat

Crisp Crust Sausage	1/2 pizza	370	20	180	4.5	4	10	890	35	2	12	2 carb, 1 med-fat meat, 3 fat
Crisp Crust Supreme	1/2 pizza	360	19	170	4.5	4	10	590	35	1	12	2 carb, 1 med-fat meat, 3 fat
Crisp Crust Triple Cheese	1/2 pizza	320	16	140	5	3	15	720	34	1	12	2 carb, 1 med-fat meat, 2 fat
Crisp Crust Triple Meat	1/2 pizza	350	18	160	4	4	10	900	34	1	12	2 carb, 1 med-fat meat, 3 fat

FROZEN SNACKS

Bagel Bites

Cheese & Pepperoni	4	220	7	60	3	0	15	480	30	2	9	2 carb, 1 med-fat meat
Three Cheese	4	210	6	60	3	0	15	400	30	2	9	2 carb, 1 med-fat meat

Delime

Taquitos, Beef	5	370	15	140	2	0	15	760	46	8	15	3 carb, 1 med-fat meat, 2 fat
Taquitos, Chicken	5	370	14	130	3	0	30	480	47	8	15	3 carb, 1 med-fat meat, 2 fat

FROZEN PIZZA, SNACKS

	Serving	Calories	Fat (g)	Cal. from Fat	Sat. Fat (g)	Trans Fat (g)	Chol. (mg)	Sod. (mg)	Carb. (g)	Fiber (g)	Prot. (g)	Servings/Exchanges
Hot Pockets												
BBQ Beef	1	340	14	130	7	0	30	670	44	2	9	3 carb, 3 fat
Ham & Cheese	1	290	12	110	5	0	30	640	36	1	10	2 1/2 carb, 1 med-fat meat, 1 fat
Meatballs & Mozzarella	1	340	16	150	7	0	30	570	37	2	10	2 1/2 carb, 1 med-fat meat, 2 fat
Pizzeria Four Cheese Pizza	1	330	13	120	6	0	25	750	39	1	13	2 1/2 carb, 1 med-fat meat, 2 fat
Pizzeria Pepperoni	1	340	17	150	8	0	25	730	37	2	10	2 1/2 carb, 1 med-fat meat, 2 fat
Jose Ole Mexi-Minis												
Beef & Cheese Mini Tacos	4	210	11	100	4	0	20	440	19	5	7	1 carb, 1 med-fat meat, 1 fat
Chicken Taquitos	3	200	8	70	1.5	0	10	390	26	3	7	2 carb, 2 fat

Shredded Steak Taquitos	3	210	9	80	2	0	10	420	25	3	6	1 1/2 carb, 2 fat
Lean Pockets												
Barbeque Recipe Beef	1	290	7	60	3.5	0	25	700	46	3	11	3 carb, 1 fat
Cheeseburger	1	290	8	70	3.5	0	25	550	41	3	12	2 1/2 carb, 1 med-fat meat, 1 fat
Chicken Parmesan	1	290	7	60	3	0	25	470	45	3	10	3 carb, 1 fat
Four Cheese Pizza	1	300	7	60	3.5	0	20	680	45	3	15	3 carb, 1 med-fat meat
Ham & Cheddar	1	270	8	70	4	0	30	540	40	3	12	2 1/2 carb, 1 med-fat meat, 1 fat
Meatball Mozzarella	1	290	9	80	4	0	25	560	40	3	12	2 1/2 carb, 1 med-fat meat, 1 fat
Mexican Style Chicken Fiesta	1	240	7	60	3	0	20	660	35	3	10	2 carb, 1 med-fat meat
Pepperoni Pizza	1	280	8	70	3.5	0	20	630	46	2	13	3 carb, 1 med-fat meat, 1 fat

FROZEN PIZZA, SNACKS

	Serving	Calories	Fat (g)	Cal. from Fat	Sat. Fat (g)	Trans Fat (g)	Chol. (mg)	Sod. (mg)	Carb. (g)	Fiber (g)	Prot. (g)	Servings/Exchanges
Philly Steak & Cheese	1	270	7	70	3.5	0	25	640	39	2	11	2 1/2 carb, 1 med-fat meat
Southwest Style Bacon, Egg & Cheese	1	250	8	70	2.5	0	50	530	33	1	11	2 carb, 1 med-fat meat, 1 fat
Stuffed Quesadilla Grilled Chicken Fajita	1	360	9	80	4	0	35	670	48	2	19	3 carb, 1 med-fat meat, 1 fat
Ling Ling Potstickers												
Chicken & Vegetable Dumplings	5	260	6	60	1.5	0	35	620	39	2	13	2 1/2 carb, 1 med-fat meat
Pork & Dumplings	5	280	8	80	2.5	0	25	640	38	2	12	2 1/2 carb, 1 med-fat meat, 1 fat
Michelina's												
Four Melt Pizza Snack Rolls	6 rolls	230	12	100	3.5	0	15	410	23	1	9	1 1/2 carb, 1 med-fat meat, 1 fat

Pepperoni Pizza Snack Rolls	6	230	11	100	3	0	10	460	24	1	8	1 1/2 carb, 1 med-fat meat, 1 fat

Poppers

Cream Cheese Jalapeños	3	220	15	130	6	0	25	470	15	1	4	1 carb, 3 fat

Totino's

Pizza Rolls, Cheese	6 rolls	200	8	70	2	1	5	440	26	1	7	2 carb, 2 fat
Pizza Rolls, Supreme	6 rolls	200	8	80	2	1.5	5	390	25	1	7	1 1/2 carb, 2 fat
Pizza Rolls, Taco	6 rolls	200	8	80	3	1	15	470	24	1	7	1 1/2 carb, 2 fat

FRUIT, FRUIT JUICES, DRINKS

FRUIT

	Serving	Calories	Fat (g)	Cal. from Fat	Sat. Fat (g)	Trans Fat (g)	Chol. (mg)	Sod. (mg)	Carb. (g)	Fiber (g)	Prot. (g)	Servings/Exchanges
Apple, Unpeeled	1 small	54	0	0	0	0	0	1	14	3	0	1 fruit
Apple, Unpeeled	1 large	125	0	0	0	0	0	0	32	6	0	2 fruit
Apples, Dried	4 rings	63	0	0	0	0	0	23	17	2	0	1 fruit
Applesauce, Sweetened	1/2 cup	97	0	0	0	0	0	35	51	2	<1	1 fruit, 2 1/2 carb
Applesauce, Unsweetened	1/2 cup	53	0	0	0	0	0	3	14	2	<1	1 fruit
Apricots, Canned, EXtra Light Syrup	1/2 cup	61	0	0	0	0	0	3	15	2	<1	1 fruit
Apricots, Canned, Heavy Syrup	1/2 cup	107	0	0	0	0	0	5	28	2	<1	1 fruit, 1 carb
Apricots, Canned, Juice Pack	1/2 cup	59	0	0	0	0	0	5	15	2	<1	1 fruit

Food	Amount	Calories								Exchanges
Apricots, Canned, Light Syrup	1/2 cup	80	0	0	0	5	21	2	<1	1 fruit, 1/2 carb
Apricots, Canned, Water Pack	1/2 cup	33	0	0	0	4	8	2	<1	1/2 fruit
Apricots, Dried	8 halves	67	0	0	0	3	18	2	0	1 fruit
Banana	6 inches	72	0	0	0	1	19	2	<1	1 fruit
Blackberries, Canned, Heavy Syrup	1/2 cup	118	0	0	0	4	29	4	2	1 fruit, 1 carb
Blackberries, Fresh	3/4 cup	56	0	0	0	0	14	6	<1	1 fruit
Blackberries, Frozen, Unsweetened	1 cup	97	0	0	0	2	24	8	2	1 1/2 fruit
Blueberries, Canned, Heavy Syrup	1/2 cup	113	0	0	0	8	28	4	<1	1 fruit, 1 carb
Blueberries, Dried	2 Tbsp	69	0	0	0	0	16	1	<1	1 fruit
Blueberries, Fresh	3/4 cup	62	0	0	0	1	16	3	<1	1 fruit
Blueberries, Frozen, Sweetened	1 cup	186	0	0	0	2	50	5	<1	1 fruit, 2 carb

FRUIT, FRUIT JUICES, DRINKS

	Serving	Calories	Fat (g)	Cal. from Fat	Sat. Fat (g)	Trans Fat (g)	Chol. (mg)	Sod. (mg)	Carb. (g)	Fiber (g)	Prot. (g)	Servings/Exchanges
Blueberries, Frozen, Unsweetened	1 cup	79	0	0	0	0	0	2	19	4	<1	1 fruit
Boysenberries, Canned, Heavy Syrup	1/2 cup	113	0	0	0	0	0	4	29	<1	2	1 fruit, 1 carb
Boysenberries, Frozen, Unsweetened	1 cup	66	0	0	0	0	0	1	16	7	1	1 fruit
Cantaloupe, Fresh	1 cup	56	0	0	0	0	0	14	13	1	1	1 fruit
Cheeries, Sour, Frozen, Unsweetened	1 cup	71	0	0	0	0	0	2	17	25	1	1 fruit
Cherries, Dried	2 Tbsp	66	0	0	0	0	0	0	16	1	0	1 fruit
Cherries, Sour, Canned, Extra Heavy Syrup	1/2 cup	149	0	0	0	0	0	9	38	1	1	1 fruit, 1 1/2 carb
Cherries, Sour, Canned, Heavy Syrup	1/2 cup	117	0	0	0	0	0	9	30	1	1	1 fruit, 1 carb

Food	Serving										Exchanges
Cherries, Sour, Canned, Light Syrup	1/2 cup	95	0	0	0	0	9	25	1	1	1 fruit, 1/2 carb
Cherries, Sour, Canned, Water Pack	1/2 cup	44	0	0	0	0	9	11	1	2	1 fruit
Cherries, Sweet, Canned, Extra Heavy Syrup	1/2 cup	133	0	0	0	0	4	34	2	<1	1 fruit, 1 carb
Cherries, Sweet, Canned, Heavy Syrup	1/2 cup	105	0	0	0	0	4	27	2	<1	1 fruit, 1 carb
Cherries, Sweet, Canned, Juice Pack	1/2 cup	68	0	0	0	0	4	18	2	<1	1 fruit
Cherries, Sweet, Canned, Light Syrup	1/2 cup	85	0	0	0	0	4	22	2	<1	1 fruit, 1/2 carb
Cherries, Sweet, Canned, Water Pack	1/2 cup	57	0	0	0	0	1	15	2	1	1 fruit
Cherries, Sweet, Fresh	12	56	0	0	0	0	0	14	2	1	1 fruit

FRUIT, FRUIT JUICES, DRINKS

	Serving	Calories	Fat (g)	Cal. from Fat	Sat. Fat (g)	Trans Fat (g)	Chol. (mg)	Sod. (mg)	Carb. (g)	Fiber (g)	Prot. (g)	Servings/Exchanges
Cherries, Sweet, Frozen, Unsweetened	1 cup	231	0	0	0	0	0	3	17	5	3	1 fruit
Cranberries	1 cup	47	<1	0	<1	0	0	<1	12	4	<1	1 fruit
Cranberries, Dried	2 Tbsp	47	0	0	0	0	0	0	13	<1	0	1 fruit
Cranberry Sauce, Canned, Sweetened	1/2 cup	209	0	0	0	0	0	40	54	1	<1	1 fruit, 2 1/2 carb
Currants, Red/White, Fresh	1 cup	63	0	0	0	0	0	1	15	5	2	1 fruit
Figs, Canned, Extra Heavy Syrup	1/2 cup	140	0	0	0	0	0	2	37	NA	<1	1 fruit, 1 1/2 carb
Figs, Canned, Heavy Syrup	1/2 cup	114	0	0	0	0	0	2	30	3	<1	1 fruit, 1 carb
Figs, Canned, Light Syrup	1/2 cup	87	0	0	0	0	0	2	23	2	<1	1 fruit, 1/2 carb

Food	Serving									
Figs, Canned, Water Pack	1/2 cup	66	0	0	0	1	18	3	<1	1 fruit
Figs, Dried	1 1/2	71	0	0	0	3	18	3	<1	1 fruit
Figs, Fresh	2 medium	74	0	0	0	1	19	3	<1	1 fruit
Fruit Cocktail, Canned, Extra Heavy Syrup	1/2 cup	114	0	0	0	8	30	1	<1	1 fruit, 1 carb
Fruit Cocktail, Canned, Extra Light Syrup	1/2 cup	55	0	0	0	5	14	1	<1	1 fruit
Fruit Cocktail, Canned, Heavy Syrup	1/2 cup	91	0	0	0	15	24	1	<1	1 fruit, 1/2 carb
Fruit Cocktail, Canned, Juice Pack	1/2 cup	104	0	0	0	5	14	1	<1	1 fruit
Fruit Cocktail, Canned, Water Pack	1/2 cup	38	0	0	0	5	10	1	<1	1 fruit
Fruit Coctail, Canned, Light Syrup	1/2 cup	69	0	0	0	8	18	1	<1	1 fruit

FRUIT, FRUIT JUICES, DRINKS

	Serving	Calories	Fat (g)	Cal. from Fat	Sat. Fat (g)	Trans Fat (g)	Chol. (mg)	Sod. (mg)	Carb. (g)	Fiber (g)	Prot. (g)	Servings/Exchanges
Fruit Salad, Canned, Extra Heavy Syrup	1/2 cup	114	0	0	0	0	0	7	30	1	<1	1 fruit, 1 carb
Fruit Salad, Canned, Heavy Syrup	1/2 cup	93	0	0	0	0	0	8	25	1	<1	1 fruit, 1/2 carb
Fruit Salad, Canned, Juice Pack	1/2 cup	62	0	0	0	0	0	6	16	1	<1	1 fruit
Fruit Salad, Canned, Light Syrup	1/2 cup	73	0	0	0	0	0	8	19	1	<1	1 fruit
Fruit Salad, Canned, Water Pack	1/2 cup	37	0	0	0	0	0	4	10	1	<1	1 fruit
Grapefruit Sections, Canned, Juice Pack	1/2 cup	46	0	0	0	0	0	9	12	<1	<1	1 fruit
Grapefruit Sections, Canned, Light Syrup	1/2 cup	76	0	0	0	0	0	3	20	<1	<1	1 fruit

Food	Serving										Exchanges
Grapefruit Sections, Canned, Water Pack	1/2 cup	44	0	0	0	0	3	11	<1	<1	1 fruit
Grapefruit, Fresh	1/2	53	0	0	0	0	0	13	2	1	1 fruit
Grapes, Canned, Heavy Syrup	1/2 cup	94	0	0	0	0	7	25	<1	<1	1 fruit, 1/2 carb
Grapes, Canned, Water Pack	1/2 cup	49	0	0	0	0	8	13	<1	<1	1 fruit
Grapes, Fresh, Seedless	17	60	0	0	0	0	2	15	<1	<1	1 fruit
Guava, Fresh	1	46	0	0	0	0	3	11	5	1	1 fruit
Honeydew Melon, Fresh	1 cup	61	0	0	0	0	31	16	1	<1	1 fruit
Kiwi	1 large	56	0	0	0	0	3	13	3	1	1 fruit
Kumquats, Fresh	2	27	0	0	0	0	4	6	2	1	1/2 fruit
Melon Balls, Mixed, Frozen	1 cup	57	<1	0	<1	0	54	14	1	2	1 fruit
Mixed Fruit, Canned, Heavy Syrup	1/2 cup	92	0	0	0	0	5	24	2	<1	1 fruit, 1/2 carb

FRUIT, FRUIT JUICES, DRINKS

	Serving	Calories	Fat (g)	Cal. from Fat	Sat. Fat (g)	Trans Fat (g)	Chol. (mg)	Sod. (mg)	Carb. (g)	Fiber (g)	Prot. (g)	Servings/Exchanges
Mixed Fruit, Frozen, Sweetened	1 cup	245	0	0	0	0	0	8	61	5	4	1 fruit, 3 carb
Nectarine, Fresh	1 small	60	0	0	0	0	0	0	14	2	1	1 fruit
Orange, Fresh	1	62	0	0	0	0	0	0	15	3	1	1 fruit
Oranges, Mandarin, Canned, Juice Pack	3/4 cup	69	<1	0	0	0	0	9	18	1	1	1 fruit
Papaya, Fresh	1 cup	55	0	0	0	0	0	4	14	3	<1	1 fruit
Peach, Fresh	1 medium	57	0	0	0	0	0	0	14	2	1	1 fruit
Peaches, Canned, Extra Heavy Syrup	1/2 cup	126	0	0	0	0	0	11	34	2	<1	1 fruit, 1 carb
Peaches, Canned, Extra Light Syrup	1/2 cup	52	0	0	0	0	0	6	14	1	<1	1 fruit
Peaches, Canned, Heavy Syrup	1/2 cup	97	0	0	0	0	0	8	26	<1	<1	1 fruit, 1 carb

Food	Serving	Cal								Exchanges
Peaches, Canned, Juice Pack	1/2 cup	55	0	0	0	5	14	1	<1	1 fruit
Peaches, Canned, Light Syrup	1/2 cup	68	0	0	0	7	18	1	<1	1 fruit
Peaches, Canned, Water Pack	1/2 cup	30	0	0	0	4	8	1	<1	1/2 fruit
Peaches, Frozen, Sweetened	1 cup	235	0	0	0	15	60	5	2	1 fruit, 2 carb
Pear, Fresh	1/2 large	61	0	0	0	1	16	3	<1	1 fruit
Pears, Canned, Extra Heavy Syrup	1/2 cup	129	0	0	0	7	34	2	<1	1 fruit, 1 carb
Pears, Canned, Extra Light Syrup	1/2 cup	58	0	0	0	3	15	2	<1	1 fruit
Pears, Canned, Heavy Syrup	1/2 cup	99	0	0	0	7	25	2	<1	1 fruit, 1/2 carb
Pears, Canned, Juice Pack	1/2 cup	62	0	0	0	5	16	2	<1	1 fruit

FRUIT, FRUIT JUICES, DRINKS

	Serving	Calories	Fat (g)	Cal. from Fat	Sat. Fat (g)	Trans Fat (g)	Chol. (mg)	Sod. (mg)	Carb. (g)	Fiber (g)	Prot. (g)	Servings/Exchanges
Pears, Canned, Light Syrup	1/2 cup	72	0	0	0	0	0	7	19	2	<1	1 fruit
Pears, Canned, Water Pack	1/2 cup	36	0	0	0	0	0	3	10	2	<1	1 fruit
Pineapple, Canned, Extra Heavy Syrup	1/2 cup	108	0	0	0	0	0	2	28	1	<1	1 fruit, 1 carb
Pineapple, Canned, Heavy Syrup	1/2 cup	99	0	0	0	0	0	2	26	1	<1	1 fruit, 1 carb
Pineapple, Canned, Juice Pack	1/2 cup	75	0	0	0	0	0	1	20	1	<1	1 fruit
Pineapple, Canned, Light Juice Pack	1/2 cup	66	0	0	0	0	0	2	17	1	<1	1 fruit
Pineapple, Canned, Water Pack	1/2 cup	40	0	0	0	0	0	1	10	1	<1	1 fruit
Pineapple, Fresh	3/4 cup	56	0	0	0	0	0	1	15	2	<1	1 fruit

Food	Serving										Exchanges
Pineapple, Frozen, Sweetened	1 cup	211	0	0	0	0	5	54	3	<1	1 fruit, 2 1/2 carb
Plum, Fresh	2	61	0	0	0	0	0	15	2	<1	1 fruit
Plums, Canned, Extra Heavy Syrup	1/2 cup	132	0	0	0	0	25	35	2	<1	1 fruit, 1 carb
Plums, Canned, Heavy Syrup	1/2 cup	115	0	0	0	0	25	30	1	<1	1 fruit, 1 carb
Plums, Canned, Juice Pack	1/2 cup	73	0	0	0	0	2	19	1	<1	1 fruit
Plums, Canned, Light Syrup	1/2 cup	80	0	0	0	0	25	21	1	<1	1 fruit, 1/2 carb
Plums, Canned, Water Pack	1/2 cup	51	0	0	0	0	1	14	1	<1	1 fruit
Plums, Dried	3	60	0	0	0	0	1	16	2	<1	1 fruit
Pomegranate, Fresh	1	105	0	0	0	0	5	26	1	1	2 fruit
Raisins, Seedless	2 Tbsp	54	0	0	0	0	2	14	<1	<1	1 fruit

FRUIT, FRUIT JUICES, DRINKS

	Serving	Calories	Fat (g)	Cal. from Fat	Sat. Fat (g)	Trans Fat (g)	Chol. (mg)	Sod. (mg)	Carb. (g)	Fiber (g)	Prot. (g)	Servings/Exchanges
Raspberries, Canned, Heavy Syrup	1/2 cup	117	0	0	0	0	0	4	30	4	1	1 fruit, 1 carb
Raspberries, Fresh	1 cup	60	0	0	0	0	0	0	14	8	1	1 fruit
Raspberries, Frozen, Sweetened	1 cup	258	0	0	0	0	0	1	65	6	2	1 fruit, 3 carb
Rhubarb, Frozen, Unsweetened	1 cup	29	0	0	0	0	0	3	7	3	<1	1/2 fruit
Star Fruit (Carambola)	2 medium	60	0	0	0	0	0	4	14	4	0	1 fruit
Strawberries, Canned, Heavy Syrup	1/2 cup	117	0	0	0	0	0	10	30	2	1	1 fruit, 1 carb
Strawberries, Fresh	1 1/4 cup	57	0	0	0	0	0	2	13	4	1	1 fruit
Strawberries, Frozen, Sweetened	1 cup	199	0	0	0	0	0	3	54	5	1	1 fruit, 2 1/2 carb

Food	Serving								Exchange
Strawberries, Frozen, Unsweetened	1 cup	52	0	0	3	14	3	<1	1 fruit
Tangerine, Fresh	2 small	81	0	0	3	20	3	1	1 fruit
Tangerines, Juice Pack	1/2 cup	36	0	0	5	9	1	<1	1/2 fruit
Tangerines, Light Syrup	1/2 cup	77	0	0	8	20	1	<1	1 fruit
Watermelon, Fresh	1 1/4 cup	57	0	0	2	14	<1	1	1 fruit
FRUIT JUICES									
Apple Juice/Cider, Canned/Bottled	1/2 cup	58	0	0	4	15	0	0	1 fruit
Apricot Nectar, Canned	1/2 cup	71	0	0	4	18	0	0	1 fruit
Cranberry Juice Cocktail, Bottled	1/3 cup	48	0	0	2	12	0	0	1 fruit
Cranberry Juice Cocktail, Reduced Calorie	1 cup	50	0	0	7	11	0	0	1 fruit
Fruit Juice Blends, 100% Juice	1/3 cup	50	0	0	10	12	0	0	1 fruit

FRUIT, FRUIT JUICES, DRINKS

	Serving	Calories	Fat (g)	Cal. from Fat	Sat. Fat (g)	Trans Fat (g)	Chol. (mg)	Sod. (mg)	Carb. (g)	Fiber (g)	Prot. (g)	Servings/Exchanges
Grape Juice	1/3 cup	50	0	0	0	0	0	3	13	0	0	1 fruit
Grapefruit Juice, Canned	1/2 cup	47	0	0	0	0	0	1	11	0	<1	1 fruit
Orange Juice, Canned	1/2 cup	52	0	0	0	0	0	3	12	0	<1	1 fruit
Orange Juice, Fresh	1/2 cup	56	0	0	0	0	0	1	13	0	<1	1 fruit
Orange Juice, Frozen	1/2 cup	56	0	0	0	0	0	1	13	<1	<1	1 fruit
Pineapple Juice, Canned	1/2 cup	70	0	0	0	0	0	1	17	<1	<1	1 fruit
Prune Juice, Bottled	1/3 cup	60	0	0	0	0	0	3	15	<1	<1	1 fruit

FRUIT JUICES

Capri Sun (Single Serving Pouch)

	Serving	Calories	Fat (g)	Cal. from Fat	Sat. Fat (g)	Trans Fat (g)	Chol. (mg)	Sod. (mg)	Carb. (g)	Fiber (g)	Prot. (g)	Servings/Exchanges
Juice Drink, Lemonade	6.6 oz	70	0	0	0	0	0	15	19	0	0	1 carb
Juice Drink, Strawberry Kiwi	6.7 oz	70	0	0	0	0	0	15	19	0	0	1 carb

Roarin' Waters, Fruit-Flavored Water	6.7 oz	35	0	0	0	0	15	9	0	0	1/2 carb
Sports Drink, Assorted Flavors	6.75 oz	60	0	0	0	0	55	16	0	0	1 carb
Dole											
Juice Blend, Orange Peach Mango	8 oz	120	0	0	0	0	25	29	0	<1	2 fruit
Juice Blend, Orange Strawberry Banana	8 oz	120	0	0	0	0	10	30	0	1	2 fruit
Juice Blend, Paradise Blend	8 oz	120	0	0	0	0	40	29	0	<1	2 fruit
Juice Blend, Piña Colada	8 oz	120	0	0	0	0	10	29	0	0	2 fruit
Juice Blend, Pineapple Peach Mango	8 oz	130	0	0	0	0	10	31	0	<1	2 fruit
Juice Blend, Strawberry Kiwi	8 oz	120	0	0	0	0	25	31	0	0	2 fruit

FRUIT, FRUIT JUICES, DRINKS

	Serving	Calories	Fat (g)	Cal. from Fat	Sat. Fat (g)	Trans Fat (g)	Chol. (mg)	Sod. (mg)	Carb. (g)	Fiber (g)	Prot. (g)	Servings/Exchanges
Pineapple Juice	8 oz	130	0	0	0	0	0	10	30	0	0	2 fruit
Donald Duck												
Orange Juice, No Pulp Plus Calcium	8 oz	110	0	0	0	0	0	20	27	0	2	2 fruit
Orange Juice, Original No Pulp	8 oz	110	0	0	0	0	0	20	27	0	2	2 fruit
Florida's Natural												
Orange Juice, Original	8 oz	110	0	0	0	0	0	0	26	0	2	2 fruit
Orange Juice, Calcium & Vitamin D	8 oz	110	0	0	0	0	0	0	26	0	2	2 fruit
Ruby Red Grapefruit Juice, Original	8 oz	90	0	0	0	0	0	0	22	0	1	1 1/2 fruit
Hansen's												
Smoothie, Assorted Flavors	11.5 oz	170–180	0	0	0	0	0	50	43–45	0	0	3 carb

Hawaiian Punch

Fruit Punch, Assorted Flavors	8 oz	120	0	0	0	0	115–120	29–30	0	0	2 carb

Hollywood

Carrot Juice	11 oz can	100	0	0	0	0	170	22	2	2	1 1/2 fruit

Kool-Aid (Single Serving)

Bursts, Soft Drink, Assorted Flavors	6.8 oz	35	0	0	0	0	30	9	0	0	1/2 carb
Jammers, Juice Drink, Cherry	5.9 oz	80	0	0	0	0	15	20	0	0	1 carb
Jammers, Juice Drink, Tropical	6.7 oz	10	0	0	0	0	25	2	0	0	free

Juicy Juice 100% Juice

Apple Juice	8 oz	110	0	0	0	0	20	28	0	0	2 fruit

Kern's

Aguas Frescas Limon Juice Drink	8 oz	120	0	0	0	0	5	31	0	0	2 carb

FRUIT, FRUIT JUICES, DRINKS

	Serving	Calories	Fat (g)	Cal. from Fat	Sat. Fat (g)	Trans Fat (g)	Chol. (mg)	Sod. (mg)	Carb. (g)	Fiber (g)	Prot. (g)	Servings/Exchanges
Apricot Nectar	8 oz	140	0	0	0	0	0	5	35	0	0	2 carb
Guava Nectar	8 oz	150	0	0	0	0	0	10	37	0	0	2 1/2 carb
Pear Nectar	8 oz	150	0	0	0	0	0	10	37	0	0	2 1/2 carb
Mango Nectar, Single Serving	11.5 oz can	210	0	0	0	0	0	25	52	0	0	3 1/2 carb
Peach Nectar, Single Serving	11.5 oz can	200	0	0	0	0	0	10	46	0	0	3 carb
Strawberry Banana	8 oz	220	0	0	0	0	0	10	52	0	0	3 1/2 carb
Langer's												
Apple Cider	8 oz	120	0	0	0	0	0	0	28	0	0	2 fruit
Apple Juice	8 oz	120	0	0	0	0	0	0	28	0	0	2 fruit
Cranberry Grape Blend	8 oz	165	0	0	0	0	0	10	41	0	0	2 1/2 fruit
Cranberry Juice Cocktail	8 oz	140	0	0	0	0	0	10	35	0	0	2 carb

Cranberry Raspberry	8 oz	150	0	0	0	0	10	36	0	0	2 1/2 fruit
Diet Low Carb Apple Juice Cocktail	8 oz	60	0	0	0	0	10	14	0	0	1 carb
Diet Low Carb Cranberry Cocktail	8 oz	30	0	0	0	0	10	8	0	0	1/2 carb
Diet Low Carb Ruby Red Grapefruit Juice Cocktail	8 oz	30	0	0	0	0	10	40	0	0	2 1/2 carb
Ruby Red Grapefruit Juice Cocktail	8 oz	130	0	0	0	0	10	33	0	0	2 carb
Martinelli's											
Apple Juice	8 oz	140	0	0	0	0	0	35	0	0	2 fruit
Apple Pomegranate Juice	8 oz	150	0	0	0	0	10	38	0	0	2 1/2 fruit
Minute Maid											
Apple Juice, Single Serving	10 oz	140	0	0	0	0	25	35	0	0	2 fruit

FRUIT, FRUIT JUICES, DRINKS

	Serving	Calories	Fat (g)	Cal. from Fat	Sat. Fat (g)	Trans Fat (g)	Chol. (mg)	Sod. (mg)	Carb. (g)	Fiber (g)	Prot. (g)	Servings/Exchanges
Apple Strawberry	6.75 oz box	100	0	0	0	0	0	15	25	0	0	1 1/2 carb
Berry Punch	8 oz	120	0	0	0	0	0	15	32	0	0	2 carb
Cherry Limeade	8 oz	120	0	0	0	0	0	15	34	0	0	2 carb
Fruit Punch	8 oz	120	0	0	0	0	0	15	31	0	0	2 carb
Lemonade	8 oz	110	0	0	0	0	0	15	31	0	0	2 carb
Light Orange Juice Beverage	8 oz	50	0	0	0	0	0	15	13	0	0	1 carb
Light Raspberry Passion	8 oz	10	0	0	0	0	0	50	2	0	0	free
Limeade	8 oz	90	0	0	0	0	0	0	25	0	0	1 1/2 carb
Mixed Berry, Single Serving	6.75 oz box	100	0	0	0	0	0	15	25	0	0	1 1/2 fruit
Orange Juice, Country Style	8 oz	110	0	0	0	0	0	15	27	0	2	2 fruit

Orange Juice, Heart Wise	8 oz	110	0	0	0	20	27	0	2	2 fruit
Orange Juice, Home Squeezed, Calcium & Vitamin D	8 oz	110	0	0	0	15	27	0	2	2 fruit
Orange Juice, Kid's +	8 oz	100	0	0	0	15	23	0	2	1 1/2 fruit
Orange Juice, Multi-Vitamin	8 oz	120	0	0	0	20	27	0	0	2 fruit
Orange Juice, Original	8 oz	110	0	0	0	15	27	0	2	2 fruit
Orange Juice, Original with Calcium	8 oz	110	0	0	0	15	27	0	0	2 fruit
Orange Juice, Original, Single Serve	8 oz	110	0	0	0	20	27	0	2	2 fruit
Pink Lemonade, Single Serving	8 oz	100	0	0	0	35	28	0	0	2 carb
Mott's										
Plus Light Juice	8 oz	130	0	0	0	35	15	0	0	1 carb

FRUIT, FRUIT JUICES, DRINKS

	Serving	Calories	Fat (g)	Cal. from Fat	Sat. Fat (g)	Trans Fat (g)	Chol. (mg)	Sod. (mg)	Carb. (g)	Fiber (g)	Prot. (g)	Servings/Exchanges
Naked												
Berry Blast	8 oz	130	0	0	0	0	0	10	29	0	1	2 fruit
Mighty Mango	8 oz	150	0	0	0	0	0	10	36	0	1	2 1/2 fruit
Power-C	8 oz	120	0	0	0	0	0	15	29	3	1	2 fruit
Protein Zone	8 oz	220	2	20	1	0	30	140	34	0	16	2 carb, 2 lean meat
Strawberry Banana	8 oz	120	0	0	0	0	0	20	29	0	1	2 fruit
Superfood Green Machine	8 oz	140	0	0	0	0	0	15	33	0	2	2 fruit
Ocean Spray												
Cran-Apple Juice Drink	8 oz	130	0	0	0	0	0	80	32	0	0	2 carb
Cranberry Juice Cocktail	8 oz	120	0	0	0	0	0	35	30	0	0	2 carb
Cranergy Juice Drink	8 oz	35	0	0	0	0	0	50	8	0	0	1/2 carb
Cran-Grape Juice Drink	8 oz	120	0	0	0	0	0	31	80	0	0	2 carb

Cran-Pomegranate	8 oz	120	0	0	0	0	0	35	30	0	0	2 carb
Cran-Raspberry Juice Drink	8 oz	110	0	0	0	0	0	70	28	0	0	2 carb
Diet Cranberry	8 oz	5	0	0	0	0	0	50	2	0	0	free
Diet Grape	8 oz	5	0	0	0	0	0	50	2	0	0	free
Light Cranberry Juice Cocktail	8 oz	40	0	0	0	0	0	75	10	0	0	1/2 carb
Light Cran-Grape Juice Drink	8 oz	40	0	0	0	0	0	75	10	0	0	1/2 carb
Light Ruby Grapefruit Juice Drink	8 oz	40	0	0	0	0	0	65	10	0	0	1/2 carb
No Sugar Added 100% Cranberry Juice Blend	8 oz	140	0	0	0	0	0	35	36	0	0	2 1/2 fruit
No Sugar Added Pink Grapefruit 100% Juice	8 oz	130	0	0	0	0	0	35	32	0	1	2 fruit
No Sugar Added White Grapefruit 100% Juice	8 oz	90	0	0	0	0	0	35	21	0	2	1 1/2 fruit

FRUIT, FRUIT JUICES, DRINKS

	Serving	Calories	Fat (g)	Cal. from Fat	Sat. Fat (g)	Trans Fat (g)	Chol. (mg)	Sod. (mg)	Carb. (g)	Fiber (g)	Prot. (g)	Servings/Exchanges
Old Orchard												
Apple Cherry Juice Cocktail	8 oz	91	0	0	0	0	0	9	21	0	0	1 1/2 carb
Apple Cranberry Juice	8 oz	130	0	0	0	0	0	25	29	0	0	2 fruit
Apple Kiwi Strawberry Juice Cocktail	8 oz	91	0	0	0	0	0	9	21	0	0	1 1/2 carb
Healthy Balance Grape Juice Cocktail	8 oz	35	0	0	0	0	0	6	9	0	0	1/2 carb
Peach Mango 100% Juice Blend	8 oz	120	0	0	0	0	0	25	29	0	0	2 fruit
SunnyD												
Fruit Punch	8 oz	80	0	0	0	0	0	160	21	0	0	1 1/2 carb
Reduced Sugar	8 oz	60	0	0	0	0	0	170	15	0	0	1 carb
Tangy Original	8 oz	90	0	0	0	0	0	170	22	0	0	1 1/2 carb

Sunsweet

Prune Juice	8 oz	180	0	0	0	0	30	43	3	2	3 fruit
Prune Juice with Pulp	8 oz	180	0	0	0	0	30	43	3	2	3 fruit

Tree Top

Apple Juice	8 oz	120	0	0	0	0	25	29	0	0	2 fruit
Fiber Rich, Apple Orange Banana	8 oz	160	0	0	0	0	30	38	6	<1	2 1/2 carb

Tropicana

Light 'n Healthy Juice Beverage	8 oz	50	0	0	0	0	10	13	0	<1	1 carb
Orange Juice, Antioxidant Advantage	8 oz	110	0	0	0	0	0	26	0	2	2 fruit
Orange Juice, Calcium & Vitamin D	8 oz	110	0	0	0	0	0	26	0	2	2 fruit
Orange Juice, Healthy Heart	8 oz	120	0.5	0	5	0	0	26	0	2	2 fruit
Orange Juice, Low Acid	8 oz	110	0	0	0	0	0	26	0	2	2 fruit

FRUIT, FRUIT JUICES, DRINKS

	Serving	Calories	Fat (g)	Cal. from Fat	Sat. Fat (g)	Trans Fat (g)	Chol. (mg)	Sod. (mg)	Carb. (g)	Fiber (g)	Prot. (g)	Servings/Exchanges
Orange Juice, Original	8 oz	110	0	0	0	0	0	0	26	0	2	2 fruit
Orange Strawberry Banana Juice	8 oz	130	0	0	0	0	0	0	30	0	2	2 fruit
Orange Tangerine Juice	8 oz	110	0	0	0	0	0	0	25	0	2	1 1/2 fruit
Ruby Red Grapefruit Juice	8 oz	90	0	0	0	0	0	0	22	0	1	1 1/2 fruit
Tropics, Orange Peach Mango	8 oz	120	0	0	0	0	0	10	29	0	1	2 fruit
Twister Juice Drink, Assorted Flavors	8 oz	120	0	0	0	0	0	25	30	0	0	2 carb
V8 Splash												
Berry Blend	8 oz	70	0	0	0	0	0	50	18	0	0	1 carb
Mango Peach	8 oz	80	0	0	0	0	0	40	19	0	0	1 carb
Tropical Blend	8 oz	70	0	0	0	0	0	30	18	0	0	1 carb

Welch's

	Serving	Calories	Fat (g)	% Cal. from Fat	Sat. Fat (g)	Chol. (mg)	Sodium (mg)	Carb. (g)	Fiber (g)	Protein (g)	Exchanges/Choices
100% Grape Juice	8 oz	170	0	0	0	0	20	42	0	0	3 fruit
100% White Grape Juice	8 oz	160	0	0	0	0	20	39	0	0	2 1/2 fruit
Blueberry Kiwi Blast Juice Drink	8 oz	160	0	0	0	0	20	40	0	0	2 1/2 carb
Concord Grape Juice Cocktail	8 oz	140	0	0	0	0	20	34	0	0	2 carb
Cranberry Juice Cocktail	8 oz	140	0	0	0	0	5	35	0	0	2 carb
Diet Berry Pomegranate	8 oz	10	0	0	0	0	20	3	0	0	free
Guava Pineapple Juice Cocktail	8 oz	140	0	0	0	0	5	36	0	0	2 1/2 carb
Light Grape Juice Cocktail	8 oz	50	0	0	0	0	80	13	0	0	1 carb
Mango Twist Juice Cocktail	8 oz	150	0	0	0	0	5	38	0	0	2 1/2 carb

FRUIT, FRUIT JUICES, DRINKS

	Serving	Calories	Fat (g)	Cal. from Fat	Sat. Fat (g)	Trans Fat (g)	Chol. (mg)	Sod. (mg)	Carb. (g)	Fiber (g)	Prot. (g)	Servings/Exchanges
Mountain Berry Juice Cocktail	8 oz	140	0	0	0	0	0	5	34	0	0	2 carb
Orange Pineapple Juice Drink	8 oz	120	0	0	0	0	0	50	31	0	0	2 carb
Passion Fruit Juice Cocktail	8 oz	150	0	0	0	0	0	5	38	0	0	2 1/2 carb
Strawberry Breeze Juice Cocktail	8 oz	130	0	0	0	0	0	5	33	0	0	2 carb
Tropical Cherry Juice Cocktail	8 oz	140	0	0	0	0	0	5	36	0	0	2 1/2 carb

GLUTEN-FREE FOODS

	Serving	Calories	Fat (g)	Cal. from Fat	Sat. Fat (g)	Trans Fat (g)	Chol. (mg)	Sod. (mg)	Carb. (mg)	Fiber (g)	Prot. (g)	Servings/Exchanges
Ancient Quinoa Harvest												
Spaghetti, Elbows, or Rotelle Pasta	2 oz	205	1	7	0	0	0	4	46	4	4	3 carb
Bakery On Main												
Granola, Extreme Fruit & Nut	2 oz	270	13	120	2	0	0	45	34	3	4	2 carb, 3 fat
Granola, Nutty Maple Cranberry	2 oz	260	12	100	1	0	0	45	35	3	4	2 carb, 2 fat
Granola, Rainforest	2 oz	290	14	120	0.5	0	0	50	38	2	4	2 1/2 carb, 3 fat
Betty Crocker (Gluten Free)												
Chocolate Chip Cookie Mix	2 cookies	150	7	60	4	0	25	160	23	<1	1	1 1/2 carb, 1 fat
Yellow Cake Mix	1/10 cake	260	11	100	6	0	90	310	37	0	3	2 1/2 carb, 2 fat

GLUTEN-FREE FOODS

	Serving	Calories	Fat (g)	Cal. from Fat	Sat. Fat (g)	Trans Fat (g)	Chol. (mg)	Sod. (mg)	Carb. (g)	Fiber (g)	Prot. (g)	Servings/Exchanges
DeBoles												
Rice Angel Hair Pasta	2 oz	210	0.5	5	0	0	0	15	46	<1	4	3 carb
Rice Angel Hair Pasta Plus Golden Flax	2 oz	210	1.5	15	0	0	0	10	44	1	4	3 carb
Rice Fettucini	2 oz	210	0.5	5	0	0	0	15	46	1	4	3 carb
Rice Lasagna	2.5 oz	260	0.5	5	0	0	0	15	56	<1	5	3 carb
Rice Spaghetti Style Pasta	2 oz	210	0.5	5	0	0	0	15	46	<1	4	3 carb
Rice Spirals	2 oz	210	0.5	5	0	0	0	15	46	<1	4	3 carb
Wheat Free Corn Spaghetti Style Pasta	2 oz	200	2	20	0	0	0	15	43	5	4	3 carb
Divine Foods												
Apricot Cashew Boomi Bar	1	190	7	60	1	0	0	75	28	3	4	2 carb, 1 fat

Cashew Almond Boomi Bar	1	260	17	150	2	0	0	55	23	4	8	1 1/2 carb, 3 fat
Fruit 'n Nut Boomi Bar	1	210	9	90	1	0	0	55	27	3	6	2 carb, 2 fat
Macadamia Paradise Boomi Bar	1	240	15	140	3	0	0	25	28	3	3	2 carb, 3 fat
Perfect Pumpkin Boomi Bar	1	230	10	100	2	0	0	45	23	1	9	1 1/2 carb, 2 fat
Walnut Date Boomi Bar	1	200	9	80	1	0	0	20	29	2	4	2 carb, 2 fat
Ener-G Foods												
Brown Rice English Muffins with Flax	1	180	5	45	0	0	0	250	35	7	2	2 carb, 1 fat
Cinnamon Crackers	10	70	5	45	0	0	0	85	12	5	0	1 carb, 1 fat
Cinnamon Rolls	1 roll	220	5	45	0.5	0	0	230	33	8	2	2 carb, 1 fat
Corn Loaf	1 slice	40	1.5	15	0	0	0	50	8	3	0	1/2 carb
Doughnut Holes, Plain	1	50	2.5	25	1	0	5	105	5	<1	1	1 fat
Four Flour Loaf	1 slice	80	2.5	20	0	0	0	100	17	3	1	1 carb, 1 fat
Gourmet Crackers	3	160	7	60	3	0	0	330	23	<1	1	1 1/2 carb, 1 fat

GLUTEN-FREE FOODS

	Serving	Calories	Fat (g)	Cal. from Fat	Sat. Fat (g)	Trans Fat (g)	Chol. (mg)	Sod. (mg)	Carb. (g)	Fiber (g)	Prot. (g)	Servings/Exchanges
Light White Rice Flax Loaf	1 slice	50	2	20	0	0	0	60	7	1	0	1/2 carb
Plain Croutons	1 Tbsp	25	1	10	0	0	0	25	3	0	0	free
Seattle Brown Hamburger Buns	1 bun	160	4.5	40	0	0	0	190	34	8	2	2 carb, 1 fat
Seattle Brown Hot Dog Buns	1 bun	160	4.5	40	0	0	0	190	34	8	2	2 carb, 1 fat
Seattle Crackers	16	80	4.5	40	0	0	0	190	9	5	0	1/2 carb, 1 fat
Tapioca Hamburger Buns	1 bun	120	3	30	0	0	0	150	21	4	1	1 1/2 carb, 1 fat
Tapioca Hot Dog Buns	1 bun	120	3	30	0	0	0	150	21	4	1	1 1/2 carb, 1 fat
Tapioca Loaf, Thin Sliced	1 slice	80	3	30	0	0	0	95	11	2	1	1 carb, 1 fat
Wylde Pretzels	40	130	3	30	1.5	0	0	230	24	3	<1	1 1/2 carb, 1 fat

Enjoy Life Foods

Food	Serving										
Caramel Apple Snack Bar	1	110	2.5	25	0	0	95	21	2	2	1 1/2 carb, 1 fat
Chewy Chocolate Chip Cookies	2	130	5	45	1	0	105	21	2	1	1 1/2 carb, 1 fat
Cinnamon Crunch Granola	1/2 cup	170	3	30	1	0	10	32	5	3	2 carb, 1 fat
Cinnamon Raisin Bagels	1	280	7	60	0	0	430	53	4	4	3 1/2 carb, 1 fat
Classic Original Bagels	1	270	7	60	0	0	380	46	3	5	3 carb, 1 fat
Crunchy Flax Cereal	3/4 cup	200	3	25	0	0	115	42	6	7	3 carb, 1 fat
Crunchy Rice Cereal	3/4 cup	210	1	20	0	0	110	46	2	4	3 carb
Gingerbread Spice Cookies	2	120	4	35	0	0	120	19	2	1	1 carb, 1 fat
No-Oats Oatmeal Cookies	2	120	3.5	30	0	0	50	21	1	1	1 1/2 carb, 1 fat
Perky's Nutty Flax Cereal	3/4 cup	220	3	30	0	0	115	44	7	5	3 carb, 1 fat

GLUTEN-FREE FOODS

	Serving	Calories	Fat (g)	Cal. from Fat	Sat. Fat (g)	Trans Fat (g)	Chol. (mg)	Sod. (mg)	Carb. (g)	Fiber (g)	Prot. (g)	Servings/Exchanges
Perky's Nutty Rice Cereal	3/4 cup	210	1.5	15	0	0	0	110	46	2	4	3 carb
General Mills Gluten Free												
Very Berry Snack Bar	1	120	2.5	20	0	0	0	95	23	2	1	1 1/2 carb, 1 fat
Corn Chex	1 cup	120	0.5	5	0	0	0	290	26	1	2	2 carb
Rice Chex	1 cup	100	0	0	0	0	0	250	23	0	2	1 1/2 carb
Gillian's Foods												
Cinnamon Raisin Rolls	1/2 roll	130	0.5	5	0	0	0	330	25	2	5	1 1/2 carb
Sesame Seed Rolls	1/2 roll	130	0.5	5	0	0	0	330	25	2	5	1 1/2 carb
French Rolls	1/2 roll	130	4	35	0.5	0	0	160	20	1	3	1 carb, 1 fat
Foods By George												
Biscotti	1	90	4.5	40	1	0	0	25	11	1	2	1 carb, 1 fat
Blueberry Muffins	1	220	8	70	1	0	25	450	33	1	3	2 carb, 2 fat
Brownies	1/9 tray	180	9	80	1	0	40	45	24	1	2	1 1/2 carb, 2 fat

Corn Muffins	1	240	9	80	1	0	30	480	36	1	4	2 1/2 carb, 2 fat
English Muffins	1	210	3.5	30	0	0	0	270	39	1	4	2 1/2 carb, 1 fat
No-Rye Rye English Muffins	1	210	4	35	0	0	0	270	40	2	4	2 1/2 carb
Pecan Tarts	1	470	28	250	7	0	95	160	51	3	6	3 1/2 carb, 6 fat
French Meadow Bakery												
Chocolate Chip Cookie	1	320	16	150	8	0	25	260	43	1	1	3 carb, 3 fat
Cinnamon Raisin Bread	1 slice	150	5	45	3	0	0	270	22	2	2	1 1/2 carb, 1 fat
Fudge Brownie	1	170	7	60	1	0	15	25	25	1	2	1 1/2 carb, 1 fat
Italian Rolls	1	340	9	80	1	0	40	470	63	8	3	4 carb, 2 fat
Muffins	1	210	8	80	1.5	0.5	45	110	31	1	2	2 carb, 2 fat
Multigrain Bread	1 slice	150	4.5	40	2	0	0	230	23	3	4	1 1/2 carb, 1 fat
Sandwich Bread	1 slice	120	4	35	2.5	0	0	310	20	1	2	1 carb, 1 fat
Tortilla	1	120	1	5	0	0	0	290	24	1	1	1 1/2 carb
Glutinos												
Apple Breakfast Bar	1	130	2	20	0	0	0	5	28	3	2	2 carb

GLUTEN-FREE FOODS

	Serving	Calories	Fat (g)	Cal. from Fat	Sat. Fat (g)	Trans Fat (g)	Chol. (mg)	Sod. (mg)	Carb. (g)	Fiber (g)	Prot. (g)	Servings/Exchanges
Breadsticks, Sesame Flavored	9	60	1.5	15	1	0	0	100	12	0	0	1 carb
Cheddar Crackers	8	140	5	45	2.5	0	10	180	21	<1	2	1 1/2 carb, 1 fat
Honey Nut Cereal	1/2 cup	120	1.5	15	0	0	0	120	26	1	1	2 carb
Lemon Wafers	3	150	6	55	4	0	0	25	24	0	0	1 1/2 carb, 1 fat
Pretzels, Sticks	33	140	6	50	2.5	0	0	420	21	0	0	1 1/2 carb, 1 fat
Vanilla Wafers	4	160	8	70	5	0	5	25	19	0	1	1 carb, 2 fat
Heartland's Finest												
All Natural Macaroni & Cheese	3 oz	340	7	65	4.5	0	20	800	53	6	14	3 1/2 carb, 1 fat
CerO's Cereal, Original	1 cup	120	0	0	0	0	0	125	24	3	5	1 1/2 carb
CerO's Cereal, Raspberry	1 cup	110	0	0	0	0	0	115	23	2	4	1 1/2 carb
Elbow Macaroni Pasta	3/4 oz	210	1.5	15	0.5	0	0	0	41	5	7	2 1/2 carb
Lasagna Pasta	2 oz	210	1.5	15	0.5	0	0	0	41	5	7	2 1/2 carb

Food	Serving											Exchanges
Linguini Pasta	2 oz	210	1.5	15	0.5	0	0	0	41	5	7	2 1/2 carb
Spaghetti Pasta	2 oz	210	1.5	15	0.5	0	0	0	41	5	7	2 1/2 carb
Hodgson Mill Brown Rice Pasta												
Elbows, Penne, Spaghetti, Angel Hair, Linguine	2 oz	209	1	12	0	0	0	0	44	2	5	3 carb
Kay's Naturals Better Balance												
Almond Delight Crisps	1 oz	120	3.5	30	0	0	0	250	14	2	10	1 carb, 1 lean meat
Apple Cinnamon Cereal	1 oz	100	1.5	10	0	0	0	140	15	3	9	1 carb, 1 lean meat
Chili Nacho Cheese Protein Chips	1 oz	110	3.5	30	0	0	0	230	14	3	10	1 carb, 1 lean meat
Crispy Parmesan Protein Chips	1 oz	110	3.5	30	0	0	0	230	14	3	10	1 carb, 1 lean meat
French Vanilla Cereal	1 oz	100	1.5	10	0	0	0	140	15	3	9	1 carb, 1 lean meat
Golden Butter Pretzels	1 oz	110	5	30	1.5	0	0	220	12	2	10	1 carb, 1 med-fat meat
Lemon Herb Protein Chips	1 oz	110	3.5	30	0	0	0	230	14	3	10	1 carb, 1 lean meat

GLUTEN-FREE FOODS

	Serving	Calories	Fat (g)	Cal. from Fat	Sat. Fat (g)	Trans Fat (g)	Chol. (mg)	Sod. (mg)	Carb. (g)	Fiber (g)	Prot. (g)	Servings/Exchanges
White Cheddar Kruncheeze	1 oz	130	6	60	0.5	0	0	200	10	2	9	1/2 carb, 1 med-fat meat
Kinnikinnick Foods												
Blueberry Muffin	1	190	7	65	2	0	10	320	32	3	1	2 carb, 1 fat
Brown Sandwich Bread	1 slice	70	2	20	<1	0	15	180	14	2	2	1 carb
Chocolate Chip Muffin	1	170	9	80	2	0	20	170	28	2	1	2 carb, 2 fat
Chocolate Dipped Donuts	1	220	6	55	3	0	0	200	41	2	2	2 1/2 carb, 1 fat
Cinnamon Sugar Donuts	1	170	4.5	40	2.5	0	0	230	30	1	2	2 carb, 1 fat
Ginger Snap Cookies	2	25	1	10	0.5	0	0	40	5	0	0	1/2 carb
Italian White Tapioca Rice Bread	1 slice	90	2.5	25	<1	0	20	190	20	1	2	1 carb, 1 fat
KinniToos Vanilla Sandwich Cookies	1	60	2.5	20	1	0	0	50	9	1	0	1/2 carb, 1 fat
Many Wonder Multigrain Rice Bread	1 slice	90	3.5	30	<1	0	20	120	18	3	2	1 carb, 1 fat

Food												
Montanas Chocolate Chip Cookies	2	115	5	45	1.5	0	15	90	15	0	1	1 carb, 1 fat
Tapioca Rice English Muffins	1	240	3.5	30	<1	0	0	260	41	2	3	2 1/2 carb, 1 fat
Tapioca Rice Hamburger Bun	1	230	7	65	0.5	0	5	330	36	4	5	2 1/2 carb, 1 fat
Tapioca Rice Hot Dog Bun	1	250	8	70	0.5	0	5	360	39	4	5	2 1/2 carb, 2 fat
Tapioca Rice New York Style Plain Bagel	1	210	7	65	2.5	0	35	430	48	3	4	3 carb, 1 fat
White Sandwich Bread	1 slice	70	2	20	<1	0	15	150	15	2	1	1 carb
La Tortilla Factory												
Dark Teff Wraps	1 wrap	180	5	45	0.5	0	0	320	31	3	2	2 carb, 1 fat
Ivory Teff Wraps	1 wrap	180	5	45	0.5	0	0	320	30	3	2	2 carb, 1 fat
Lundberg Organic Brown Rice Pasta												
Rotini, Penne, Spaghetti	2 oz	190	3	30	0.5	0	0	0	40	4	4	2 1/2 carb

GLUTEN-FREE FOODS

	Serving	Calories	Cal. from Fat	Fat (g)	Sat. Fat (g)	Trans Fat (g)	Chol. (mg)	Sod. (mg)	Carb. (g)	Fiber (g)	Prot. (g)	Servings/Exchanges
Mary's Gone Crackers												
Black Pepper Crackers	13	140	45	5	0.5	0	0	180	21	3	3	1 1/2 carb, 1 fat
Original Crackers	13	140	45	5	0.5	0	0	190	21	3	3	1 1/2 carb, 1 fat
Sticks & Twigs, Chipotle Tomato	15	150	45	5	0.5	0	0	160	20	4	4	1 carb, 1 fat
Sticks & Twigs, Sea Salt Crackers	15	150	45	5	0.5	0	0	300	21	4	4	1 1/2 carb, 1 fat
Mi-Del												
Arrowroot Cookies	10	130	35	6	1	NA	10	85	23	2	2	1 1/2 carb, 1 fat
Chocolate Chip Cookies	5	130	40	4.5	1.5	0	0	130	21	1	2	1 1/2 carb, 1 fat
Ginger Snaps	5	140	50	6	0	0	0	85	21	1	2	1 1/2 carb, 1 fat
Pecan Cookies	5	140	60	6	1.5	0	5	150	19	1	2	1 carb, 1 fat
Royal Vanilla Sandwich Cookies	3	170	70	8	0.5	0	5	85	24	1	2	1 1/2 carb, 2 fat

Nature's Path

Crunchy Maple Sunrise	2/3 cup	110	1	10	0	0	130	25	3	2	1 1/2 carb
Crunchy Vanilla Sunrise	2/3 cup	110	1	10	0	0	130	25	3	2	1 1/2 carb
EnviroKidz Panda Puffs	3/4 cup	130	2.5	25	0	0	130	24	2	2	1 1/2 carb, 1 fat
Whole O's Cereal	2/3 cup	110	1.5	10	0	0	115	25	3	2	1 1/2 carb

Nu-World Foods

Amaranth Berry Delicious Hot Cereal	1 cup	90	1	10	<1	0	10	16	3	4	1 carb
Flatbread, Amaranth-Garbanzo	1 piece	165	4	35	0.5	0	100	28	6	8	2 carb, 1 fat
Puffed Amaranth Cereal	1 cup	120	1	15	0	0	1	15	3	6	1 carb

Pamela's Products

Almond Anise Biscotti	1	120	6	50	2.5	0	150	18	1	1	1 carb, 1 fat
Butter Shortbread Cookies	1	110	7	60	4	0	70	13	1	1	1 carb, 1 fat
Chocolate Chip Walnut Cookies	1	120	7	70	1	0	80	13	0.5	1	1 carb, 1 fat

GLUTEN-FREE FOODS

	Serving	Calories	Fat (g)	Cal. from Fat	Sat. Fat (g)	Trans Fat (g)	Chol. (mg)	Sod. (mg)	Carb. (g)	Fiber (g)	Prot. (g)	Servings/Exchanges
Chunky Chocolate Chip Cookies	1	120	6	60	1	0	10	80	14	0.5	1	1 carb, 2 fat
Lemon Shortbread Cookies	1	120	6	50	4	0	15	50	15	0	0.5	1 carb, 1 fat
Peanut Butter Cookies	1	100	5	45	1	0	15	120	11	0.5	3	1 carb, 1 fat
Shortbread Swirl Cookies	1	120	7	60	4	0	15	70	14	0.5	0	1 carb, 1 fat
Schär												
Chocolate-Dipped Cookies	3	150	7	70	3.5	0	0	60	21	1	1	1 1/2 carb, 1 fat
Classic White Bread	1 slice	70	1.5	15	1	0	0	130	12	1	<1	1 carb
Classic White Rolls	1	170	5	45	1	0	0	370	30	0	2	2 carb, 1 fat
Crispbread	4 slices	100	0.5	5	0	0	0	250	22	<1	2	1 1/2 carb
Italian Breadsticks	7	120	2.5	25	0.5	0	0	310	24	1	<1	1 1/2 carb, 1 fat
Ladyfingers	3	110	2	20	0.5	0	40	40	22	1	2	1 1/2 carb

Multigrain Bread	1 slice	70	1.5	15	0.5	0	0	140	12	2	2	1 carb
Shortbread Cookies	4	130	5	45	2.5	0	10	20	20	<1	2	1 carb, 1 fat
Table Crackers	3	120	3.5	35	1.5	0	0	220	21	1	<1	1 1/2 carb, 1 fat
Vanilla Wafers	4	160	8	70	7	0	0	160	20	1	1	1 carb, 2 fat

Tinkyada Brown Rice Pasta

Fettucini, Lasagne, Penne, Spaghetti, Shells, Spirals	2 oz	210	2	15	0	0	0	15	43	2	4	3 carb

Trader Joe's

Brown Rice Tortillas	1 tortilla	130	2.5	25	0	0	0	160	24	2	2	1 1/2 carb, 1 fat
Organic Brown Rice Penne Pasta	2 oz	200	0	0	0	0	0	0	45	1	5	3 carb
Rice Sticks	1/4 cup	210	0.5	5	0	0	0	10	46	1	4	3 carb

Whole Foods Gluten Free Bakehouse

Almond Cookies	1	270	12	110	1	0	0	20	34	<1	6	2 carb, 2 fat
Apple Pie	2 oz	120	5	45	3	0	20	70	20	1	1	1 carb, 1 fat

GLUTEN-FREE FOODS

	Serving	Calories	Fat (g)	Cal. from Fat	Sat. Fat (g)	Trans Fat (g)	Chol. (mg)	Sod. (mg)	Carb. (g)	Fiber (g)	Prot. (g)	Servings/Exchanges
Banana Bread	2 oz	220	11	100	4.5	0	55	170	28	0	3	2 carb, 2 fat
Blueberry Muffins	1	330	13	110	1	0	60	380	53	1	4	3 1/2 carb, 3 fat
Chocolate Chip Cookies	1	160	8	80	4.5	0	30	95	22	0	2	1 1/2 carb, 2 fat
Cornbread	2 oz	160	7	70	1	0	50	320	21	2	3	1 1/2 carb, 1 fat
Cream Biscuits	1	220	13	120	8	0	50	400	24	<1	2	1 1/2 carb, 1 fat
Hamburger Buns	1	330	10	90	6	0	65	300	55	1	4	3 1/2 carb, 2 fat
Honey Oat Bread	2 oz	140	3.5	35	0	0	35	200	24	1	2	1 1/2 carb, 1 fat
Lemon Poppy Seed Muffin	1	390	20	180	0	0	120	300	48	<1	5	3 carb, 4 fat
Morning Glory Muffin	1	310	18	160	1.5	0	70	310	36	1	4	2 1/2 carb, 4 fat
Prairie Bread	1 slice	150	5	45	0	0	35	180	23	<1	3	1 1/2 carb, 1 fat
Sandwich Bread	1 slice	150	4.5	40	0	0	40	190	24	0	3	1 1/2 carb, 1 fat
Walnut Brownies	2 oz	270	16	140	6	0	65	150	31	<1	5	2 carb, 3 fat

ICE CREAM, FROZEN YOGURT, PUDDING, GELATIN

	Serving	Calories	Fat (g)	Cal. from Fat	Sat. Fat (g)	Trans Fat (g)	Chol. (mg)	Sod. (mg)	Carb. (g)	Fiber (g)	Prot. (g)	Servings/Exchanges
Frozen Yogurt, Fat Free	1/3 cup	66	0	0	0	0	0	43	13	0	3	1 carb
Frozen Yogurt, Regular	1/2 cup	110	3	30	2	0	10	40	19	0	3	1 carb, 1 fat
Fruit Juice Bar, Frozen, 100% Juice	3 oz	75	<1	0	0	0	0	4	19	0	1	1 carb
Gelatin, Dessert	1/2 cup	84	0	0	0	0	0	101	19	0	2	1 carb
Ice Cream	1/2 cup	165	10	90	5	0	23	102	15	0	3	1 carb, 2 fat
Ice Cream, Fat Free	1/2 cup	90	0	0	0	0	0	55	22	4	3	1 1/2 carb
Ice Cream, Light	1/2 cup	120	5	45	2	0	15	90	16	0	3	1 carb, 1 fat
Ice Cream, No Sugar Added	1/2 cup	115	6	55	2	0	10	93	15	3	3	1 carb, 1 fat
Ice Pops	1	27	0	0	0	0	0	4	7	0	0	1/2 carb
Pudding, Chocolate	1/2 cup	153	5	45	1	0	1	164	25	0	2	1 1/2 carb, 1 fat
Pudding, Fat Free	3.5 oz	88	0	0	0	0	0	189	20	0	2	1 carb

ICE CREAM, FROZEN YOGURT, PUDDING, GELATIN

	Serving	Calories	Fat (g)	Cal. from Fat	Sat. Fat (g)	Trans Fat (g)	Chol. (mg)	Sod. (mg)	Carb. (g)	Fiber (g)	Prot. (g)	Servings/Exchanges
Pudding, Tapioca	1/2 cup	143	4	35	1	0	1	160	24	0	2	1 1/2 carb, 1 fat
Pudding, Vanilla	1/2 cup	143	4	35	1	0	1	156	25	0	2	1 1/2 carb, 1 fat
Sherbet, Orange	1/2 cup	138	2	20	1	0	0	44	29	3	1	2 carb
Sorbet	1/2 cup	130	0	0	0	0	0	21	31	1	<1	2 carb
Topping, Butterscotch	2 Tbsp	103	0	0	0	0	<1	143	27	<1	<1	2 carb
Topping, Hot Fudge	2 Tbsp	147	6	55	2	0	5	28	25	<1	2	1 1/2 carb, 1 fat
Topping, Marshmallow	2 Tbsp	118	0	0	0	0	0	18	30	<1	<1	2 carb
Topping, Whipped	2 Tbsp	24	2	20	1	0	0	0	2	0	0	free
Topping, Whipped, Light	2 Tbsp	19	1	10	<1	0	0	0	2	0	0	free
ICE CREAM/FROZEN YOGURT BRANDS												
Ben & Jerry's												
Frozen Yogurt, Cherry Garcia	1/2 cup	160	3	30	2	0	15	15	31	1	4	2 carb, 1 fat

Food	Serving											
Frozen Yogurt, Chocolate Fudge Brownie	1/2 cup	170	2.5	25	0.5	0	15	95	34	1	5	2 carb, 1 fat
Frozen Yogurt, Half Baked	1/2 cup	180	3	25	1.5	0	20	95	35	1	4	2 carb, 1 fat
Ice Cream, Cherry Garcia	1/2 cup	200	14	100	8	0	45	50	23	0	3	1 1/2 carb, 3 fat
Ice Cream, Chocolate Chip Cookie Dough	1/2 cup	220	12	110	7	0	55	70	26	0	4	2 carb, 2 fat
Ice Cream, Chocolate Fudge Brownie	1/2 cup	220	11	100	6	0	25	70	27	1	3	2 carb, 2 fat
Ice Cream, Chubby Hubby	1/2 cup	330	20	180	11	0	55	150	31	1	7	2 carb, 4 fat
Ice Cream, Chunky Monkey	1/2 cup	240	14	130	8	0	45	35	24	0	4	1 1/2 carb, 3 fat
Ice Cream, Coffee Heath Bar Crunch	1/2 cup	280	16	150	10	1	60	115	29	0	4	2 carb, 3 fat

ICE CREAM, FROZEN YOGURT, PUDDING, GELATIN

	Serving	Calories	Fat (g)	Cal. from Fat	Sat. Fat (g)	Trans Fat (g)	Chol. (mg)	Sod. (mg)	Carb. (g)	Fiber (g)	Prot. (g)	Servings/Exchanges
Ice Cream, Light, Chocolate Chip Cookie Dough	1/2 cup	200	6	50	3.5	0	35	80	35	2	4	2 carb, 1 fat
Ice Cream, Light, Phish Food	1/2 cup	210	6	60	4.5	0	25	90	37	1	4	2 1/2 carb, 1 fat
Ice Cream, Light, Raspberry Chocolate	1/2 cup	180	5	50	4	0	25	60	32	2	3	2 carb, 1 fat
Ice Cream, Mint Chocolate Cookie	1/2 cup	250	14	130	8	0	60	100	26	0	4	2 carb, 3 fat
Ice Cream, No Sugar Added, Vanilla Fudge Chip	1/2 cup	180	13	120	10	0	45	40	20	3	3	1 carb, 3 fat
Ice Cream, Original Butter Pecan	1/2 cup	260	20	180	8	0	50	105	17	0	4	1 carb, 4 fat

Ice Cream, Original Vanilla	1/2 cup	230	14	130	9	0	70	60	22	0	4	1 1/2 carb, 3 fat
Ice Cream, Peanut Butter Cup	1/2 cup	340	24	220	12	0	55	125	28	1	6	2 carb, 5 fat
Ice Cream, Vanilla Caramel Fudge	1/2 cup	270	14	130	10	0	65	100	31	0	4	2 carb, 3 fat
Sorbet, Berried Treasure	1/2 cup	110	0	0	0	0	0	5	29	1	0	2 carb
Sorbet, Jamaican Me Crazy	1/2 cup	130	0	0	0	0	0	10	33	1	0	2 carb
Blue Bunny												
Sweet Freedom No Sugar Added, Lite Chocolate Ice Cream	1 bar	100	7	60	5	0	<5	25	12	2	2	1 carb, 1 fat
Breyers												
Carb Smart, Chocolate	1/2 cup	90	6	50	3.5	0	15	75	13	4	2	1 carb, 1 fat
Carb Smart, Vanilla	1/2 cup	90	6	50	3.5	0	15	45	13	4	2	1 carb, 1 fat
Ice Cream, Chocolate	1/2 cup	140	7	60	4.5	0	20	45	17	1	2	1 carb, 1 fat

ICE CREAM, FROZEN YOGURT, PUDDING, GELATIN

	Serving	Calories	Fat (g)	Cal. from Fat	Sat. Fat (g)	Trans Fat (g)	Chol. (mg)	Sod. (mg)	Carb. (g)	Fiber (g)	Prot. (g)	Servings/Exchanges
Ice Cream, Heath English Toffee	1/2 cup	160	6	50	3.5	0	10	130	25	0	2	1 1/2 carb, 1 fat
Ice Cream, Natural Vanilla	1/2 cup	130	7	60	4	0	20	35	14	0	3	1 carb, 1 fat
Ice Cream, Reese's Peanut Butter Cup	1/2 cup	160	6	50	2.5	0	10	110	25	1	3	1 1/2 carb, 1 fat
Ice Cream, Smooth & Dreamy	1/2 cup	110	3.5	30	2	0	10	50	16	0	3	1 carb, 1 fat
Ice Cream, Smooth & Dreamy, 1/2 Fat Creamy Chocolate	1	110	3.5	35	2	0	10	55	17	1	3	1 carb, 1 fat
Ice Cream, Smooth & Dreamy, Chocolate Cookies & Cream	1/2 cup	110	0	0	0	0	0	70	25	3	3	1 1/2 carb

Ice Cream, Smooth & Dreamy, French Chocolate	1/2 cup	90	0	0	0	0	55	22	4	3	1 1/2 carb
Ice Cream, No Sugar Added, Chocolate Fudge Brownie	1/2 cup	90	1.5	15	1	0	5	85	20	4	3	1 carb
Ice Cream, Smooth & Dreamy, No Sugar Added, French Vanilla	1/2 cup	90	4.5	40	2.5	0	30	45	14	4	2	1 carb, 1 fat
Ice Cream, Snickers	1/2 cup	170	8	70	4.5	0	20	80	20	0	3	1 carb, 2 fat
Ice Cream, Strawberry	1/2 cup	120	5	45	3	0	15	35	15	0	2	1 carb, 1 fat
Häagen-Dazs												
Frozen Yogurt, Coffee	1/2 cup	200	4.5	40	2.5	0	65	50	31	0	8	2 carb, 1 fat
Frozen Yogurt, Dulce de Leche	1/2 cup	190	2.5	25	2	0	5	75	35	2	6	2 carb, 1 fat
Frozen Yogurt, Vanilla	1/2 cup	200	4.5	40	2.5	0	65	55	31	0	9	2 carb, 1 fat

ICE CREAM, FROZEN YOGURT, PUDDING, GELATIN

	Serving	Calories	Fat (g)	Cal. from Fat	Sat. Fat (g)	Trans Fat (g)	Chol. (mg)	Sod. (mg)	Carb. (g)	Fiber (g)	Prot. (g)	Servings/Exchanges
Frozen Yogurt, Vanilla Raspberry Swirl	1/2 cup	170	2.5	25	1.5	0	25	35	32	0	4	2 carb, 1 fat
Ice Cream, Butter Pecan	1/2 cup	310	23	210	11	0.5	110	110	21	<1	5	1 1/2 carb, 5 fat
Ice Cream, Chocolate	1/2 cup	270	18	160	11	0.5	115	60	22	1	5	1 1/2 carb, 4 fat
Ice Cream, Chocolate Chocolate Chip	1/2 cup	300	20	180	12	0.5	105	55	26	2	5	2 carb, 4 fat
Ice Cream, Rocky Road	1/2 cup	300	18	160	9	0	90	75	29	1	5	2 carb, 4 fat
Sorbet, Mango	1/2 cup	120	0	0	0	0	0	10	37	0	0	2 1/2 carb
Kraft												
Cool Whip Free Whipped Topping	2 Tbsp	15	0	0	0	0	0	5	3	0	0	free
Cool Whip Lite Whipped Topping	2 Tbsp	15	1	10	1	0	0	0	2	0	0	free
Cool Whip Sugar Free Whipped Topping	2 Tbsp	20	1	10	1	0	0	0	3	0	0	free

Cool Whip Whipped Topping, Regular	2 Tbsp	25	1.5	15	1.5	0	0	0	2	0	0	free
Dream Whip Whipped Topping Mix	2 Tbsp	15	0	0	0	0	0	0	2	0	0	free
Marshmallow Creme, Jet Puffed	2 Tbsp	40	0	0	0	0	0	10	11	0	0	1 carb
Marshmallows, Jet Puffed	4	100	0	0	0	0	0	25	24	0	1	1 1/2 carb
Marshmallows, Miniature	2/3 cup	100	0	0	0	0	0	25	24	0	1	1 1/2 carb
Smuckers											
Topping, Butterscotch	2 Tbsp	120	2	20	1	0	0	105	30	0	0	2 carb
Topping, Hot Fudge	2 Tbsp	130	4.5	40	1.5	0	0	45	22	<1	2	1 1/2 carb, 1 fat
Topping, Magic Shell, Chocolate Fudge	2 Tbsp	210	16	140	7	0	0	45	17	0	1	1 carb, 3 fat
Topping, Strawberry	2 Tbsp	100	0	0	0	0	0	15	26	0	0	2 carb

ICE CREAM, FROZEN YOGURT, PUDDING, GELATIN

	Serving	Calories	Fat (g)	Cal. from Fat	Sat. Fat (g)	Trans Fat (g)	Chol. (mg)	Sod. (mg)	Carb. (g)	Fiber (g)	Prot. (g)	Servings/Exchanges
Topping, Sugar Free Caramel	2 Tbsp	90	0	0	0	0	0	65	24	0	2	1 1/2 carb
Topping, Sugar Free Hot Fudge	2 Tbsp	90	0.5	5	0	0	0	40	23	1	1	1 1/2 carb
FROZEN NOVELTIES												
Blue Bunny												
Banana Pop	1	35	0	0	0	0	0	5	9	0	0	1/2 carb
Big Star Bar	1	130	8	70	7	0	5	40	13	0	2	1 carb, 2 fat
Champ! Banana Split Ice Cream Cone	1	220	8	80	6	0	10	65	33	<1	3	2 carb, 2 fat
Champ! Caramel Lovers Ice Cream Cone	1	350	19	170	12	0	35	140	40	1	7	2 1/2 carb, 4 fat
Champ! Chocolate Lovers Ice Cream	1	290	15	130	10	0.5	30	110	37	2	4	2 1/2 carb, 3 fat

Food												
Chips Galore! Ice Cream Sandwich	1	310	16	150	8	0	35	170	40	1	3	2 1/2 carb, 3 fat
Chips Galore! Ice Cream Sandwich	1	310	16	150	8	0	35	170	40	1	3	2 1/2 carb, 3 fat
Chocolate Raspberry Ice Cream Bar	1	270	18	160	12	0	35	45	25	1	3	1 1/2 carb, 4 fat
Classic Sundae Cone	1	270	14	130	9	0	25	105	32	1	4	2 carb, 3 fat
Cookies 'N Cream Ice Cream Sandwich	1	250	10	90	5	0	20	310	36	2	4	2 1/2 carb, 2 fat
Health Smart FrozFruit Chunky Strawberry Bar	1	35	0	0	0	0	0	10	15	3	0	1 carb
Hot Fudge Bar	1	370	25	220	14	0	30	90	33	2	7	2 carb, 5 fat
Jolly Rancher Bomb Pop	1	40	0	0	0	0	0	15	11	0	0	1 carb
Krunch Bar	1	190	13	120	10	0	20	55	17	0	2	1 carb, 3 fat
Malt Cup	1	330	11	100	7	0	45	160	52	0	6	3 1/2 carb, 2 fat

ICE CREAM, FROZEN YOGURT, PUDDING, GELATIN

	Serving	Calories	Fat (g)	Cal. from Fat	Sat. Fat (g)	Trans Fat (g)	Chol. (mg)	Sod. (mg)	Carb. (g)	Fiber (g)	Prot. (g)	Servings/Exchanges
Neapolitan Sandwich	1	150	3.5	30	1.5	0	10	170	27	<1	3	2 carb, 1 fat
Orange Dream Bar	1	80	1.5	15	1	0	5	35	16	0	1	1 carb
Original Bomb Pop	1	50	0	0	0	0	0	5	11	0	0	1 carb
Root Beer Float Bar	1	80	2	20	1.5	0	10	25	14	0	<1	1 carb
Slush Pop	1	45	0	0	0	0	0	10	11	0	0	1 carb
Sour Power Bomb Pop	1	50	0	0	0	0	0	5	12	0	0	1 carb
Star Bar	1	110	7	60	6	0	5	30	11	0	1	1 carb, 1 fat
Sugar Free Bomb Pop	1	25	0	0	0	0	0	5	8	2	0	1/2 carb
Sweet Freedom No Sugar Added Ice Cream Bar, Almond	1	150	11	100	7	0	5	45	16	2	3	1 carb, 2 fat
Sweet Freedom No Sugar Added Krunch Lites	1	100	7	70	6	0	<5	30	11	1	2	1 carb, 1 fat

Sweet Freedom No Sugar Added, Ice Cream Bar, Lites	1	100	8	70	6	0	5	30	11	1	2	1 carb, 2 fat
Sweet Freedom Sugar Free Pops	1	20	0	0	0	0	0	15	7	<1	0	1/2 carb
Turtle Bar	1	360	24	220	14	0	30	80	33	<1	5	2 carb, 5 fat
Twin Pops	1	70	0	0	0	0	0	10	18	0	0	1 carb
Vanilla Ice Cream Sandwich	1	140	3	30	1.5	0	5	170	25	<1	3	1 1/2 carb, 1 fat
Breyers												
All Natural No Sugar Added Pure Fruit Bar	1	25	0	0	0	0	0	0	5	0	0	free
All Natural Pure Fruit Bar, All Varieties	1	40	0	0	0	0	0	0	10	0	0	1 carb
Carb Smart Fudge Ice Cream Bar	1	100	7	60	4.5	0	20	50	9	1	2	1/2 carb, 1 fat

ICE CREAM, FROZEN YOGURT, PUDDING, GELATIN

	Serving	Calories	Fat (g)	Cal. from Fat	Sat. Fat (g)	Trans Fat (g)	Chol. (mg)	Sod. (mg)	Carb. (g)	Fiber (g)	Prot. (g)	Servings/Exchanges
Carb Smart Vanilla Ice Cream Bar	1	170	15	130	11	0	15	45	9	2	2	1/2 carb, 3 fat
Double Churn Creamy Vanilla Ice Cream Bar	1	160	8	70	5	0	5	45	21	3	3	1 1/2 carb, 2 fat
Double Churn Rocky Road Ice Cream Bar	1	180	9	90	5	0	5	80	23	3	4	1 1/2 carb, 2 fat
Oreo Ice Cream Sandwich	1	170	6	60	2.5	0	10	190	26	1	2	2 carb, 1 fat
Dole												
Fruit Juice Bar, All Varieties	1	70	0	0	0	0	0	15	17	0	0	1 carb
Dove												
Dove Bar, Dark Chocolate with Vanilla	1	330	21	190	14	0	35	40	31	2	4	2 carb, 4 fat

Dove Bar, Milk Chocolate with Almonds	1	340	23	200	13	0	35	135	28	1	6	2 carb, 5 fat
Dove Bar, Milk Chocolate with Vanilla	1	330	21	190	14	0	35	40	31	2	4	2 carb, 4 fat

Dreyer's

Fruit Bar, Creamy Coconut	1	120	3	25	2	0	0	40	21	1	3	1 1/2 carb, 1 fat
Fruit Bar, Strawberry	1	80	0	0	0	0	0	0	21	1	0	1 1/2 carb

Eskimo Pie

No Sugar Added Vanilla with Dark Chocolatey Coating	1	150	10	90	7	NA	5	45	13	2	2	1 carb, 2 fat
Vanilla with Dark Chocolatey Coating	1	150	10	90	7	NA	10	40	15	1	1	1 carb, 2 fat
Vanilla with Nestlé Crunch Coating	1	200	13	120	9	NA	10	55	19	0	1	1 carb, 3 fat

ICE CREAM, FROZEN YOGURT, PUDDING, GELATIN

	Serving	Calories	Fat (g)	Cal. from Fat	Sat. Fat (g)	Trans Fat (g)	Chol. (mg)	Sod. (mg)	Carb. (g)	Fiber (g)	Prot. (g)	Servings/Exchanges
Good Humor												
Chocolate Chip Cookie Sandwich	1	270	10	90	6	0	5	200	44	1	3	3 carb, 2 fat
Chocolate Eclair Bar	1	220	10	90	5	0	10	55	30	1	2	2 carb, 2 fat
Cookies & Cream Bar	1	90	1.5	15	1	0	5	55	18	2	2	1 carb
Premium Sundae Cone	1	260	15	140	9	0	15	80	29	1	4	2 carb, 3 fat
Strawberry Shortcake Bar	1	230	12	110	5	0	10	55	31	1	2	2 carb, 2 fat
Toasted Almond Bar	1	240	12	110	4	0.5	10	40	30	1	2	2 carb, 2 fat
Vanilla Ice Cream Sandwich	1	160	5	45	3	0	10	90	26	0	2	2 carb, 1 fat
Häagen-Dazs												
Chocolate & Dark Chocolate Ice Cream Bar	1	290	20	180	12	0	65	30	24	2	4	1 1/2 carb, 4 fat

Vanilla & Almonds Ice Cream Bar	1	310	22	200	13	0	65	40	22	<1	5	1 1/2 carb, 4 fat
Vanilla & Dark Chocolate Ice Cream Bar	1	300	21	190	13	0	70	45	23	<1	4	1 1/2 carb, 4 fat
Vanilla & Milk Chocolate Ice Cream Bar	1	290	21	190	14	0	75	55	22	0	4	1 1/2 carb, 4 fat
Healthy Choice											
Caramel Swirl Sandwich	1	150	2	20	1	0	10	115	30	1	3	2 carb
Fudge Bar	1	80	1	10	0.5	0	5	60	13	0	4	1 carb
Ice Cream Sandwich	1	130	2	20	1	0	5	115	25	2	3	1 1/2 carb
Mocha Swirl Bar	1	90	1.5	15	1	0	5	50	17	1	2	1 carb
Sorbet & Cream Bar	1	90	1	10	0.5	0	5	35	17	1	1	1 carb
Klondike											
Caramel Pretzel Bar	1	260	15	130	12	0	10	170	29	1	3	2 carb, 3 fat

ICE CREAM, FROZEN YOGURT, PUDDING, GELATIN

	Serving	Calories	Fat (g)	Cal. from Fat	Sat. Fat (g)	Trans Fat (g)	Chol. (mg)	Sod. (mg)	Carb. (g)	Fiber (g)	Prot. (g)	Servings/Exchanges
Choco Taco	1	290	15	140	11	0	10	120	36	1	4	2 1/2 carb, 3 fat
Dark Chocolate Bar	1	250	14	130	11	0	10	55	29	1	3	2 carb, 3 fat
Double Chocolate Bar	1	240	14	130	11	0	10	75	27	1	3	2 carb, 3 fat
Heath Bar	1	230	15	130	11	0	10	70	24	1	3	1 1/2 carb, 3 fat
Krunch Bar	1	250	14	130	11	0	10	55	30	1	3	2 carb, 3 fat
Neapolitan Bar	1	250	14	120	11	0	10	75	29	1	3	2 carb, 3 fat
Oreo Cookie Sandwich	1	260	17	150	12	0	15	115	26	1	2	2 carb, 3 fat
Reese's Bar	1	260	16	150	11	0	10	90	26	1	3	2 carb, 3 fat
Slim-a-Bear 100 Calorie Chocolate Fudge Bar	1	100	3	25	2	0	5	90	20	4	3	1 carb, 1 fat
Slim-a-Bear 100 Calorie English Toffee Bar	1	100	6	60	5	0	5	30	12	2	1	1 carb, 1 fat
Slim-a-Bear 100 Calorie Vanilla Sandwich	1	100	1.5	15	1	0	0	65	21	2	2	1 1/2 carb

Slim-a-Bear No Sugar Added Krunch Bar	1	170	10	90	8	0	5	85	22	4	4	1 1/2 carb, 2 fat
Slim-a-Bear No Sugar Added Vanilla Bar	1	170	9	90	8	0	5	65	21	4	4	1 1/2 carb, 2 fat
Triple Chocolate Bar	1	230	14	120	11	0	10	55	26	1	3	2 carb, 3 fat
Vanilla Cone	1	280	14	130	9	0	0	95	35	1	5	2 carb, 3 fat
Whitehouse Cherry Bar	1	250	14	120	15	0	10	75	31	1	3	2 carb, 3 fat
Luigi's											
Italian Ice, All Varieties	6 oz cup	120	0	0	0	0	0	10	31–32	<1	0	2 carb
Italian Ice, No Sugar Added	6 oz cup	60	0	0	0	0	0	10	20	0	0	1 carb
Nestlé											
Drumstick, Classic, Vanilla	1	290	16	140	9	0	15	100	33	2	4	2 carb, 3 fat
Drumstick, Classic, Vanilla Caramel	1	320	17	150	9	0	15	125	37	2	4	2 1/2 carb, 3 fat

ICE CREAM, FROZEN YOGURT, PUDDING, GELATIN

	Serving	Calories	Fat (g)	Cal. from Fat	Sat. Fat (g)	Trans Fat (g)	Chol. (mg)	Sod. (mg)	Carb. (g)	Fiber (g)	Prot. (g)	Servings/Exchanges
Drumstick, Simply Dipped, Cookies & Cream	1	300	14	130	10	0	15	115	39	1	3	2 1/2 carb, 3 fat
Drumstick, Simply Dipped, Vanilla	1	270	13	120	9	0	15	115	37	1	2	2 1/2 carb, 3 fat
Lil' Drums Cone, Cookie Dough	1	140	7	80	4	0	5	60	18	0	1	1 carb, 1 fat
Popsicle All Natural Ice Pop	1.8 oz pop	50	0	0	0	0	0	5	12	0	0	1 carb
Big Stick Cherry Pineapple Ice Pop	1	70	0	0	0	0	0	5	17	0	0	1 carb
Cotton Candy Swirl Bar	1	45	0	0	0	0	0	5	12	0	0	1 carb
Creamsicle 100 Calorie	1	100	2	20	0.5	0	<5	30	20	0	1	1 carb
Fat Free Fudgsicle	1	60	0	0	0	0	0	60	13	1	2	1 carb

Food											
Firecracker Ice Pop	1	35	0	0	0	0	0	9	0	0	1/2 carb
Fudgsicle 100 Calorie Pop	1	100	2	20	1	0	80	17	<1	2	1 carb
Fudgsicle Triple Chocolate Bar	1	60	1.5	15	1	0	60	11	0	1	1 carb
Lemon Lime Shots	1	80	1	10	1	0	0	17	0	0	1 carb
Lick-A-Color Ice Pop	1	90	0	0	0	0	10	22	0	0	1 1/2 carb
Lowfat Creamsicle Bar	1	70	1	10	0	<5	20	13	0	<1	1 carb
No Sugar Added Creamsicle Pop	1	25	0	0	0	0	10	5	<1	<1	free
Orange Burst Pop-Ups	1	90	1	10	1	5	20	18	0	1	1 carb
Rainbow Ice Pops	1	45	0	0	0	0	0	11	0	0	1 carb
Root Beer, Banana & Lemon Lime Ice Pop	1	45	0	0	0	0	0	11	0	0	1 carb
Scribblers Ice Pop	1	30	0	0	0	0	0	8	0	0	1/2 carb
Slow Melt Ice Age	1	40	0	0	0	0	0	10	0	2	1/2 carb

ICE CREAM, FROZEN YOGURT, PUDDING, GELATIN

	Serving	Calories	Fat (g)	Cal. from Fat	Sat. Fat (g)	Trans Fat (g)	Chol. (mg)	Sod. (mg)	Carb. (g)	Fiber (g)	Prot. (g)	Servings/Exchanges
Slow Melt Swirlwinds	1	40	0	0	0	0	0	0	10	0	0	1/2 carb
Snow Cone	1	30	0	0	0	0	0	0	8	0	0	1/2 carb
Spider Man Bar	1	100	0	0	0	0	0	20	25	0	0	1 1/2 carb
SpongeBob SquarePants Pop Ups	1	80	1	10	0	0	5	10	16	0	<1	1 carb
Sugar Free Fudgsicle	1	40	1	10	0	0	0	50	10	2	2	1/2 carb
Sugar Free Ice Pop, All Varieties	1	15	0	0	0	0	0	0	4	0	0	free
Super Heroes Ice Pop	1	40	0	0	0	0	0	0	11	0	0	1 carb
The Skinny Cow/Silhouette												
Chocolate With Fudge Cone	1	150	3	25	2	0	4	95	28	3	4	2 carb, 1 fat
Fudge Bar	1	100	1	10	0.5	0	3	45	22	4	4	1 1/2 carb
Ice Cream Sandwich, Vanilla	1	140	2	15	1	0	1	95	30	3	4	2 carb

Ice Cream Sandwich, Vanilla, No Sugar Added	1	140	2	20	1	0	0	95	28	4	4	2 carb

Snickers

Snickers Ice Cream Bar	1	180	11	100	6	0	10	60	18	1	3	1 carb, 2 fat

Weight Watchers

Smart Ones Chocolate Chip Cookie Dough	1	170	3	30	1.5	0	5	100	32	1	3	2 carb, 1 fat
Smart Ones Mocha Fudge Sundae	1	160	4	35	2	0	5	85	27	1	3	2 carb, 1 fat
Smart Ones Peanut Butter Cup Sundae	1	170	5	50	2.5	0	5	90	28	3	4	2 carb, 1 fat

PUDDING & GELATIN

Jell-O Gelatin

Gelatin Desserts, Dry Mix, All Varieties	1/2 cup	80	0	0	0	0	0	80–120	19	0	2	1 carb

ICE CREAM, FROZEN YOGURT, PUDDING, GELATIN

	Serving	Calories	Fat (g)	Cal. from Fat	Sat. Fat (g)	Trans Fat (g)	Chol. (mg)	Sod. (mg)	Carb. (g)	Fiber (g)	Prot. (g)	Servings/Exchanges
Gelatin Desserts, Dry Mix, Sugar Free	1/2 cup	55	0	0	0	0	0	45–80	0	0	1	free
Gelatin Snacks, All Flavors	3.5 oz	70	0	0	0	0	0	40	17	0	1	1 carb
Sugar-Free Snacks, All Flavors	3.5 oz	10	0	0	0	0	0	45–80	0	0	1	free
Jell-O Pudding Snacks												
Cheesecake	3.5 oz	130	2	20	1.5	0	5	120	26	0	2	2 carb
Chocolate	4 oz	140	4	35	1.5	0	0	170	26	1	2	2 carb, 1 fat
Chocolate Fudge Sundae	4 oz	140	3.5	30	1.5	0	0	170	25	0	2	1 1/2 carb, 1 fat
Chocolate Vanilla Swirl	4 oz	140	4	35	1.5	0	0	170	26	1	2	2 carb, 1 fat
Fat Free Chocolate	4 oz	100	0	0	0	0	0	180	23	1	2	1 1/2 carb
Fat Free Chocolate Vanilla Swirl	4 oz	100	0	0	0	0	0	200	23	1	2	1 1/2 carb

Fat Free Devil's Food	4 oz	100	0	0	0	0	0	190	22	1	2	1 1/2 carb
Fat Free Tapioca	4 oz	100	0	0	0	0	0	230	23	0	1	1 1/2 carb
Oreo	4 oz	120	1.5	15	1.5	0	0	200	25	1	2	1 1/2 carb
Sugar Free Double Chocolate	3.8 oz	60	1.5	10	1	0	0	170	14	1	2	1 carb
Sugar Free Vanilla	3.8 oz	60	1	10	1	0	0	190	13	0	1	1 carb
Tapioca	4 oz	130	3	25	1	0	0	150	25	0	1	1 1/2 carb, 1 fat
Vanilla	4 oz	130	3.5	30	1.5	0	0	160	24	0	1	1 1/2 carb, 1 fat

Jell-O Smoothie Snacks

Mixed Berry	4 oz	100	2.5	25	1.5	0	10	40	18	0	1	1 carb, 1 fat
Strawberry Banana	4 oz	100	2.5	25	1.5	0	10	40	18	0	1	1 carb, 1 fat

Kozy Shack

Chocolate Pudding	1/2 cup	140	3.5	30	2	0	15	140	24	<1	4	1 1/2 carb, 1 fat
Cinnamon Raisin Rice Pudding	1/2 cup	140	3	30	2	0	20	130	24	0	4	1 1/2 carb, 1 fat
Créme Caramel Flan	1/2 cup	150	3.5	35	2	0	35	85	27	0	4	2 carb, 1 fat

ICE CREAM, FROZEN YOGURT, PUDDING, GELATIN

	Serving	Calories	Fat (g)	Cal. from Fat	Sat. Fat (g)	Trans Fat (g)	Chol. (mg)	Sod. (mg)	Carb. (g)	Fiber (g)	Prot. (g)	Servings/Exchanges
Dulce De Leche Flan	1 cup	190	6	50	3	0	50	135	28	0	5	2 carb, 1 fat
European Style Rice Pudding	1/2 cup	130	3.5	30	2	0	25	130	22	0	4	1 1/2 carb, 1 fat
No Sugar Added Chocolate Pudding	1/2 cup	90	3	30	1.5	0	10	120	10	4	3	1/2 carb, 1 fat
No Sugar Added Rice Pudding	1/2 cup	90	3	30	2	0	15	115	14	3	4	1 carb, 1 fat
No Sugar Added Tapioca Pudding	1/2 cup	90	3	30	2	0	15	140	11	4	3	1 carb, 1 fat
Original Rice Pudding	1/2 cup	130	3	30	2	0	20	135	22	0	4	1 1/2 carb, 1 fat
Tapioca Pudding	1/2 cup	130	3	25	2	0	15	140	23	0	3	1 1/2 carb, 1 fat
Kraft Handi-Snacks Pudding Cups												
Butterscotch	3.5 oz	90	1	10	1	0	0	160	21	0	1	1 1/2 carb
Chocolate	3.5 oz	100	1	10	1	0	0	150	23	1	1	1 1/2 carb

Fat Free Chocolate	3.5 oz	90	0	0	0	0	0	170	21	0	2	1 1/2 carb
Rice	3.5 oz	140	6	50	1	0	0	130	19	0	3	1 carb, 1 fat
Vanilla	3.5 oz	90	0	0	0	0	0	160	20	0	1	1 carb
Snack Pack												
Gel Snack	3.5 oz	100	0	0	0	0	0	45	25	0	0	1 1/2 carb
Gel Snack, Sugar Free	3.5 oz	10	0	0	0	0	0	65	2	<1	0	free
Pudding Cups, Banana	3.5 oz	110	3.5	30	2	0	0	150	19	0	1	1 carb, 1 fat
Pudding Cups, Banana Creme Pie	3.5 oz	110	3.5	30	2	0	0	150	19	0	1	1 carb, 1 fat
Pudding Cups, Butterscotch	3.5 oz	120	3.5	30	1.5	0	0	150	21	0	1	1 1/2 carb, 1 fat
Pudding Cups, Caramel Creme	3.5 oz	120	3.5	30	1.5	0	0	160	21	0	1	1 1/2 carb, 1 fat
Pudding Cups, Chocolate	3.5 oz	120	3.5	30	2	0	0	135	21	<1	2	1 1/2 carb, 1 fat
Pudding Cups, Chocolate Fudge	3.5 oz	120	3.5	30	2	0	0	135	22	<1	2	1 1/2 carb, 1 fat

ICE CREAM, FROZEN YOGURT, PUDDING, GELATIN

	Serving	Calories	Fat (g)	Cal. from Fat	Sat. Fat (g)	Trans Fat (g)	Chol. (mg)	Sod. (mg)	Carb. (g)	Fiber (g)	Prot. (g)	Servings/Exchanges
Pudding Cups, Chocolate Lover's	3.5 oz	120	3.5	30	2	0	0	135	22	0	2	1 1/2 carb, 1 fat
Pudding Cups, Fat Free Chocolate	3.5 oz	90	0	0	0	0	0	140	20	0	2	1 carb
Pudding Cups, Fat Free Tapioca	3.5 oz	80	0	0	0	0	0	150	19	0	1	1 carb
Pudding Cups, Fat Free Vanilla	3.5 oz	80	0	0	0	0	0	140	18	0	1	1 carb
Pudding Cups, Ice Cream Sandwich	3.5 oz	120	3.5	30	2	0	0	135	21	0	2	1 1/2 carb, 1 fat
Pudding Cups, Lemon Meringue	3.5 oz	120	2.5	25	1.5	0	0	60	25	0	0	1 1/2 carb, 1 fat
Pudding Cups, No Sugar Added Chocolate	3.5 oz	60	3	30	1	0	0	110	8	<1	1	1/2 carb, 1 fat

Pudding Cups, No Sugar Added Vanilla	3.5 oz	60	3.5	30	1.5	0	0	115	8	0	<1	1/2 carb, 1 fat
Pudding Cups, Tapioca	3.5 oz	120	3.5	30	2	0	0	140	20	0	2	1 carb, 1 fat
Pudding Cups, Vanilla	3.5 oz	120	3.5	30	2	0	0	130	20	0	1	1 carb, 1 fat
Swiss Miss Pudding Cups												
Banana Cream	1	130	3.5	30	3.5	0	<5	170	23	0	2	1 1/2 carb, 1 fat
Chocolate Cream	1	150	4	35	3.5	0	<5	170	26	<1	3	2 carb, 1 fat
Chocolate Dream	1	150	4	35	3.5	0	<5	170	26	<1	3	2 carb, 1 fat
Chocolate Vanilla	1	140	3.5	30	3	0	0	160	27	0	2	2 carb, 1 fat
Classic Butterscotch	1	130	3.5	30	3	0	0	180	22	0	2	1 1/2 carb, 1 fat
Creamy Milk Chocolate	1	150	3.5	30	3	0	0	190	27	0	3	2 carb, 1 fat
Creamy Vanilla	1	140	3.5	30	3	0	0	180	24	0	2	1 1/2 carb, 1 fat
Lemon Meringue	1	140	3	30	3.5	0	0	600	28	0	0	2 carb, 1 fat
Low Fat Creamy Chocolate	1	130	2	20	2	0	0	180	26	0	3	2 carb
Old Fashioned Tapioca	1	140	3.5	30	3	0	0	180	24	0	2	1 1/2 carb, 1 fat

MEAT, POULTRY, FISH, SEAFOOD (FRESH, COOKED)

	Serving	Calories	Fat (g)	Cal. from Fat	Sat. Fat (g)	Trans Fat (g)	Chol. (mg)	Sod. (mg)	Carb. (g)	Fiber (g)	Prot. (g)	Servings/Exchanges
BEEF (Trimmed)												
Brisket												
Brisket, Flat Cut	3 oz	181	7	63	3	0	34	46	0	0	28	4 lean meat
Brisket, Whole	3 oz	247	17	153	6	0	79	55	0	0	23	3 med-fat meat
Chuck												
Arm Pot Roast	3 oz	238	14	126	6	0	85	53	0	0	25	3 med-fat meat
Blade Roast	3 oz	284	21	189	8	0	88	55	0	0	23	3 high-fat meat
Clod Roast	3 oz	176	9	81	3	0	59	60	0	0	22	3 lean meat
Flank Steak	3 oz	160	7	63	3	0	38	48	0	0	24	3 lean meat
Mock Tender Steak	3 oz	136	5	45	2	0	54	60	0	0	22	3 lean meat
Top Blade Steak	3 oz	184	10	90	3	0	52	57	0	0	22	3 lean meat
Ground Beef												
80% Lean Ground Beef	3 oz	230	15	135	6	0	77	64	0	0	22	3 med-fat meat

85% Lean Ground Beef	3 oz	213	13	117	5	0	77	61	0	22	3 med-fat meat
90% Lean Ground Beef	3 oz	184	10	90	4	0	72	58	0	22	3 lean meat
95% Lean Ground Beef	3 oz	145	6	54	3	0	65	55	0	22	3 lean meat
Plate											
Inside Skirt Steak	3 oz	187	10	90	4	0	51	64	0	22	3 lean meat
Round											
Bottom Round	3 oz	159	7	63	2	0	73	31	0	23	3 lean meat
Eye of Round	3 oz	145	5	45	2	0	59	53	0	24	3 lean meat
Tip Round	3 oz	162	7	63	2	0	69	54	0	24	3 lean meat
Top Round	3 oz	178	5	45	2	0	77	38	0	30	4 lean meat
Ribs											
Rib Eye	3 oz	210	13	117	5	0	94	48	0	23	3 med-fat meat
Short Ribs	3 oz	400	36	324	15	0	80	45	0	18	3 high-fat meat
Shank											
Shank Crosscuts, Trimmed to 1/4 inch	3 oz	224	12	108	5	0	68	52	0	26	3 med-fat meat

MEAT, POULTRY, FISH, SEAFOOD

	Serving	Calories	Fat (g)	Cal. from Fat	Sat. Fat (g)	Trans Fat (g)	Chol. (mg)	Sod. (mg)	Carb. (g)	Fiber (g)	Prot. (g)	Servings/Exchanges
Short Loin												
Porterhouse Steak	3 oz	235	16	144	6	0	57	55	0	0	20	3 med-fat meat
T-bone Steak	3 oz	210	14	126	5	0	51	57	0	0	21	3 med-fat meat
Tenderloin	3 oz	200	11	99	4	0	72	53	0	0	23	3 med-fat meat
Top Loin	3 oz	180	9	81	3	0	65	57	0	0	24	3 lean meat
Sirloin												
Bottom Sirloin Roast	3 oz	177	9	81	3	0	71	45	0	0	22	3 lean meat
Top Sirloin	3 oz	183	8	72	3	0	76	55	0	0	25	3 lean meat
Variety Cuts												
Liver	3 oz	162	4	36	1	0	337	67	0	0	25	3 lean meat
Tongue	3 oz	236	19	171	7	0	112	55	0	0	16	2 high-fat meat
BUFFALO	3 oz	120	2	18	<2	0	69	48	0	0	24	3 lean meat
LAMB												
Ground, Broiled	3 oz	240	17	153	7	0	81	69	0	0	21	3 med-fat meat

Leg, Sirloin, Roast, Lean	3 oz	174	8	70	3	0	78	60	0	0	24	3 lean meat
Rib, Roasted	3 oz	198	11	99	3	0	75	69	0	0	22	3 med-fat meat
Loin, Roast/Chop, Cooked	3 oz	183	8	72	3	0	81	72	0	0	26	4 lean meat
VEAL												
Breast	3 oz	226	14	126	6	0	96	55	0	0	23	3 med-fat meat
Ground Veal	3 oz	146	6	54	3	0	88	71	0	0	21	3 lean meat
Leg (Top Round)	3 oz	136	4	36	2	0	88	58	0	0	24	3 lean meat
Loin	3 oz	184	10	90	4	0	88	79	0	0	21	3 lean meat
Rib	3 oz	194	12	108	5	0	94	78	0	0	20	3 med-fat meat
Shank	3 oz	162	5	45	2	0	105	79	0	0	27	4 lean meat
Shoulder	3 oz	156	7	63	3	0	96	82	0	0	22	3 lean meat
Sirloin	3 oz	172	9	81	4	0	87	71	0	0	21	3 lean meat
PORK												
Ground Pork	3 oz	252	18	162	7	0	80	62	0	0	22	3 high-fat meat
Leg (Ham)	3 oz	232	15	135	5	0	80	51	0	0	23	3 med-fat meat

MEAT, POULTRY, FISH, SEAFOOD

	Serving	Calories	Fat (g)	Cal. from Fat	Sat. Fat (g)	Trans Fat (g)	Chol. (mg)	Sod. (mg)	Carb. (g)	Fiber (g)	Prot. (g)	Servings/Exchanges
Loin												
Back Ribs	3 oz	315	25	225	9	0	100	86	0	0	21	3 high-fat meat
Blade Chops	3 oz	272	21	189	8	0	73	60	0	0	19	3 high-fat meat
Center Loin Chops	3 oz	210	12	108	5	0	73	50	0	0	24	3 med-fat meat
Center Rib Roast	3 oz	214	13	117	5	0	69	41	0	0	23	3 med-fat meat
Country-Style Ribs	3 oz	279	22	198	8	0	78	44	0	0	20	3 high-fat meat
Sirloin Roast	3 oz	222	14	126	5	0	74	51	0	0	23	3 med-fat meat
Tenderloin	3 oz	147	5	45	2	0	67	47	0	0	24	3 lean meat
Top Loin Roast	3 oz	192	10	90	4	0	66	37	0	0	24	3 lean meat
Whole Loin	3 oz	211	12	108	5	0	70	50	0	0	23	3 med-fat meat
Shoulder												
Arm Picnic	3 oz	269	20	180	7	0	80	60	0	0	20	3 high-fat meat
Blade Boston Roast	3 oz	229	16	144	6	0	73	57	0	0	20	3 med-fat meat
Whole Shoulder	3 oz	248	18	162	7	0	77	58	0	0	20	3 med-fat meat

POULTRY

Food	Serving										Exchanges
Chicken Back, No Skin, Roasted	3 oz	203	11	99	3	0	76	82	0	0	24	3 med-fat meat
Chicken Breast, No Skin, Roasted	3 oz	141	3	27	1	0	72	63	0	0	26	3 lean meat
Chicken Drumstick, No Skin, Roasted	3 oz	146	5	45	1	0	79	81	0	0	24	3 lean meat
Chicken Leg, No Skin, Roasted	3 oz	162	7	63	2	0	80	77	0	0	23	3 lean meat
Chicken Thigh, No Skin, Roasted	3 oz	178	9	81	3	0	81	75	0	0	22	3 lean meat
Chicken Wing, No Skin, Roasted	3 oz	173	7	63	2	0	72	78	0	0	26	4 lean meat
Chicken, Capon	3 oz	195	10	90	3	0	73	42	0	0	25	3 lean meat
Chicken, Dark Meat with Skin, Roasted	3 oz	216	14	126	3.6	0	78	75	0	0	22	3 med-fat meat

MEAT, POULTRY, FISH, SEAFOOD

	Serving	Calories	Fat (g)	Cal. from Fat	Sat. Fat (g)	Trans Fat (g)	Chol. (mg)	Sod. (mg)	Carb. (g)	Fiber (g)	Prot. (g)	Servings/Exchanges
Chicken, Dark Meat, No Skin, Roasted	3 oz	174	8	76	2	0	78	78	0	0	23	3 lean meat
Chicken, Light Meat with Skin, Roasted	3 oz	189	9	81	3	0	72	63	0	0	25	3 lean meat
Cornish Game Hen, Whole Bird, Cooked, No Skin	3 oz	114	3	27	1	0	90	54	0	0	20	3 lean meat
Duck, Domestic, No Skin, Roasted	3 oz	171	10	86	3	0	75	54	0	0	20	3 lean meat
Goose, No Skin, Roasted	3 oz	201	11	97	3	0	81	66	0	0	25	3 med-fat meat
Ostrich, cooked	3 oz	120	2	18	0	0	81	66	0	0	23	3 lean meat
Pheasant, No Skin	3 oz	114	3	27	0	0	57	30	0	0	20	3 lean meat

Turkey Back, No Skin, Roasted	3 oz	144	5	45	2	0	81	62	0	0	24	3 lean meat
Turkey Breast, Roasted	3 oz	114	1	9	0	0	69	45	0	0	26	3 lean meat
Turkey Dark Meat, No Skin, cooked	3 oz	159	6	54	3	0	72	66	0	0	24	3 lean meat
Turkey Leg, No Skin, Roasted	3 oz	135	3	27	1	0	101	69	0	0	25	3 lean meat
Turkey Wing, No Skin, Roasted	3 oz	139	3	27	1	0	87	66	0	0	26	4 lean meat
Turkey, Ground, Cooked	3 oz	201	11	99	3	0	87	90	0	0	23	3 med-fat meat
FISH/SEAFOOD											
Bluefish, Baked	3 oz	130	5	35	1	0	65	65	0	0	22	3 lean meat
Carfish, Baked	3 oz	129	7	63	2	0	54	68	0	0	16	2 lean meat
Catfish, Baked	3 oz	129	6	54	2	0	54	69	0	0	15	3 lean meat
Caviar, Black/Red, Granular	2 Tbsp	81	6	54	1	0	188	480	1	0	8	1 med-fat meat

MEAT, POULTRY, FISH, SEAFOOD

	Serving	Calories	Fat (g)	Cal. from Fat	Sat. Fat (g)	Trans Fat (g)	Chol. (mg)	Sod. (mg)	Carb. (g)	Fiber (g)	Prot. (g)	Servings/Exchanges
Clams, Fresh, Steamed	1 oz	42	<1	5	<1	0	19	32	1	0	7	1 lean meat
Cod, Baked	3 oz	89	1	9	0	0	47	66	0	0	19	3 lean meat
Crab	3 oz	114	6	54	2	0	81	453	2	0	15	3 lean meat
Escargot/Snails	1 oz	51	<1	5	<1	0	28	34	1	0	9	1 lean meat
Flounder/Sole, Baked	3 oz	99	1	14	0	0	58	89	0	0	21	3 lean meat
Haddock, Baked	3 oz	95	1	7	0	0	63	74	0	0	21	3 lean meat
Halibut, Baked	3 oz	119	2	22	0	0	35	59	0	0	23	3 lean meat
Herring, Atlantic, Baked	3 oz	173	10	89	2	0	65	98	0	0	20	3 lean meat
Imitation Shellfish, from Surimi	1 oz	29	<1	0	<1	0	6	238	3	0	3	1 lean meat
Lobster, Fresh, Steamed	1 oz	28	<1	0	<1	0	20	108	<1	0	6	1 lean meat
Mackerel, Atlantic/ Pacific, Baked	3 oz	223	15	120	4	0	64	71	0	0	20	3 med-fat meat
Mackerel, King, Baked	3 oz	114	2	20	0	0	58	173	0	0	22	3 lean meat

Food	Serving											Exchanges
Ocean Perch, Baked	3 oz	102	2	16	0	0	46	82	0	0	20	3 lean meat
Octopus	1 oz	46	<1	0	<1	0	27	130	1	0	9	1 lean meat
Orange Roughy, Baked	3 oz	76	1	7	0	0	22	69	0	0	16	2 lean meat
Oyster, Medium	6	58	2	18	<1	0	44	177	3	0	6	1 lean meat
Pollock, Baked	3 oz	100	1	9	0	0	77	94	0	0	21	3 lean meat
Rainbow Trout, Baked	3 oz	144	6	55	2	0	58	36	0	0	21	3 lean meat
Rockfish, Baked	3 oz	103	2	15	0	0	37	65	0	0	20	3 lean meat
Sablefish, Baked	3 oz	212	17	152	3	0	54	61	0	0	15	2 high-fat meat
Salmon, Atlantic/Coho, Baked	3 oz	175	10	94	2	0	54	52	0	0	19	3 lean meat
Salmon, Chum/Pink, Baked	3 oz	130	4	32	0	0	81	54	0	0	22	3 lean meat
Salmon, Sockeye, Baked	3 oz	184	9	84	2	0	75	55	0	0	23	3 lean meat
Scallops, Fresh, Steamed	1 oz	32	<1	0	<1	0	15	78	0	0	7	1 lean meat

MEAT, POULTRY, FISH, SEAFOOD

	Serving	Calories	Fat (g)	Cal. from Fat	Sat. Fat (g)	Trans Fat (g)	Chol. (mg)	Sod. (mg)	Carb. (g)	Fiber (g)	Prot. (g)	Servings/Exchanges
Sea Bass, Baked	3 oz	105	2	20	0	0	45	74	0	0	20	3 lean meat
Shark, Baked	3 oz	140	5	22	1	0	50	85	0	0	22	3 lean meat
Shrimp, Fresh, Cooked in Water	1 oz	28	<1	0	<1	0	56	64	0	0	6	1 lean meat
Swordfish, Baked	3 oz	130	4	39	1	0	43	98	0	0	22	3 lean meat
Tilefish, Baked	3 oz	125	4	36	1	0	54	50	0	0	20	3 lean meat
Trout	3 oz	162	6	54	2	0	63	57	0	0	24	3 lean meat
Tuna, Yellowfin, Baked	3 oz	118	1	9	0	0	49	40	0	0	25	3 lean meat
Whiting, Baked	3 oz	98	1	13	0	0	71	112	0	0	20	3 lean meat
RABBIT	3 oz	174	6	54	2	0	72	30	0	0	27	3 lean meat
VENISON	3 oz	135	2	18	2	0	96	45	0	0	27	3 lean meat

MILK, YOGURT, NON-DAIRY MILK

	Serving	Calories	Fat (g)	Cal. from Fat	Sat. Fat (g)	Trans Fat (g)	Chol. (mg)	Sod. (mg)	Carb. (g)	Fiber (g)	Prot. (g)	Servings/Exchanges
Buttermilk, 1%, Low Fat	1 cup	98	2	20	1	0	10	257	12	0	8	1 low-fat milk
Buttermilk, Fat Free	1 cup	98	0	0	0	0	0	257	12	0	8	1 fat-free milk
Eggnog, Whole	1/2 cup	171	10	90	6	0	75	69	17	0	5	1 whole milk
Kefir, 2%	1 cup	120	5	45	3	0	19	70	13	2	9	1 reduced-fat milk
Milk, 1%, Low Fat	1 cup	110	2.5	23	1.5	0	15	125	13	0	8	1 lowfat milk
Milk, 2% Reduced Fat, Lactaid	1 cup	130	5	45	3	0	19	125	13	0	8	1 reduced-fat milk
Milk, 2%, Low Fat, Acidophilus	1 cup	128	5	45	3	0	19	123	11	0	8	1 reduced-fat milk
Milk, 2%, Reduced Fat	1 cup	130	5	45	3	0	20	130	12	0	8	1 reduced-fat milk
Milk, Evaporated, Fat Free	1 cup	100	0	0	0	0	5	147	15	0	10	1 fat-free milk
Milk, Evaporated, Whole	1/2 cup	169	10	90	6	0	37	134	13	0	8	1 whole milk

MILK, YOGURT, NON-DAIRY MILK

	Serving	Calories	Fat (g)	Cal. from Fat	Sat. Fat (g)	Trans Fat (g)	Chol. (mg)	Sod. (mg)	Carb. (g)	Fiber (g)	Prot. (g)	Servings/Exchanges
Milk, Fat Free, Chocolate	1 cup	160	0	0	0	0	5	220	31	0	9	1 fat-free milk, 1 carb
Milk, Fat Free, Lactaid	1 cup	80	0	0	0	0	0	125	13	0	8	1 fat-free milk
Milk, Fat Free, Nonfat, Skim	1 cup	90	0	0	0	0	4	130	13	0	9	1 fat-free milk
Milk, Goat, Whole	1 cup	168	10	90	7	0	27	122	11	0	9	1 whole milk
Milk, Whole	1 cup	150	8	70	5	0	33	120	12	0	8	1 whole milk
Milk, Whole, Chocolate	1 cup	208	9	81	5	0	30	150	26	2	8	1 whole milk, 1 carb
Rice Drink, Fat Free or 1%, Plain	1 cup	90	1.5	14	0	0	0	70	18	0	1	1 carb
Rice Drink, Low Fat, Flavored	1 cup	122	2	20	0	0	0	70	25	0	1	1 1/2 carb
Smoothie, Regular, Yogurt Based, Flavored	10 oz	260	3	25	2	0	12	130	50	0	8	1 reduced-fat milk, 2 1/2 carb

Soy Milk, Light	1 cup	100	2	20	0	0	0	90	15	0	5	1 low-fat milk
Soy Milk, Regular, Plain	1 cup	115	4	35	0.5	0	0	107	11	1.5	8	1 reduced-fat milk
Yogurt & Juice Blend	1 cup	150	0	0	0	0	0	55	34	0	3	2 carb
Yogurt with Fruit, Low Fat	6 oz	150	1.5	14	1	0	5	100	28	0	6	1 low-fat milk, 1 carb
Yogurt, Low Fat, Plain	1 cup	107	2.5	23	1.5	0	10	119	12	0	9	1 low-fat milk
Yogurt, Nonfat, Plain	6 oz	82	<1	0	<1	0	12	112	12	0	8	1 fat-free milk
Yogurt, Whole Milk, Plain	1 cup	160	8	70	5	0	20	120	12	0	9	1 whole milk

YOGURT

Breyers Yogurt

Creme Savers, Strawberry & Creme	6 oz	170	1.5	15	1	0	10	180	33	0	6	1 low-fat milk, 1 1/2 carb
Fruit on the Bottom, Strawberry	6 oz	170	1.5	15	1	0	10	85	33	<1	6	1 low-fat milk, 1 1/2 carb
Inspirations, Natural Strawberry	4 oz	110	1	10	0.5	0	5	55	22	<1	4	1 low-fat milk, 1/2 carb

MILK, YOGURT, NON-DAIRY MILK

	Serving	Calories	Fat (g)	Cal. from Fat	Sat. Fat (g)	Trans Fat (g)	Chol. (mg)	Sod. (mg)	Carb. (g)	Fiber (g)	Prot. (g)	Servings/Exchanges
Light, Nonfat, Strawberry	6 oz	80	0	0	0	0	<5	105	12	<1	6	1 fat-free milk
Smooth & Creamy, Strawberry	6 oz	170	1.5	15	1	0	10	90	34	0	6	1 low-fat milk, 1 1/2 carb
Dannon Yogurt												
Activia Fiber, Strawberry & Cereal	4 oz	110	2	15	1	0	5	80	19	3	5	1 low-fat milk, 1/2 carb
Activia Light, Strawberry	4 oz	70	0	0	0	0	<5	80	13	3	5	1 fat-free milk
Activia, Strawberry	4 oz	110	2	20	1	0	5	75	19	0	5	1 low-fat milk, 1/2 carb
All Natural, Blended, Strawberry	4 oz	120	1	10	1	0	5	70	21	0	5	1 low-fat milk, 1/2 carb
All Natural, Lowfat, Plain	6 oz	100	2.5	25	1.5	0	10	115	12	0	8	1 low-fat milk

All Natural, Nonfat, Plain	6 oz	80	0	0	0	5	120	12	0	9	1 fat-free milk
All Natural, Plain	8 oz	160	8	5	70	20	120	12	0	9	1 whole milk
DanActive, Strawberry	3.1-oz bottle	80	1.5	1	15	5	40	13	0	3	1 carb
Danimals Drinkable, Swingin' Strawberry/ Banana	3.1 oz	70	0.5	0	5	<5	30	15	0	2	1 carb
Fruit on the Bottom, Strawberry	6 oz	150	1.5	1	15	5	110	28	<1	6	1 low-fat milk, 1 carb
Light & Fit 0% Plus, Assorted Flavors	4 oz	60	0	0	0	<5	55	10	0	3	1/2 fat-free milk
Light & Fit 0% Plus, Strawberry	6 oz	80	0	0	0	<5	80	16	0	5	1 fat-free milk
Light & Fit Cup, Carb & Sugar Control	4 oz	50	1.5	1	15	5	25	3	0	5	1/2 low-fat milk
Light & Fit Smoothie, Carb & Sugar Control	7 oz	60	2.5	1.5	25	15	35	4	0	6	1/2 low-fat milk

MILK, YOGURT, NON-DAIRY MILK

	Serving	Calories	Fat (g)	Cal. from Fat	Sat. Fat (g)	Trans Fat (g)	Chol. (mg)	Sod. (mg)	Carb. (g)	Fiber (g)	Prot. (g)	Servings/Exchanges
Yoplait Yogurt												
Delights	4 oz	100	1.5	10	1	0	5	90	18	0	5	1 low-fat milk, 1/2 carb
Fiber One, Fat Free	4 oz	50	0	0	0	0	<5	55	13	5	3	1 carb
GoGurt, Fruit Flavors	2.25-oz tube	70	0.5	5	0	0	<5	30	13	0	2	1 carb
Light, Fruit Flavors	6 oz	100	0	0	0	0	<5	85	19	0	5	1 low-fat milk
Original, Fruit Flavors	6 oz	170	1.5	15	1	0	10	80	33	0	5	1 low-fat milk, 1 1/2 carb
Smoothie, Prepared	8 oz	110	1.5	15	0.5	0	<5	20	14	2	1	1 carb
Thick & Creamy, Fruit Flavors	6 oz	190	3.5	30	2	0	10	100	32	0	7	1 reduced-fat milk, 1 carb
Tri Yogurt, Fruit Flavors	4 oz	90	0.5	5	0.5	0	<5	50	18	0	4	1 low-fat milk, 1/2 carb
Yoplait Kids, Strawberry	4 oz	100	2	20	1.5	0	10	75	17	1	5	1 low-fat milk
Yo-Plus	4 oz	110	1.5	10	1	0	10	70	21	3	4	1 low-fat milk, 1/2 carb

	Serving	Calories	Fat (g)	% Cal. Fat	Sat. Fat (g)	Chol. (mg)	Sodium (mg)	Carb. (g)	Fiber (g)	Protein (g)	Exchanges/Choices
Yo-Plus Light	4 oz	70	0	0	0	5	65	15	3	4	1 low-fat milk
NON-DAIRY MILK											
Almond Milk											
Blue Diamond Almond Breeze (Shelf Stable)											
Chocolate	1 cup	110	3	25	0	0	150	22	1	1	1 1/2 carb, 1 fat
Chocolate, Unsweetened	1 cup	45	3.5	30	0	0	180	3	1	2	1 fat
Original	1 cup	60	2.5	25	0	0	150	8	<1	1	1/2 carb, 1 fat
Original, Unsweetened	1 cup	40	3	30	0	0	150	2	1	1	1 fat
Vanilla	1 cup	90	2.5	25	0	0	150	16	<1	1	1 carb, 1 fat
Vanilla, Unsweetened	1 cup	45	3.5	30	0	0	180	3	1	2	1 fat
Pacific (Shelf Stable)											
Original, Unsweetened	1 cup	35	2.5	25	0	0	180	2	0	1	1 fat
Grain Milk											
Pacific (Shelf Stable)											
Organic Oat, Low Fat, Vanilla	1 cup	130	2.5	20	0	0	110	24	2	4	1 1/2 carb, 1 fat

MILK, YOGURT, NON-DAIRY MILK

	Serving	Calories	Fat (g)	Cal. from Fat	Sat. Fat (g)	Trans Fat (g)	Chol. (mg)	Sod. (mg)	Carb. (g)	Fiber (g)	Prot. (g)	Servings/Exchanges
Hazelnut Milk												
Pacific (Shelf Stable)												
Original	1 cup	110	3.5	30	0	0	0	120	18	<1	2	1 carb, 1 fat
Rice Milk												
Pacific (Shelf Stable)												
Plain, Low Fat	1 cup	130	2	20	0	0	0	60	27	0	1	2 carb
Rice Dream (Refrigerated)												
Original, Enriched	1 cup	120	2.5	20	0	0	0	80	23	0	1	1 1/2 carb, 1 fat
Vanilla, Enriched	1 cup	130	2.5	20	0	0	0	80	26	0	1	2 carb, 1 fat
Rice Dream (Shelf Stable)												
Carob	1 cup	150	2.5	25	0	0	0	80	30	<1	1	2 carb, 1 fat
Chocolate, Enriched	1 cup	160	3	25	0	0	0	90	34	<1	2	2 carb, 1 fat
Horchata	1 cup	160	2.5	25	0	0	0	150	32	0	1	2 carb, 1 fat
Original	1 cup	120	2.5	20	0	0	0	100	24	0	1	1 1/2 carb, 1 fat

Original, Enriched	1 cup	120	2.5	20	0	0	100	23	0	1	1 1/2 carb, 1 fat
Original, Heartwise	1 cup	130	2	20	0	0	80	27	3	1	2 carb
Vanilla	1 cup	130	2.5	25	0	0	105	27	0	1	2 carb, 1 fat
Vanilla, Enriched	1 cup	130	2.5	20	0	0	105	26	0	1	2 carb, 1 fat
Vanilla, Heartwise	1 cup	140	2	20	0	0	80	30	3	1	2 carb
WestSoy (Shelf Stable)											
Rice Beverage, Plain	1 cup	110	2.5	25	0	0	105	20	0	1	1 carb, 1 fat
Rice Beverage, Vanilla	1 cup	110	2.5	25	0	0	105	20	0	1	1 carb, 1 fat
Soy Milk											
Pacific (Shelf Stable)											
Organic Soy, Unsweetened, Original	1 cup	90	4.5	40	0.5	0	15	4	2	9	1 med-fat meat
Select Soy, Low Fat, Plain	1 cup	70	2.5	20	0	0	115	9	<1	5	1/2 carb, 1 lean meat
Select Soy, Low Fat, Vanilla	1 cup	80	2.5	20	0	0	115	11	1	5	1 carb, 1 fat

MILK, YOGURT, NON-DAIRY MILK

	Serving	Calories	Fat (g)	Cal. from Fat	Sat. Fat (g)	Trans Fat (g)	Chol. (mg)	Sod. (mg)	Carb. (g)	Fiber (g)	Prot. (g)	Servings/Exchanges
Ultra Soy, Plain	1 cup	120	4	35	0.5	0	0	150	12	<1	10	1 carb, 1 med-fat meat
Ultra Soy, Vanilla	1 cup	130	4	35	0.5	0	0	150	14	<1	10	1 carb, 1 med-fat meat
Silk (Refrigerated)												
Silk Light, Chocolate	1 cup	120	1.5	15	0	0	0	100	22	2	5	1 1/2 carb
Silk Light, Original	1 cup	70	2	20	0	0	0	120	8	1	6	1/2 carb, 1 lean meat
Silk Light, Vanilla	1 cup	80	2	20	0	0	0	95	10	1	6	1/2 carb, 1 lean meat
Simply Silk, Chocolate	1 cup	140	3.5	30	0.5	0	0	100	23	2	5	1 1/2 carb, 1 med-fat meat
Simply Silk, Original	1 cup	100	4	35	0.5	0	0	120	8	1	7	1/2 carb, 1 med-fat meat
Simply Silk, Unsweetened	1 cup	80	4	35	0.5	0	0	85	4	1	7	1 med-fat meat
Simply Silk, Vanilla	1 cup	100	3.5	30	0.5	0	0	95	10	1	6	1/2 carb, 1 med-fat meat

Simply Silk, Very Vanilla	1 cup	130	4	35	0.5	0	140	19	1	6	1 carb, 1 med-fat meat
Silk (Shelf Stable)											
Plain Original	1 cup	100	4	35	0.5	0	120	8	1	7	1/2 carb, 1 med-fat meat
Unsweetened	1 cup	80	4	35	0.5	0	85	4	1	7	1 med-fat meat
Vanilla	1 cup	100	3.5	30	0.5	0	95	10	1	6	1/2 carb, 1 lean meat
Soy Dream (Refrigerated)											
Classic Original	1 cup	130	4	35	0.5	0	150	16	2	7	1 carb, 1 med-fat meat
Vanilla, Enriched	1 cup	120	3.5	30	0.5	0	130	14	2	8	1 carb, 1 med-fat meat
Soy Dream (Shelf Stable)											
Chocolate, Enriched	1 cup	150	4	40	0.5	0	125	21	3	7	1 1/2 carb, 1 med-fat meat
Classic Vanilla	1 cup	140	4	25	0.5	0	135	18	2	7	1 carb, 1 med-fat meat
Original, Enriched	1 cup	100	4	35	0.5	0	135	8	2	7	1/2 carb, 1 med-fat meat
Vanilla, Enriched	1 cup	120	4	35	0.5	0	135	14	2	7	1 carb, 1 med-fat meat

MILK, YOGURT, NON-DAIRY MILK

	Serving	Calories	Fat (g)	Cal. from Fat	Sat. Fat (g)	Trans Fat (g)	Chol. (mg)	Sod. (mg)	Carb. (g)	Fiber (g)	Prot. (g)	Servings/Exchanges
WestSoy (Shelf Stable)												
Lite, Plain	1 cup	60	2	20	0	0	0	85	6	<1	4	1/2 carb
Lite, Vanilla	1 cup	70	2	20	0	0	0	75	8	<1	5	1/2 carb, 1 lean meat
Low Fat, Plain	1 cup	90	1.5	15	0	0	0	90	14	2	4	1 carb
Low Fat, Vanilla	1 cup	120	1.5	15	0	0	0	90	21	2	4	1 1/2 carb
Non Fat, Plain	1 cup	70	0	0	0	0	0	105	10	<1	6	1/2 carb, 1 lean meat
Non Fat, Vanilla	1 cup	80	0	0	0	0	0	105	12	<1	6	1 carb, 1 lean meat
Organic Plus, Plain	1 cup	90	3.5	30	0.5	0	0	125	7	<1	7	1/2 carb, 1 lean meat
Organic Plus, Vanilla	1 cup	100	3.5	30	0.5	0	0	125	10	<1	7	1/2 carb, 1 lean meat
Organic, Unsweetened Original	1 cup	90	4.5	40	0.5	0	0	30	5	4	9	1 med-fat meat
Organic, Unsweetened, Vanilla	1 cup	100	4.5	40	0.5	0	0	30	5	4	9	1 med-fat meat

NUTS, SEEDS, NUT/SEED PRODUCTS

	Serving	Calories	Fat (g)	Cal. from Fat	Sat. Fat (g)	Trans Fat (g)	Chol. (mg)	Sod. (mg)	Carb. (g)	Fiber (g)	Prot. (g)	Servings/Exchanges
Almond Butter, Plain	1 Tbsp	91	10	90	<1	0	0	17	3	<1	2	2 fat
Almond Butter, Salted	1 Tbsp	98	9	80	<1	0	0	70	3	<1	2	2 fat
Almonds, Dried, Whole	1 oz	165	15	135	1	0	0	3	6	4	5	1 med-fat meat, 2 fat
Almonds, Dry Roasted, Salted	1 oz	166	15	135	1	0	0	221	7	4	5	1 med-fat meat, 2 fat
Almonds, Dry Roasted, Whole, Unsalted	1 oz	166	15	135	1	0	0	3	7	4	5	1 med-fat meat, 2 fat
Almonds, Oil Roasted	1 oz	175	16	145	2	0	0	221	5	3	6	1 med-fat meat, 2 fat
Almonds, Toasted	1 oz	167	14	125	1	0	0	3	7	3	6	1 med-fat meat, 2 fat
Beechnuts, Dried	1 oz	164	14	125	2	0	0	11	10	<1	2	1/2 starch, 3 fat
Brazil Nuts, Dried	1 oz	186	19	170	5	0	0	<1	4	2	4	1 med-fat meat, 3 fat
Cashew Butter, Plain	1 Tbsp	86	7	65	2	0	0	2	4	<1	3	1 fat
Cashews, Dry Roasted	1 oz	161	13	115	3	0	0	179	9	<1	5	1/2 starch, 3 fat

NUTS, SEEDS, NUT/SEED PRODUCTS

	Serving	Calories	Fat (g)	Cal. from Fat	Sat. Fat (g)	Trans Fat (g)	Chol. (mg)	Sod. (mg)	Carb. (g)	Fiber (g)	Prot. (g)	Servings/Exchanges
Cashews, Oil Roasted	1 oz	163	14	125	3	0	0	178	8	1	5	1/2 starch, 3 fat
Chinese Chestnuts, Dried	1 oz	103	<1	0	<1	0	0	1	23	<1	2	1 1/2 starch
Chinese Chestnuts, Roasted	1 oz	68	<1	0	<1	0	0	1	15	<1	1	1 starch
Coconut Milk, Raw	1 cup	552	57	515	51	0	0	36	13	5	6	1 starch, 11 fat
Coconut, Dried, Shredded, Sweetened	1/4 cup	117	8	60	7	0	0	61	11	1	<1	1 starch, 2 fat
Coconut, Fresh	2.52-inch piece	159	15	135	13	0	0	9	7	4	2	1/2 starch, 3 fat
Coconut, Toasted	1 oz	168	13	115	12	0	0	11	13	2	2	1 starch, 3 fat
English Walnut Halves, Dried	1 oz	182	18	160	2	0	0	3	5	1	4	1 med-fat meat, 3 fat
European Chestnuts, Roasted	1 oz	69	<1	0	<1	0	0	<1	15	2	<1	1 starch

Food	Serving											Exchanges
Filberts/Hazelnuts, Dried, Whole	1 oz	177	18	160	1	0	0	<1	4	2	4	1 med-fat meat, 3 fat
Filberts/Hazelnuts, Dry Roasted, Salted	1 oz	188	18	160	1	0	0	221	5	2	3	3 fat
Filberts/Hazelnuts, Oil Roasted, Salted	1 oz	187	18	160	1	0	0	223	6	2	4	1/2 starch, 3 fat
Flaxseed, Whole	1 Tbsp	55	4	35	<1	0	0	3	3	3	2	1 fat
Ginkgo Nuts	1 oz	52	0	0	0	0	0	2	11	NA	1	1 carb
Hickory Nuts, Dried	1 oz	186	18	160	2	0	0	<1	5	2	4	4 fat
Japanese Chestnuts, Dried	1 oz	101	<1	0	<1	0	0	10	23	<1	2	1 1/2 starch
Japanese Chestnuts, Roasted	1 oz	57	<1	0	<1	0	0	5	13	<1	<1	1 starch
Macadamia Nuts	1 oz	199	21	190	3	0	0	1	4	3	2	4 fat
Macadamia Nuts, Oil Roasted	1 oz	204	22	200	3	0	0	74	4	3	2	4 fat

NUTS, SEEDS, NUT/SEED PRODUCTS

	Serving	Calories	Fat (g)	Cal. from Fat	Sat. Fat (g)	Trans Fat (g)	Chol. (mg)	Sod. (mg)	Carb. (g)	Fiber (g)	Prot. (g)	Servings/Exchanges
Mixed Nuts, Dry Roasted	1 oz	168	15	135	2	0	0	190	7	3	5	1/2 starch, 3 fat
Mixed Nuts, Oil Roasted	1 oz	175	16	145	4	0	0	185	6	3	5	1/2 starch, 3 fat
Mixed Nuts, Oil Roasted, No Peanuts	1 oz	172	16	145	3	0	0	196	6	2	4	1/2 starch, 3 fat
Mixed Nuts, Oil Roasted, Unsalted	1 oz	173	16	145	2	0	0	3	6	2	4	1 med-fat meat, 2 fat
Peanut Butter, Chunky or Creamy	1 Tbsp	96	8	70	2	0	0	80	3	<1	4	1 med-fat meat, 1 fat
Peanut Butter, Natural, Salted	1 Tbsp	94	8	70	1	0	0	40	3	1	4	1 high-fat meat
Peanut Butter, Natural, Unsalted	1 Tbsp	94	8	70	1	0	0	<1	3	1	4	1 high-fat meat
Peanuts, Dry Roasted, Unsalted	1 oz	166	14	125	2	0	0	2	6	2	7	1 high-fat meat, 1 fat

Peanuts, Oil Roasted	1 oz	165	14	125	2	0	0	123	5	3	8	1 high-fat meat, 1 fat
Peanuts, Spanish, Raw	1 oz	167	14	125	2	0	0	6	5	3	8	1 high-fat meat, 1 fat
Pecans, Dried Halves	1 oz	189	19	170	2	0	0	<1	5	2	2	4 fat
Pecans, Dry Roasted	1 oz	187	18	160	2	0	0	222	6	3	2	3 fat
Pecans, Oil Roasted	1 oz	194	20	180	2	0	0	214	5	2	2	4 fat
Pine Nuts (Pignoli), Dried	1 oz	178	17	155	3	0	0	20	6	3	3	1/2 carb, 1 high-fat meat, 1 fat
Pistachio Nuts, Dry Roasted	1 oz	170	15	135	2	0	0	218	8	3	4	1/2 starch, 3 fat
Pumpkin Kernels, Roasted	1 oz	148	12	110	2	0	0	163	4	1	9	1 med-fat meat, 1 fat
Pumpkin Seeds, Roasted	1 oz	126	6	55	1	0	0	163	15	2	5	1 starch, 1 fat
Sesame Seeds, Dried, Whole	1 Tbsp	52	5	45	1	0	0	1	2	1	2	1 fat
Soy Nut Butter	1 Tbsp	96	8	70	1	0	0	70	3	2	4	1 high-fat meat

NUTS, SEEDS, NUT/SEED PRODUCTS

	Serving	Calories	Fat (g)	Cal. from Fat	Sat. Fat (g)	Trans Fat (g)	Chol. (mg)	Sod. (mg)	Carb. (g)	Fiber (g)	Prot. (g)	Servings/Exchanges
Soy Nuts, Dry Roasted, No Salt	3/4 oz	96	5	45	<1	0	0	0	7	2	8	1/2 carb, 1 med-fat meat
Sunflower Seeds, Dry	1 oz	162	14	125	2	0	0	<1	5	3	7	1 high-fat meat, 1 fat
Sunflower Seeds, Dry Roasted	1 oz	163	14	125	2	0	0	<1	7	3	6	1 high-fat meat, 1 fat
Sunflower Seeds, Oil Roasted	1 oz	174	16	145	2	0	0	171	4	2	6	1 high-fat meat, 1 fat
Tahini/Sesame Butter	2 Tbsp	60	5	45	<1	0	0	12	2	<1	2	1 fat
BRANDS												
Fifty50												
Peanut Butter, Creamy, No Added Sugar	2 Tbsp	190	16	140	2	0	0	0	7	3	7	1 high-fat meat, 1 fat
Peanut Butter, Crunchy, No Added Sugar	2 Tbsp	190	16	140	2	0	0	0	7	3	7	1 high-fat meat, 1 fat

Jif

	Serving	Cal	Fat								Exchanges
Creamy	2 Tbsp	190	16	145	3	0	150	7	2	7	1 high-fat meat, 1 fat
Extra Crunchy	2 Tbsp	190	16	145	3	0	130	7	2	7	1 high-fat meat, 1 fat
Omega-3	2 Tbsp	190	16	140	2.5	0	160	8	2	7	1/2 carb, 1 high-fat meat, 1 fat
Peanut Butter & Honey	2 Tbsp	180	14	130	2.5	0	120	10	2	6	1/2 carb, 1 high-fat meat, 1 fat
Reduced Fat, Creamy	2 Tbsp	190	12	111	2.5	0	250	15	2	8	1 carb, 1 high-fat meat, 1 fat
Reduced Fat, Crunchy	2 Tbsp	190	12	110	2.5	0	210	15	2	8	1 carb, 1 high-fat meat, 1 fat
Simply Jif, Creamy	2 Tbsp	190	16	130	3	0	65	6	2	8	1/2 carb, 1 high-fat meat, 1 fat

Laura Scudder's

	Serving	Cal	Fat								Exchanges
Peanut Butter, Nutty	2 Tbsp	210	16	144	2.5	0	120	6	2	8	1 high-fat meat, 2 fat
Peanut Butter, Smooth	2 Tbsp	210	16	144	2.5	0	120	6	2	8	1 high-fat meat, 2 fat

NUTS, SEEDS, NUT/SEED PRODUCTS

	Serving	Calories	Fat (g)	Cal. from Fat	Sat. Fat (g)	Trans Fat (g)	Chol. (mg)	Sod. (mg)	Carb. (g)	Fiber (g)	Prot. (g)	Servings/Exchanges
Peter Pan												
Creamy	2 Tbsp	210	17	150	3	0	0	140	6	2	8	1/2 carb, 1 high-fat meat, 1 fat
Crunchy	2 Tbsp	190	16	140	3	0	0	110	6	3	8	1/2 carb, 1 high-fat meat, 1 fat
Creamy Spread, Reduced Fat	2 Tbsp	200	13	120	2	0	0	150	14	2	8	1 carb, 1 high-fat meat, 1 fat
Creamy Honey Roast	2 Tbsp	200	15	140	3	0	0	125	10	2	8	1/2 carb, 1 high-fat meat, 1 fat
Creamy Plus	2 Tbsp	210	17	150	3	0	0	140	7	2	7	1/2 carb, 1 high-fat meat, 1 fat
Creamy Whipped	2 Tbsp	150	12	110	2.5	0	0	105	5	2	6	1 high-fat meat
Chunky Reduced Fat	2 Tbsp	200	13	120	2.5	0	0	150	14	2	8	1 carb, 1 high-fat meat, 1 fat

Skippy

Creamy	2 Tbsp	190	16	140	3	0	3	150	7	2	7	1/2 carb, 1 high-fat meat, 1 fat
Natural Creamy	2 Tbsp	180	17	150	3.5	0	0	125	6	2	7	1/2 carb, 1 high-fat meat, 1 fat
Reduced Fat Creamy	2 Tbsp	180	12	110	2	0	0	170	15	2	7	1 carb, 1 high-fat meat, 1 fat
Reduced Fat Super Chunk	2 Tbsp	180	12	110	2	0	0	160	15	2	7	1 carb, 1 high-fat meat, 1 fat
Roasted Honey Nut	2 Tbsp	190	16	140	3	0	0	125	7	2	7	1/2 carb, 1 high-fat meat, 1 fat
Roasted Honey Nut Super Chunk	2 Tbsp	190	16	140	3	0	0	105	6	2	7	1/2 carb, 1 high-fat meat, 1 fat

Smart Balance

Chunky	2 Tbsp	200	18	160	3	0	0	110	6	2	7	1/2 carb, 1 high-fat meat, 2 fat

PASTA, PASTA MIXES, PASTA SAUCE

	Serving	Calories	Fat. (g)	Cal. from Fat	Sat. Fat (g)	Trans Fat (g)	Chol. (mg)	Sod. (mg)	Carb. (g)	Fiber (g)	Prot. (g)	Servings/Exchanges
Lasagna, Cut, Cooked	1/2 cup	99	<1	0	<1	0	0	<1	20	<1	3	1 starch
Linguine, Cooked	1/2 cup	99	<1	0	<1	0	0	<1	20	2	3	1 starch
Macaroni, Cooked	1/2 cup	99	<1	0	<1	0	0	<1	20	<1	3	1 starch
Macaroni, Vegetable, Cooked	1/2 cup	86	<1	0	<1	0	0	4	18	1	3	1 starch
Macaroni, Whole Wheat, Cooked	1/2 cup	87	<1	0	<1	0	0	2	19	2	4	1 starch
Noodles, Chow Mein	1/2 cup	119	7	63	1	0	0	99	13	<1	2	1 starch, 1 fat
Noodles, Egg, Cooked	1/2 cup	107	1	9	<1	0	26	6	20	<1	4	1 starch
Noodles, Ramen, Cooked	1 cup	156	2	18	<1	0	38	1349	29	3	6	2 starch
Noodles, Rice, Cooked	1/2 cup	80	<1	0	<1	0	0	5	20	<1	<1	1 starch
Noodles, Spinach Egg, Cooked	1/2 cup	106	1	9	<1	0	27	10	20	2	4	1 starch

Food	Serving										
Pasta/Noodles, Fresh, Cooked	2 oz	74	<1	0	<1	19	3	14	<1	3	1 starch
Pasta/Noodles, Homemade, No Egg, Cooked	2 oz	70	<1	0	<1	0	42	14	<1	3	1 starch
Pasta/Noodles, Homemade, with Egg, Cooked	2 oz	74	<1	0	<1	23	47	13	2	3	1 starch
Pasta/Noodles, Spinach, Fresh, Cooked	2 oz	74	<1	0	<1	19	3	14	1	3	1 starch
Rotini, Cooked	1/2 cup	99	<1	0	<1	0	<1	20	<1	3	2 starch
Shells, Jumbo, Cooked	2	65	<1	0	<1	0	<1	13	<1	2	1 starch
Shells, Small, Cooked	1/2 cup	81	<1	0	<1	0	<1	17	<1	3	1 starch
Shells, Whole Wheat, Cooked	1/2 cup	87	<1	0	<1	0	2	19	2	4	1 starch
Spaghetti, Cooked	1/2 cup	99	<1	0	<1	0	<1	20	3	3	1 starch

PASTA, PASTA MIXES, PASTA SAUCE

	Serving	Calories	Fat (g)	Cal. from Fat	Sat. Fat (g)	Trans Fat (g)	Chol. (mg)	Sod. (mg)	Carb. (g)	Fiber (g)	Prot. (g)	Servings/Exchanges
Spaghetti, Whole Wheat, Cooked	1/2 cup	87	<1	0	<1	0	0	2	19	3	4	1 starch
Spirals Pasta, Cooked	1/2 cup	95	<1	0	<1	0	0	<1	19	<1	3	1 starch
Vermicelli, Cooked	1/2 cup	99	<1	0	<1	0	0	<1	20	2	3	1 starch
Wagon Wheels Pasta, Cooked	1/2 cup	99	<1	0	<1	0	0	<1	20	<1	3	1 starch
BRANDS												
Pasta Mixes												
Knorr/Lipton												
Pasta Sides, Alfredo	1 cup	310	12	90	4.5	0	15	890	43	1	11	3 starch, 2 fat
Pasta Sides, Chicken	1 cup	250	6	50	1	0	<5	720	43	1	8	3 starch, 1 fat
Pasta Sides, Parmesan	1 cup	280	12	80	4.5	0	15	760	42	1	10	3 starch, 2 fat
Kraft												
Macaroni & Cheese	1 cup	410	19	170	5	4	15	710	49	1	9	3 starch, 4 fat

Macaroni & Cheese, Deluxe Original	1 cup	320	10	90	3	0	15	930	45	1	12	3 starch, 2 fat
Macaroni & Cheese, Easy Mac, Original	1 pouch	230	4	35	2.5	0	5	550	42	1	7	3 starch, 1 fat
Macaroni & Cheese, Thick 'n Creamy	1 cup	380	15	140	4	3	5	740	52	2	10	3 1/2 starch, 3 fat
Macaroni & Cheese, Three Cheese	1 cup	380	15	130	4	3	5	760	51	2	9	3 1/2 starch, 3 fat
Velveeta Shells & Cheese, Original	1 cup	360	12	110	4	0	20	940	49	2	13	3 starch, 1 med-fat meat, 1 fat

Asian Pasta

Dynasty

Maifun Rice Sticks	2 oz	200	0.5	5	0	0	0	130	48	1	0	3 starch
Saifun Bean Threads	1 bundle	170	0	0	0	0	0	10	42	0	0	3 starch

Eden

100% Buckwheat Soba	2 oz	200	1	10	0	0	0	5	43	3	6	3 starch

PASTA, PASTA MIXES, PASTA SAUCE

	Serving	Calories	Fat (g)	Cal. from Fat	Sat. Fat (g)	Trans Fat (g)	Chol. (mg)	Sod. (mg)	Carb. (g)	Fiber (g)	Prot. (g)	Servings/Exchanges
40% Buckwheat Soba	2 oz	190	1	5	0	0	0	490	37	3	8	2 1/2 starch
Bifun (Rice) Pasta	2 oz	200	0.5	0	0	0	5	5	44	0	5	3 starch
Brown Rice Udon	2 oz	190	1	5	0	0	0	510	38	2	8	2 1/2 starch
Kamut Soba, Organic	1/2 cup	200	1	10	0	0	0	60	38	3	7	2 1/2 starch
Kamut Udon, Organic	1/2 cup	200	1.5	15	0	0	0	55	37	3	10	2 1/2 starch
Kuzu Pasta	2 oz	200	0	0	0	0	0	0	48	2	0	3 starch
Lotus Root Soba	2 oz	190	1	5	0	0	0	470	37	4	9	2 1/2 starch
Mugwort Soba	2 oz	190	0.5	5	0	0	0	550	37	2	8	2 1/2 starch
Mung Bean Pasta	2 oz	190	0	0	0	0	0	5	47	0	0	3 starch
Soba, Organic	1/2 cup	200	1.5	15	0	0	0	70	38	2	8	2 1/2 starch
Spelt Soba, Organic	1/2 cup	200	1.5	15	0	0	0	50	37	2	9	2 1/2 starch
Udon	2 oz	190	1.5	15	0	0	0	660	37	3	8	2 1/2 starch
La Choy												
Chow Mein Noodles	1/2 cup	130	5	50	1.5	NA	0	230	19	0	3	1 starch, 1 fat

	Serving	Cal.	Fat (g)	% Fat Cal.	Sat. Fat (g)	Chol. (mg)	Sod. (mg)	Carb. (g)	Fiber (g)	Prot. (g)	Exchanges
Rice Noodles	1/2 cup	130	4	36	1	NA	0	21	0	2	1 1/2 starch, 1 fat
Thai Kitchen											
Stir-Fry Rice Noodles	2 oz	195	0	0	0	0	0	46	2	3	3 starch
Thin Rice Noodles	2 oz	196	0	0	0	0	0	46	2	3	3 starch
Wel-Pac											
Chinese Noodles	2 oz	200	0	0	0	0	400	42	1	7	3 starch
Chow Mein Stir-Fry Noodles	2 oz	200	1	5	0	0	125	42	0	7	3 starch
Japanese Udon Noodles	2 oz	180	0.5	0	0	0	115	40	1	5	2 1/2 starch
Dry Pasta											
Al Dente											
Carba-Nada	1 1/2 cup	140	1	10	0	10	20	24	6	12	1 1/2 starch
Garlic Parsley Fettucini	2 oz	220	2	20	0.5	33	15	41	2	8	2 1/2 starch
American Beauty											
Angel Hair	2 oz	210	1	10	0	0	0	42	2	7	3 starch
Ditalini	2 oz	210	1	10	0	0	0	42	2	7	3 starch

PASTA, PASTA MIXES, PASTA SAUCE

	Serving	Calories	Fat (g)	Cal. from Fat	Sat. Fat (g)	Trans Fat (g)	Chol. (mg)	Sod. (mg)	Carb. (g)	Fiber (g)	Prot. (g)	Servings/Exchanges
Elbow Macaroni	2 oz	210	1	10	0	0	0	0	42	2	7	3 starch
Extra Wide Egg Noodles	2 oz	210	2.5	25	1	0	70	15	40	2	8	2 1/2 starch
Fettuccine	2 oz	210	1	10	0	0	0	0	42	2	7	3 starch
Fideo Cortado (Fino)	2 oz	210	1	10	0	0	0	0	42	2	7	3 starch
Jumbo Shells	2 oz	210	1	10	0	0	0	0	42	2	7	3 starch
Large Elbows	2 oz	210	1	10	0	0	0	0	42	2	7	3 starch
Large Shells	2 oz	210	1	10	0	0	0	0	42	2	7	3 starch
Manicotti	2 oz	210	1	10	0	0	0	0	42	2	7	3 starch
Oven Ready Lasagna	2 oz	210	1	10	0	0	0	0	42	2	7	3 starch
Penne Rigate	2 oz	210	1	10	0	0	0	0	42	2	7	3 starch
Rainbow Twirls	2 oz	210	1	10	0	0	0	30	42	2	7	3 starch
Rice & Spinach Tortelloni	2 oz	220	5	45	2.5	0	30	560	35	2	8	2 starch, 1 fat
Rotini	2 oz	210	1	10	0	0	0	0	42	2	7	3 starch

Sea Shells	2 oz	210	1	10	0	0	0	42	2	7	3 starch
Small Shells	2 oz	210	1	10	0	0	0	42	2	7	3 starch
Spaghetti	2 oz	210	1	10	0	0	0	42	2	7	3 starch
Thin Spaghetti	2 oz	210	1	10	0	0	0	42	2	7	3 starch
Three Cheese Tortelloni	2 oz	210	4	40	2	30	0	35	2	7	2 starch, 1 fat
Vermicelli	2 oz	210	1	10	0	0	0	42	2	7	3 starch
Wide Egg Noodles	2 oz	210	2.5	25	1	70	15	40	2	8	2 1/2 starch, 1 fat
Barilla											
Angel Hair	2 oz	200	1	10	0	0	0	42	2	7	3 starch
Elbows	2 oz	200	1	10	0	0	0	42	2	7	3 starch
Farfalle	2 oz	200	1	10	0	0	0	42	2	7	3 starch
Fetuccine	2 oz	200	1	10	0	0	0	42	2	7	3 starch
Lasagna	2 pieces	180	1	10	0	0	0	38	2	6	2 1/2 starch
Lasagna, No Boil	3 pieces	190	2	20	0.5	0	50	36	2	7	2 starch
Linguine	2 oz	200	1	10	0	0	0	42	2	7	3 starch
Medium Shells	2 oz	200	1	10	0	0	0	42	2	7	3 starch

PASTA, PASTA MIXES, PASTA SAUCE

	Serving	Calories	Fat (g)	Cal. from Fat	Sat. Fat (g)	Trans Fat (g)	Chol. (mg)	Sod. (mg)	Carb. (g)	Fiber (g)	Prot. (g)	Servings/Exchanges
Mini Penne	2 oz	200	1	10	0	0	0	0	42	2	7	3 starch
Mostaccioli	2 oz	200	1	10	0	0	0	0	42	2	7	3 starch
Penne	2 oz	200	1	10	0	0	0	0	42	2	7	3 starch
Rigatoni	2 oz	200	1	10	0	0	0	0	42	2	7	3 starch
Rotini	2 oz	200	1	10	0	0	0	0	42	2	7	3 starch
Spaghetti	2 oz	200	1	10	0	0	0	0	42	2	7	3 starch
Spaghetti Rigati	2 oz	200	1	10	0	0	0	0	42	2	7	3 starch
Thin Spaghetti	2 oz	200	1	10	0	0	0	0	42	2	7	3 starch
Tortellini Ricotta & Spinach	3/4 cup	230	8	70	2.5	0	60	340	32	5	8	2 starch
Tortellini Three Cheese	2/3 cup	230	8	70	2.5	0	40	475	33	3	8	2 starch
Tri-Color Rotini	2 oz	200	1	10	0	0	0	15	42	2	7	3 starch
Barilla Plus												
Angel Hair	2 oz	200	1	10	0	0	0	25	38	4	10	2 1/2 starch

	Serving	Cal.	Fat				Chol.	Sod.	Carb.		Prot.	Exchanges
Elbows	2 oz	200	1	10	0	0	0	25	38	4	10	2 1/2 starch
Penne	2 oz	200	1	10	0	0	0	25	38	4	10	2 1/2 starch
Spaghetti	2 oz	200	1	10	0	0	0	25	38	4	10	2 1/2 starch
Thin Spaghetti	2 oz	210	1	10	0	0	0	25	38	4	10	2 1/2 starch
Buitoni (Refrigerated)												
Chicken & Prosciutto Tortelloni	1 cup	330	9	80	3	0	40	610	46	2	15	3 carb, 2 fat
Four Cheese Ravioli	1 1/4 cup	340	12	110	4	0	55	650	42	3	15	3 carb, 2 fat
Linguine	1 1/4 cup	240	2.5	25	1	0	50	20	45	2	10	3 carb, 1 fat
Mixed Cheese Tortellini	1 cup	320	7	60	3.5	0	40	490	50	1	15	3 carb, 1 fat
Spinach Cheese Tortellini	1 cup	320	7	60	3.5	0	55	510	49	3	15	3 carb, 1 fat
Colavita												
Angel Hair	2 oz	210	1	10	0	0	0	0	44	2	7	3 starch
Bow Ties	3/4 cup	210	1	10	0	0	0	0	44	2	7	3 starch
Fettuccine Nests	2 nests	210	1	10	0	0	0	0	44	2	7	3 starch

PASTA, PASTA MIXES, PASTA SAUCE

	Serving	Calories	Fat (g)	Cal. from Fat	Sat. Fat (g)	Trans Fat (g)	Chol. (mg)	Sod. (mg)	Carb. (g)	Fiber (g)	Prot. (g)	Servings/Exchanges
Linguine	2 oz	210	1	10	0	0	0	0	44	2	7	3 starch
Long Fusilli	2 oz	210	1	10	0	0	0	0	44	2	7	3 starch
Creamette												
Angel Hair	2 oz	210	1	10	0	0	0	0	42	2	7	3 starch
Elbow Macaroni	2 oz	210	1	10	0	0	0	0	42	2	7	3 starch
Extra Wide Egg Noodles	2 oz	210	2.5	25	1	0	70	15	40	2	8	2 1/2 starch
Lasagna	2 oz	210	1	10	0	0	0	0	42	2	7	3 starch
Spaghetti	2 oz	210	1	10	0	0	0	0	42	2	7	3 starch
Da Vinci												
100% Whole Wheat Elbows	1/2 cup	180	1.5	10	0	0	<5	0	44	5	7	3 starch
100% Whole Wheat Penne	3/4 cup	170	1	10	0	0	<5	0	42	5	7	3 starch
Angel Hair	2 oz	210	1	5	0	0	0	0	43	2	6	3 starch

Bowties	1 cup	210	1	10	0	0	0	41	2	7	2 1/2 starch
Cut Ziti	3/4 cup	210	1	5	0	0	0	43	2	6	3 starch
Fettuccine	2 oz	210	1	10	0	0	0	43	2	6	3 starch
Fusilli Springs	3/4 cup	210	1	10	0	0	0	43	2	6	3 starch
Penne Rigate	3/4 cup	210	1	10	0	0	0	41	2	7	2 1/2 starch
Potato Gnocchi	3/4 cup	200	0	0	0	0	440	44	2	4	3 starch
Rotini	1 cup	210	1	10	0	0	0	41	2	6	2 1/2 starch
Spaghetti	2 oz	210	1	10	0	0	0	41	2	6	2 1/2 starch
DeBoles											
Organic Whole Wheat Spaghetti Style Pasta	2 oz	210	1.5	10	0	0	10	42	5	7	3 carb
Rice Spaghetti Style Pasta	2 oz	210	0.5	5	0	0	15	46	<1	4	3 carb
Rice Spirals	2 oz	210	0.5	5	0	0	15	46	<1	4	3 carb
Tomato & Basil Angel Hair Pasta	2 oz	210	1	10	0	0	0	41	2	7	2 1/2 carb

PASTA, PASTA MIXES, PASTA SAUCE

	Serving	Calories	Fat (g)	Cal. from Fat	Sat. Fat (g)	Trans Fat (g)	Chol. (mg)	Sod. (mg)	Carb. (g)	Fiber (g)	Prot. (g)	Servings/Exchanges
DeCecco												
Farfalle	1 cup	200	1	10	0	0	0	0	41	2	7	2 1/2 starch
Fusilli	3/4 cup	200	1	10	0	0	0	0	41	2	7	2 1/2 starch
Linguine	2 oz	200	1	10	0	0	0	0	41	2	7	2 1/2 starch
Penne Rigate	1/2 cup	200	1	10	0	0	0	0	41	2	7	2 1/2 starch
Spaghetti	2 oz	200	1	10	0	0	0	0	41	2	7	2 1/2 starch
Zita Cut	2/3 cup	200	1	10	0	0	0	0	41	2	7	2 1/2 starch
Dreamfields												
Elbows	2 oz	190	1	10	0	0	0	10	41	4	7	2 1/2 starch
Lasagna	2 oz	190	1	10	0	0	0	10	41	5	7	2 1/2 starch
Linguine	2 oz	190	1	10	0	0	0	10	41	2	7	2 1/2 starch
Penne Rigate	2 oz	190	1	10	0	0	0	10	41	4	7	2 1/2 starch
Spaghetti	2 oz	190	1	10	0	0	0	10	41	5	7	2 1/2 starch
Fiber Wise												

High Fiber Elbows	2 oz	170	1	10	0	0	0	25	41	12	8	2 1/2 starch
High Fiber Penne	2 oz	170	1	10	0	0	0	25	41	12	8	2 1/2 starch
High Fiber Spaghetti	2 oz	170	1	10	0	0	0	25	41	12	8	2 1/2 starch

Hodgson Mill

Organic Whole Wheat Fettuccine with Milled Flax Seed	2 oz	200	2	20	0	0	0	10	40	6	9	2 1/2 starch
Organic Whole Wheat Penne with Milled Flax Seed	2 oz	215	2	20	0	0	0	0	40	6	9	2 1/2 starch
Organic Whole Wheat Spaghetti with Milled FlaX Seed	2 oz	200	2	20	0	0	0	10	40	6	9	2 1/2 starch
Organic Whole Wheat Spirals with Milled Flax Seed	2 oz	200	2	20	0	0	0	10	40	6	9	2 1/2 starch
Veggie Rotini	2 oz	200	1	5	0	0	0	15	41	1	8	2 1/2 starch

PASTA, PASTA MIXES, PASTA SAUCE

	Serving	Calories	Fat (g)	Cal. from Fat	Sat. Fat (g)	Trans Fat (g)	Chol. (mg)	Sod. (mg)	Carb. (g)	Fiber (g)	Prot. (g)	Servings/Exchanges
Whole Wheat Fettuccine	2 oz	210	1	15	0	0	0	0	41	6	9	2 1/2 starch
Whole Wheat Spaghetti	2 oz	210	1	15	0	0	0	0	41	6	9	2 1/2 starch
Whole Wheat Spirals	2 oz	190	1	15	1	0	0	10	34	6	9	2 starch
No Yolks (Cholesterol Free)												
Dumplings	2 oz	210	0.5	5	0	0	0	30	41	3	8	2 1/2 starch
Extra Broad Noodles	2 oz	210	0.5	5	0	0	0	30	41	3	8	2 1/2 starch
Rao's												
Fusilli	1/2 cup	200	1	10	0	0	0	10	41	2	7	2 1/2 starch
Penne Rigate	1/2 cup	200	1	10	0	0	0	10	41	2	7	2 1/2 starch
Ronzoni												
Healthy Harvest Whole-Grain Thin Spaghetti	2 oz	180	2	15	0	0	0	0	41	6	7	2 1/2 starch
Healthy Harvest 7 Grain Fusilli	2 oz	180	2	20	0	0	0	0	40	5	8	2 1/2 starch

Pasta Sauce

Amy's Organic

Family Marinara	1/2 cup	80	4.5	40	0.5	0	0	590	10	3	1	1/2 carb, 1 fat
Low Sodium Marinara	1/2 cup	40	1	10	0	0	0	100	7	1	1	1/2 carb
Puttanesca	1/2 cup	45	2	20	0	0	0	680	6	1	2	1/2 carb
Roasted Garlic	1/2 cup	130	8	70	1	0	0	470	13	3	2	1 carb, 2 fat
Tomato Basil	1/2 cup	110	6	50	1	0	0	580	11	3	2	1 carb, 1 fat

Barilla

Marinara	1/2 cup	70	1.5	15	0	0	0	460	12	2	2	1 carb
Roasted Garlic	1/2 cup	60	1	10	0	0	0	460	12	2	2	1/2 carb
Tomato & Basil	1/2 cup	60	1	10	0	0	0	460	12	2	2	1/2 carb

Bertolli

Alfredo	1/4 cup	110	10	90	5	0	40	460	3	0	2	2 fat
Marinara	1/2 cup	80	2	20	0	0	0	530	13	1	2	1 carb
Mushroom Alfredo	1/2 cup	80	6	50	3	0	30	420	3	0	2	1 fat
Olive Oil & Garlic	1/2 cup	90	3	25	0	0	0	500	14	3	3	1 carb, 1 fat

PASTA, PASTA MIXES, PASTA SAUCE

	Serving	Calories	Fat (g)	Cal. from Fat	Sat. Fat (g)	Trans Fat (g)	Chol. (mg)	Sod. (mg)	Carb. (g)	Fiber (g)	Prot. (g)	Servings/Exchanges
Portobello Mushroom	1/2 cup	80	2.5	25	0	0	0	470	12	1	2	1 carb, 1 fat
Buitoni												
Alfredo Sauce	1/4 cup	130	11	100	7	0	35	390	4	0	4	2 fat
Arrabiata Sauce	1/2 cup	90	6	50	1	0	0	610	8	2	1	1/2 carb, 1 fat
Light Alfredo Sauce	1/4 cup	90	6	50	3.5	0	15	350	5	0	4	1 fat
Marinara	1/2 cup	70	3	25	0.5	0	0	560	10	2	1	1/2 carb, 1 fat
Pesto with Basil	1/4 cup	300	28	250	5	0	20	540	6	2	7	1/2 carb, 6 fat
Reduced Fat Pesto with Basil	1/4 cup	240	19	170	4	0	15	540	9	2	7	1/2 carb, 4 fat
Roasted Garlic Marinara	1/2 cup	60	1.5	15	0.5	0	0	530	10	2	2	1/2 carb
Tomato Herb Parmesan	1/2 cup	130	8	70	2.5	0	10	740	10	2	4	1/2 carb, 2 fat
Vodka Sauce	1/2 cup	100	7	60	4	0	20	610	7	1	2	1/2 carb, 1 fat
Classico												
Creamy Alfredo	1/4 cup	100	9	80	5	0	50	410	3	0	2	2 fat

Florentine Spinach & Cheese	1/2 cup	80	5	45	1	0	5	560	7	2	3	1/2 carb, 1 fat
Four Cheese	1/2 cup	90	3.5	30	1	0	0	490	11	3	3	1 carb, 1 fat
Four Cheese Alfredo	1/4 cup	80	7	60	4	0	35	350	3	0	2	1 fat
Mushroom & Olives	1/2 cup	60	1	10	0.5	0	0	390	11	2	2	1 carb
Organic Tomato, Herbs & Spices	1/2 cup	70	1	10	0	0	0	350	12	2	2	1 carb
Roasted Garlic	1/2 cup	60	1	10	0	0	0	220	11	2	2	1 carb
Spicy Red Pepper	1/2 cup	60	1.5	15	0	0	0	300	7	2	2	1/2 carb
Sun-Dried Tomato	1/2 cup	80	3	25	1	0	0	390	11	2	2	1 carb, 1 fat
Sun-Dried Tomato & Pesto	1/4 cup	90	5	45	1	0	0	630	8	1	3	1/2 carb
Tomato & Basil	1/2 cup	60	1	10	0	0	0	310	11	2	2	1 carb
Vodka Sauce	1/2 cup	150	10	90	3.5	0	10	500	12	3	3	1 carb, 2 fat
Eden Organic												
No Salt Added Spaghetti Sauce	1/2 cup	70	2.5	25	0	0	0	10	9	5	2	1/2 carb, 1 fat

PASTA, PASTA MIXES, PASTA SAUCE

	Serving	Calories	Fat (g)	Cal. from Fat	Sat. Fat (g)	Trans Fat (g)	Chol. (mg)	Sod. (mg)	Carb. (g)	Fiber (g)	Prot. (g)	Servings/Exchanges
Spaghetti Sauce	1/2 cup	70	2.5	25	0	0	0	300	9	5	2	1/2 carb, 1 fat
Emeril's												
Eggplant Gaaahlic	1/2 cup	90	4.5	40	0	0	0	510	12	2	2	1 carb, 1 fat
Home Style Marinara	1/2 cup	90	3	25	0	0	0	640	12	1	2	1 carb, 1 fat
Tomato & Basil	1/2 cup	80	2.5	25	0	0	0	640	13	1	2	1 carb, 1 fat
Healthy Choice												
Garlic & Herb Sauce	1/2 cup	60	0	0	0	0	0	370	12	3	2	1 carb
Traditional	1/2 cup	60	0	0	0	0	0	400	13	3	2	1 carb
Hunt's												
Four Cheese Spaghetti Sauce	1/2 cup	50	1	10	0	0	0	580	10	3	3	1/2 carb
Meat Sauce	1/2 cup	60	1	10	0	0	0	610	11	3	3	1 carb
Traditional Spaghetti Sauce	1/2 cup	60	1	1	0	0	0	580	10	2	2	1/2 carb

	Serving	Cal.	Fat (g)		Sat. Fat (g)	Chol. (mg)	Sod. (mg)	Carb. (g)	Fiber (g)	Prot. (g)	Choices/Exchanges
Traditional Spaghetti Sauce (Pouch)	1/2 cup	50	1	10	0	0	580	10	2	2	1/2 carb
Zesty & Spicy Spaghetti Sauce	1/2 cup	60	2	15	0	0	700	10	3	1	1/2 carb
Maruchan											
Instant Lunch, Beef	1 container	290	12	110	6	0	1200	38	2	7	2 1/2 carb, 2 fat
Ramen Noodle Soup, Chicken	1/2 pkg	190	7	70	3.5	0	830	26	1	5	2 carb, 1 fat
Muir Glen Organic											
Beef Bolognese	1/2 cup	70	2	20	0.5	0	<5	410	10	2	3	1/2 carb
Cabernet Marinara	1/2 cup	60	1	10	0	0	360	11	2	2	1 carb
Chunky Tomato & Herb	1/2 cup	60	0.5	5	0	0	350	11	2	2	1 carb
Fire Roasted Tomato	1/2 cup	70	2	0	0	0	390	12	2	2	1 carb
Four Cheese	1/2 cup	80	2.5	20	1	5	380	11	2	4	1 carb
Garden Vegetable	1/2 cup	60	1	5	0	0	350	10	2	2	1/2 carb

PASTA, PASTA MIXES, PASTA SAUCE

	Serving	Calories	Fat (g)	Cal. from Fat	Sat. Fat (g)	Trans Fat (g)	Chol. (mg)	Sod. (mg)	Carb. (g)	Fiber (g)	Prot. (g)	Servings/Exchanges
Garlic Roasted Garlic	1/2 cup	60	0.5	5	0	0	0	380	12	2	2	1 carb
Italian Herb	1/2 cup	60	0.5	5	0	0	0	350	11	2	2	1 carb
Italian Sausage with Peppers	1/2 cup	80	3	25	1	0	<5	420	10	2	3	1/2 carb, 1 fat
Portabello Mushroom	1/2 cup	50	0	0	0	0	0	350	10	2	2	1/2 carb
Tomato Basil	1/2 cup	60	1	10	0	0	0	370	12	2	2	1 carb
Newman's Own												
Five Cheese	1/2 cup	80	3	30	1.5	0	5	610	10	<1	3	1/2 carb, 1 fat
Italian Sausage & Peppers	1/2 cup	90	4	35	1	0	10	630	11	<1	4	1 carb, 1 fat
Marinara	1/2 cup	70	2	20	0	0	0	510	12	<1	2	1 carb
Marinara with Mushrooms	1/2 cup	70	2	20	0	0	0	520	12	<1	2	1 carb
Sockarooni	1/2 cup	70	2	20	0	0	0	520	12	<1	2	1 carb

Nissin

	Serving	Cal					Sodium	Carb			Exchanges
Top Ramen, Chicken	1/2 pkg	190	7	60	3.5	0	0	910	26	2	5	2 carb, 1 fat

Prego

	Serving	Cal					Sodium	Carb			Exchanges
Flavored with Meat	1/2 cup	130	5	45	1	0	5	570	19	3	2	1 carb, 1 fat
Garden Combo	1/2 cup	70	1.5	15	0.5	0	0	470	13	3	2	1 carb
Heart Smart Mushroom Italian	1/2 cup	100	3	30	0.5	0	0	410	15	3	2	1 carb, 1 fat
Heart Smart Traditional Italian	1/2 cup	90	3	30	1	0	0	430	13	3	2	1 carb, 1 fat
Marinara	1/2 cup	100	5	45	1	0	0	550	11	4	2	1 carb, 1 fat
Mini Meatball	1/2 cup	110	5	45	1.5	0	5	650	13	3	4	1 carb, 1 fat
Mushroom & Garlic	1/2 cup	80	2.5	25	0.5	0	0	470	13	3	2	1 carb, 1 fat
Organic Mushroom Italian	1/2 cup	70	2.5	25	0.5	0	0	470	13	4	2	1 carb, 1 fat
Organic Tomato & Basil Italian	1/2 cup	80	2.5	25	0.5	0	0	470	13	4	2	1 carb, 1 fat

PASTA, PASTA MIXES, PASTA SAUCE

	Serving	Calories	Fat (g)	Cal. from Fat	Sat. Fat (g)	Trans Fat (g)	Chol. (mg)	Sod. (mg)	Carb. (g)	Fiber (g)	Prot. (g)	Servings/Exchanges
Three Cheese	1/2 cup	80	1.5	15	0.5	0	<5	430	14	3	3	1 carb
Traditional	1/2 cup	80	3	30	0	0	0	580	13	3	2	1 carb, 1 fat
Ragu												
Cheesy, Classic Alfredo	1/4 cup	110	10	90	3.5	0	30	350	2	0	1	2 fat
Chunky, Garden Combination	1/2 cup	80	2.5	25	0	0	0	530	12	2	2	1 carb, 1 fat
Chunky, Sundried Tomato & Sweet Basil	1/2 cup	90	2.5	25	0	0	0	580	14	3	2	1 carb, 1 fat
Chunky, Super Chunk Mushroom	1/2 cup	80	2.5	25	0	0	0	620	13	2	2	1 carb, 1 fat
Chunky, Super Vegetable Primavera	1/2 cup	80	2.5	25	0	0	0	490	13	3	2	1 carb, 1 fat
Chunky, Tomato, Garlic & Onion	1/2 cup	80	2.5	25	0	0	0	510	13	2	2	1 carb, 1 fat
Old World Style, Meat	1/2 cup	70	3	25	0.5	0	0	570	10	2	2	1/2 carb, 1 fat

Food	Serving	Cal	Fat				Sodium				Exchanges
Old World Style, Mushroom	1/2 cup	70	2.5	25	0	0	580	10	2	2	1/2 carb, 1 fat
Old World Style, Traditional	1/2 cup	70	2.5	25	0	0	580	10	2	2	1/2 carb, 1 fat
Organic, Traditional	1/2 cup	80	3	25	0	0	510	11	2	2	1 carb, 1 fat
Robusto, 7-Herb Tomato	1/2 cup	80	3	25	0	0	550	12	2	2	1 carb, 1 fat
Robusto, Roasted Garlic	1/2 cup	80	2.5	25	0	0	550	13	3	2	1 carb, 1 fat
Robusto, Si Cheese	1/2 cup	90	3	25	1	0	580	12	2	3	1 carb, 1 fat
Rao's Homemade											
Arrabbiata	1/2 cup	70	5	45	0.5	0	350	6	2	1	1/2 carb, 1 fat
Filetto Sauce with Tomato, Prosciutto & Onion	1/2 cup	90	6	60	1	5	390	5	2	2	1 fat
Marinara	1/2 cup	70	4.5	40	0.5	0	350	6	2	1	1/2 carb, 1 fat
Puttanesca	1/2 cup	80	5	50	0.5	0	250	6	2	2	1/2 carb, 1 fat
Roasted Eggplant Siciliana Sauce	1/2 cup	70	5	45	0.5	0	320	6	1	1	1/2 carb, 1 fat

PASTA, PASTA MIXES, PASTA SAUCE

	Serving	Calories	Fat (g)	Cal. from Fat	Sat. Fat (g)	Trans Fat (g)	Chol. (mg)	Sod. (mg)	Carb. (g)	Fiber (g)	Prot. (g)	Servings/Exchanges
Southern Italian Pepper & Mushroom	1/2 cup	70	5	45	0.5	0	0	430	6	2	1	1/2 carb, 1 fat
Tomato & Basil	1/2 cup	70	4.5	40	0.5	0	0	350	6	2	1	1/2 carb, 1 fat
Vodka Sauce	1/2 cup	80	5	45	1	0	5	450	6	2	2	1/2 carb, 1 fat
Trader Joe's												
Alfredo	1/4 cup	90	8	70	4.5	0	0	320	2	0	4	2 fat
Bolognese Meat Pasta Sauce	1/2 cup	80	4.5	40	1	0	5	490	8	2	3	1/2 carb, 1 fat
Italian Sausage	1/2 cup	50	2.5	20	0.5	0	0	570	6	<1	3	1/2 carb, 1 fat
Organic Marinara	1/2 cup	50	2	20	0	0	0	490	8	2	1	1/2 carb
Organic Marinara No Added Salt	1/2 cup	50	0.5	5	0	0	0	25	11	<1	2	1 carb
Organic Spaghetti with Mushrooms	1/2 cup	45	0	0	0	0	0	350	10	2	1	1/2 carb

Organic Tomato Basil Marinara	1/2 cup	60	3	25	0	0	440	8	2	1	1/2 carb, 1 fat
Roasted Garlic Spaghetti Sauce	1/2 cup	70	2.5	20	0	0	450	10	1	2	1/2 carb, 1 fat
Rustico Pasta Sauce	1/2 cup	45	1.5	15	0	0	360	6	2	1	1/2 carb
Tomato Basil Marinara	1/2 cup	80	4.5	40	0.5	0	540	10	2	2	1/2 carb, 1 fat
Traditional Marinara	1/2 cup	50	1	10	0	0	530	9	2	1	1/2 carb
Walnut Acres Organic											
Garlic-Garlic	1/2 cup	50	1	10	0	0	280	10	1	2	1/2 carb
Low Sodium Tomato & Basil, Fat Free	1/2 cup	40	0	0	0	0	20	9	<1	2	1/2 carb
Marinara with Herbs	1/2 cup	50	1	10	0	0	330	9	1	2	1/2 carb
Roasted Garlic	1/2 cup	60	1	10	0	0	280	11	1	2	1 carb
Sweet Pepper & Onion	1/2 cup	50	1	10	0	0	280	9	1	2	1/2 carb
Tomato & Basil	1/2 cup	50	1	10	0	0	330	9	1	2	1/2 carb
Zesty Basil	1/2 cup	50	1	10	0	0	330	9	1	2	1/2 carb

PASTA, PASTA MIXES, PASTA SAUCE

	Serving	Calories	Fat (g)	Cal. from Fat	Sat. Fat (g)	Trans Fat (g)	Chol. (mg)	Sod. (mg)	Carb. (g)	Fiber (g)	Prot. (g)	Servings/Exchanges
Whole Foods 365 Everyday												
Marinara	1/2 cup	50	1.5	10	0	0	0	430	9	2	2	1/2 carb
Pesto & Sundried Tomato	1/2 cup	60	1.5	15	0.5	0	0	460	10	3	2	1/2 carb
Roasted Garlic	1/2 cup	60	1.5	15	0	0	0	480	10	2	2	1/2 carb
Roasted Red Pepper	1/2 cup	50	1	10	0	0	0	420	10	2	1	1/2 carb
Roasted Vegetable	1/2 cup	25	1	10	0	0	0	490	3	<1	0	free
Whole Foods 365 Everyday Organic												
Classic Pasta Sauce	1/2 cup	70	4	35	0.5	0	0	500	9	2	1	1/2 carb, 1 fat
Eggplant Marinara	1/2 cup	40	1	10	0	0	0	470	7	2	1	1/2 carb
Fat Free Pasta Sauce	1/2 cup	35	0	0	0	0	0	470	7	2	1	1/2 carb
Four Cheese	1/2 cup	70	4	35	1.5	0	<5	480	7	<1	3	1/2 carb, 1 fat
Italian Herb	1/2 cup	50	1	10	0	0	0	480	8	<1	2	1/2 carb
Mushroon Marinara	1/2 cup	45	1.5	15	0	0	0	450	6	<1	2	1/2 carb

PROCESSED MEAT, BREAKFAST MEAT, LUNCH MEAT, HOT DOGS, CANNED TUNA AND CHICKEN

	Serving	Calories	Fat (g)	Cal. from Fat	Sat. Fat (g)	Trans Fat (g)	Chol. (mg)	Sod. (mg)	Carb. (g)	Fiber (g)	Prot. (g)	Servings/Exchanges
Applegate Farms	1 Tbsp	98	9	80	<1	0	0	70	3	<1	2	2 fat
Chicken & Apple Sausage	1 link	140	6	60	1.5	0	65	500	6	1	14	2 lean meat
Fire Roasted Red Pepper Sausage	1 link	120	6	60	1.5	0	65	500	2	1	14	2 lean meat
Natural Canadian Bacon	2 slices	90	4	35	1.5	0	35	500	1	0	12	2 lean meat
Natural Dry Cured Bacon	2 slices	60	5	45	2	0	10	290	0	0	4	1 med-fat meat
Natural Sunday Bacon	2 slices	60	5	45	2	0	10	290	0	0	4	1 med-fat meat
Natural Turkey Bacon	2 slices	35	1.5	15	0	0	25	200	0	0	6	1 lean meat
Organic Sunday Bacon	2 slices	60	5	45	2	0	10	290	0	0	4	1 med-fat meat
Organic Turkey Bacon	1 slice	35	1.5	15	0	0	25	200	0	0	6	1 lean meat

PROCESSED MEAT, BREAKFAST MEAT, LUNCH MEAT

	Serving	Calories	Fat (g)	Cal. from Fat	Sat. Fat (g)	Trans Fat (g)	Chol. (mg)	Sod. (mg)	Carb. (g)	Fiber (g)	Prot. (g)	Servings/Exchanges
Pork Andouille Sausage	1 link	200	15	140	5	0	50	510	2	1	12	2 high-fat meat
Pork Bratwurst Sausage	1 link	170	12	110	4	0	45	660	2	0	12	2 med-fat meat
Pork Kielbasa Sausage	1 link	190	14	130	5	0	50	600	2	0	12	2 med-fat meat, 1 fat
Spinach & Feta Sausage	1 link	120	7	60	2.5	0	60	470	2	0	13	2 lean meat
Sweet Italian Sausage	1 link	130	7	60	2	0	70	500	2	1	15	2 lean meat
Banquet Brown 'N Serve												
Beef Fully Cooked Sausage Links	3	190	17	160	8	1	15	420	1	0	7	1 high-fat meat, 1 fat
Original Fully Cooked Sausage Links	3	200	18	160	6	0	30	490	2	1	8	1 high-fat meat, 1 fat
Turkey Fully Cooked Sausage Links	3	110	7	60	2	0	40	390	2	0	9	1 med-fat meat
Bob Evans												

Brown Sugar and Honey Links	3	140	11	100	NA	0	25	290	4	0	9	1 high-fat meat
Canadian Bacon	4 slices	60	1.5	14	NA	0	20	700	1	0	11	2 lean meat
Country Pepper Bacon	2 slices	100	8	72	NA	0	20	510	0	0	6	1 high-fat meat
Express Fully Cooked Bacon	3 slices	80	6	55	NA	0	15	280	1	0	5	1 med-fat meat
Express Fully Cooked Lite	2	80	5	45	NA	0	15	220	0	0	8	1 med-fat meat
Express Fully Cooked Original Links	2	130	10	90	NA	0	25	290	0	0	8	1 high-fat meat
Hickory Smoked Bacon	2 slices	80	7	63	NA	0	15	270	0	0	5	1 med-fat meat
Original Sausage Links	3	140	11	100	NA	0	25	330	0	0	9	1 high-fat meat
Original Sausage Patties	2	160	13	117	NA	0	30	380	0	0	11	2 med-fat meat, 1 fat
Celebrity												
Healthy Canadian Style Bacon	3 slices	60	1	15	0.5	0	30	350	1	0	10	1 lean meat

PROCESSED MEAT, BREAKFAST MEAT, LUNCH MEAT

	Serving	Calories	Fat (g)	Cal. from Fat	Sat. Fat (g)	Trans Fat (g)	Chol. (mg)	Sod. (mg)	Carb. (g)	Fiber (g)	Prot. (g)	Servings/Exchanges
Farmer John												
Premium Bacon Links	2	70	5	45	3	0	15	280	0	0	6	1 med-fat meat
Premium Pork Links	2	140	12	110	4	0	30	400	<1	0	6	1 high-fat meat, 1 fat
Farmland												
Hickory Smoked Bacon	2 slices	80	7	60	3	0	15	260	0	0	4	1 med-fat meat
Original Pork Sausage Links	3	250	23	210	9	0	60	510	1	0	10	1 high-fat meat, 3 fat
Pork & Bacon Sausage Links	3	270	25	220	9	0	60	640	1	0	10	1 high-fat meat, 3 fat
Thick Sliced Bacon	1 slice	70	6	50	2.5	0	10	230	0	0	3	1 med-fat meat
Hormel												
Little Sizzlers Pork Sausage	3	200	19	170	7	0	40	580	0	0	8	1 high-fat meat, 2 fat
Jennie-O Turkey Store												

Breakfast Bacon	1/2 oz	35	3	25	1	0	13	150	1	0	2	1 fat
Breakfast Lover's Turkey Sausage	2 oz	130	10	100	3	0	45	310	0	0	8	1 high-fat meat
Breakfast Sausage Rolls	4 oz	270	21	190	6	0.5	80	720	0	0	16	2 high-fat meat
Extra Lean Turkey Bacon	1/2 oz	20	0.5	5	0	0	10	140	0	0	3	1 lean meat
Fully Cooked Turkey Breakfast Sausage Patties	1.2 oz	65	4	35	1	0	30	250	0	0	6	1 med-fat meat
Fully Cooked Turkey Sausage Breakfast Links	2.1 oz	110	7	60	2	0	50	430	0	0	11	2 lean meat
Maple Turkey Breakfast Sausage Links	2 oz	140	11	100	3	0	40	340	3	0	8	1 high-fat meat
Turkey Breakfast Sausage Links	2 oz	140	11	100	3	0	45	360	0	0	9	1 high-fat meat

PROCESSED MEAT, BREAKFAST MEAT, LUNCH MEAT

	Serving	Calories	Fat (g)	Cal. from Fat	Sat. Fat (g)	Trans Fat (g)	Chol. (mg)	Sod. (mg)	Carb. (g)	Fiber (g)	Prot. (g)	Servings/Exchanges
Jimmy Dean (Uncooked)												
All Natural Regular Pork Sausage	2 oz	190	15	130	5	0	55	520	1	0	12	2 high-fat meat
Hardwood Smoked Turkey Premium Bacon	1 slice	25	2	20	1	0	15	200	0	0	2	1 fat
Lower Sodium Premium Bacon	1 slice	50	4	40	1.5	0	10	105	0	0	4	1 med-fat meat
Maple Sausage Links	2 oz	170	14	130	5	0	35	400	2	0	7	1 high-fat meat, 1 fat
Maple Sausage Patties	2 patties	170	14	130	5	0	35	410	2	0	7	1 high-fat meat, 1 fat
Original Premium Bacon	1 slice	50	4	40	1.5	0	10	230	0	0	4	1 med-fat meat
Original Sausage Links	3	170	14	130	5	0	35	350	1	0	7	1 high-fat meat, 1 fat
Original Sausage Patties	2 patties	240	23	200	8	0	50	610	1	0	9	1 high-fat meat, 3 fat

Premium Pork Bold Country Sausage	2 oz	190	17	150	6	0	40	340	2	0	8	1 high-fat meat, 1 fat
Premium Pork Maple Sausage	2 oz	180	16	140	5	0	40	450	1	1	8	1 high-fat meat, 1 fat
Premium Pork Regular Sausage	2 oz	180	16	140	5	0	40	450	1	0	8	1 high-fat meat, 1 fat
Thick Sliced Premium Bacon	1 slice	80	6	50	2	0	15	320	0	0	5	1 med-fat meat
Jimmy Dean (Fully Cooked)												
Maple Bacon Links	3	80	7	60	3	0	15	105	0	0	4	1 med-fat meat
Maple Sausage Patties	2	250	22	200	8	0	45	510	3	0	8	1 high-fat meat, 2 fat
Original Sausage Links	3	240	22	200	8	0	45	450	1	0	9	1 high-fat meat, 2 fat
Original Sausage Patties	2	240	23	200	8	0	50	610	1	0	9	1 high-fat meat, 3 fat
Turkey Sausage Patties	2	120	7	70	2	0	55	490	1	0	13	2 lean meat
Jimmy Dean (Heat 'N Serve)												
Sausage Links	3	250	24	220	8	0	45	200	2	0	7	1 high-fat meat, 3 fat

PROCESSED MEAT, BREAKFAST MEAT, LUNCH MEAT

	Serving	Calories	Fat (g)	Cal. from Fat	Sat. Fat (g)	Trans Fat (g)	Chol. (mg)	Sod. (mg)	Carb. (g)	Fiber (g)	Prot. (g)	Servings/Exchanges
Sausage Patties	2	190	18	160	6	0	30	250	1	0	6	1 high-fat meat, 2 fat
Jones												
Light Pork Sausage & Rice Links	2	110	7	60	2.5	0	30	440	4	0	8	1 med-fat meat
Little Pork Sausages	3	190	17	150	7	0	45	420	1	0	8	1 high-fat meat, 1 fat
Pork Sausage Patties	1	120	11	100	4	0	30	250	0	0	6	1 high-fat meat
Land O'Frost												
Canadian Bacon	5 slices	60	1.5	10	0	0	30	750	1	0	10	1 lean meat
Oscar Mayer												
Bacon	2 slices	60	5	45	1.5	0	10	250	0	0	4	1 med-fat meat
Bacon, Center Cut	2 slices	50	4	35	2	0	15	270	0	0	4	1 med-fat meat
Bacon, Lower Sodium	2 slices	70	6	50	2.5	0	10	170	0	0	4	1 med-fat meat
Bacon, Smoked, Uncured	2 slices	70	5	50	2	15	15	250	0	0	6	1 med-fat meat

Trader Joe's

	Serving	Calories	Fat (g)	Sat. Fat (g)	Cal. from Fat	Cholesterol (mg)	Sodium (mg)	Carb. (g)	Protein (g)	Exchanges
Uncured Apple Smoked Bacon	1 slice	90	7	2.5	70	15	240	0	5	1 med-fat meat
Uncured Turkey Bacon	1 slice	30	0.5	0	5	25	180	0	6	1 lean meat

LUNCH MEAT & HOT DOGS

Applegate Farms

	Serving	Calories	Fat (g)	Sat. Fat (g)	Cal. from Fat	Cholesterol (mg)	Sodium (mg)	Carb. (g)	Protein (g)	Exchanges
Honey & Maple Turkey Breast	2 oz	60	1	0	10	20	450	0	11	2 lean meat
Organic Herb Turkey Breast	2 oz	50	0.5	0	5	30	420	0	11	2 lean meat
Organic Roasted Chicken Breast	2 oz	60	1.5	0.5	15	30	580	1	10	1 lean meat
Organic Roasted Turkey Breast	2 oz	50	0	0	0	30	360	0	12	2 lean meat
Organic Uncured Ham	2 oz	50	1.5	0.5	15	35	530	0	10	1 lean meat
Roasted Turkey Breast	2 oz	50	0	0	0	30	360	0	12	2 lean meat

PROCESSED MEAT, BREAKFAST MEAT, LUNCH MEAT

	Serving	Calories	Fat (g)	Cal. from Fat	Sat. Fat (g)	Trans Fat (g)	Chol. (mg)	Sod. (mg)	Carb. (g)	Fiber (g)	Prot. (g)	Servings/Exchanges
Slow Cooked Ham	2 oz	60	1.5	15	0.5	0	35	480	0	0	11	2 lean meat
Uncured Black Forest Ham	2 oz	50	1.5	10	0.5	0	35	480	0	0	10	1 lean meat
Uncured Turkey Bologna	2 oz	90	5.5	50	1.5	0	30	400	0	0	9	1 med-fat meat
Armour Healthy Ones 97% Fat Free												
Deli Thin-Sliced												
Honey Ham	1.9 oz	60	1.5	15	0.5	0	25	450	0	3	9	1 lean meat
Oven Roasted Turkey Breast	1.9 oz	60	1.5	15	0.5	0	25	450	0	2	9	1 lean meat
Smoked Ham	1.9 oz	60	1.5	15	0.5	0	25	450	0	2	9	1 lean meat
Deluxe Thin-Sliced												
Honey Ham	2 oz	60	1.5	15	0.5	0	25	470	0	4	10	1 lean meat
Turkey Breast	2 oz	60	1.5	15	0.5	0	25	470	0	2	10	1 lean meat
Ball Park Franks												

Food	Serving											Exchanges
Beef Franks	1	190	16	150	7	1	35	550	4	0	6	1 high-fat meat, 1 fat
Bun Size Beef Franks	1	180	16	140	6	0	45	550	4	0	6	1 high-fat meat, 1 fat
Meat Franks	1	180	16	140	6	0	45	550	4	0	6	1 high-fat meat, 1 fat
Bar-S												
Beef Bologna	1 oz	110	9	80	3.5	0	20	350	0	2	4	1 high-fat meat
Bologna	1 oz	100	8	70	2.5	0	35	350	0	2	3	1 high-fat meat
Chicken Bologna	1 oz	80	7	60	2	0	35	360	0	3	3	1 med-fat meat
Cooked Ham	1.3 oz	45	1.5	15	0	0	15	510	0	2	5	1 lean meat
Cotto Salami	1 oz	90	8	70	2.5	0	40	360	0	2	3	1 high-fat meat
Deli Thin Cut Ham	2 oz	80	2.5	25	1	0	30	700	0	5	9	1 lean meat
Deli Thin Cut Turkey Breast	2 oz	60	1.5	15	0	0	30	540	0	3	9	1 lean meat
Extra Lean Cooked Ham	1 oz	40	1	10	0	0	20	420	0	1	5	1 lean meat
Extra Lean Honey Cured Ham	1 oz	45	1.5	15	0	0	20	450	0	3	5	1 lean meat
Oven Roasted Turkey	1 oz	35	0.5	5	0	0	15	350	0	2	5	1 lean meat

PROCESSED MEAT, BREAKFAST MEAT, LUNCH MEAT

	Serving	Calories	Fat (g)	Cal. from Fat	Sat. Fat (g)	Trans Fat (g)	Chol. (mg)	Sod. (mg)	Carb. (g)	Fiber (g)	Prot. (g)	Servings/Exchanges
Thick Sliced Bologna	2 oz	180	15	140	5	0	60	620	0	4	5	1 high-fat meat, 1 fat
Turkey Bologna	1 oz	60	4.5	40	1.5	0	25	370	0	3	3	1 med-fat meat
Buddig												
Beef	2 oz	90	5	45	2	0	40	790	0	1	10	1 med-fat meat
Chicken	2 oz	90	5	45	1.5	0	30	530	0	2	10	1 med-fat meat
Corned Beef	2 oz	90	5	45	2	0	40	760	0	1	10	1 med-fat meat
Ham	2 oz	90	5	45	2	0	35	760	0	1	10	1 med-fat meat
Honey Ham	2 oz	90	5	45	2	0	35	590	0	2	10	1 med-fat meat
Honey Turkey	2 oz	100	5	45	2	0	30	600	0	3	9	1 med-fat meat
Pastrami	2 oz	90	5	45	2	0	40	790	0	1	10	1 med-fat meat
Turkey	2 oz	90	5	45	2	0	30	600	0	2	10	1 med-fat meat
Deli Cuts												
Honey Ham	2 oz	80	2.5	25	1	0	20	460	0	3	10	1 lean meat
Honey-Roasted Turkey	2 oz	80	2.5	25	1	0	20	460	0	4	9	1 lean meat

Oven-Roasted Turkey	2 oz	70	2.5	25	1	0	20	460	0	2	10	1 lean meat
Butterball												
All Natural Oven Roasted Turkey Breast	2 oz	60	1	10	0	0	35	280	0	0	13	2 lean meat
Extra Thin Sliced Oven Roasted Turkey Breast	2 oz	70	1.5	15	0.5	0	25	580	0	3	10	1 lean meat
Extra Thin Sliced Rotisserie Flavored Turkey Breast	2 oz	50	0.5	5	0	0	20	510	0	1	11	2 lean meat
Thin Sliced Honey Turkey Breast	2 oz	70	1	10	0	0	25	550	0	4	10	1 lean meat
Thin Sliced Oven Roasted Chicken Breast	2 oz	50	0.5	5	0	0	25	480	0	1	11	2 lean meat
Thin Sliced Oven Roasted Turkey Breast	2 oz	70	1.5	10	0.5	0	2	570	0	3	10	1 lean meat

PROCESSED MEAT, BREAKFAST MEAT, LUNCH MEAT

	Serving	Calories	Fat (g)	Cal. from Fat	Sat. Fat (g)	Trans Fat (g)	Chol. (mg)	Sod. (mg)	Carb. (g)	Fiber (g)	Prot. (g)	Servings/Exchanges
Thin Sliced Smoked Turkey Breast	2 oz	70	1.5	10	0.5	0	25	560	0	4	7	1 lean meat
Deep Fried Lunchmeat												
Extra Thin Sliced Original Deep Fried Turkey Lunchmeat	2 oz	60	1.5	15	0	0	25	510	0	3	9	1 lean meat
Thick Sliced Original Deep Fried Turkey Lunchmeat	1 oz	30	0.5	5	0	0	15	260	0	1	5	1 lean meat
Deli Premium												
Honey Roasted & Smoked Turkey Breast	2 oz	50	0	10	0	0	25	400	0	2	9	1 lean meat
Oven Roasted Chicken Breast	2 oz	60	0	10	0	0	25	440	0	1	11	2 lean meat

Oven Roasted Turkey Breast	2 oz	50	0.5	5	0	0	40	440	0	0	12	2 lean meat

Celebrity

Black Forest Smoked Ham 99% Fat Free	1 oz	25	0	0	0	0	15	180	0	<1	5	1 lean meat
Ham 99% Fat Free	1 oz	20	0	0	0		15	180	0		5	1 lean meat
Columbus Salame												
Choice Roast Beef	2 oz	90	3	25	1	0	40	310	1	0	13	2 lean meat
Italian Style Salame	1 oz	110	9	80	4	0	10	420	0	0	6	1 high-fat meat
Maple Honey Turkey	2 oz	70	1	10	0	0	20	340	3	0	13	2 lean meat
Pan Roasted Turkey Breast	2 oz	50	0.5	5	0	0	25	480	0	0	12	2 lean meat
Peppered Salami	1 oz	110	9	80	4	0	10	420	0	0	6	1 high-fat meat

Farmer John Sliced Deli Meats

Bologna	2 oz	160	14	130	4.5	0	25	520	2	2	6	1 high-fat meat, 1 fat
Cotto Salami	2 oz	140	11	100	4	0	45	470	3	3	7	1 high-fat meat

PROCESSED MEAT, BREAKFAST MEAT, LUNCH MEAT

	Serving	Calories	Fat (g)	Cal. from Fat	Sat. Fat (g)	Trans Fat (g)	Chol. (mg)	Sod. (mg)	Carb. (g)	Fiber (g)	Prot. (g)	Servings/Exchanges
Ham Roll	2 oz	60	1.5	15	1	0	25	450	0	1	10	1 lean meat
Head Cheese	1.4 oz	100	7	60	4	0	30	400	0	0	8	1 med-fat meat
Mission Loaf	2 oz	60	1.5	15	1	0	25	450	0	1	10	1 lean meat
Oven Roasted Turkey Breast	1 oz	25	0	0	0	0	10	270	0	1	5	1 lean meat
Foster Farms												
Mesquite Smoked Turkey Breast	2 oz	60	1.5	10	0	0	10	520	0	2	9	1 lean meat
Oven Roasted Turkey Breast	2 oz	60	2	20	0.5	0	15	440	0	1	9	1 lean meat
Hebrew National												
Beef Bologna	1 oz	80	8	70	3.5	0	15	240	0	0	3	1 high-fat meat
Beef Salami	2 oz	150	13	120	6	0	35	420	0	0	8	1 high-fat meat, 1 fat
Corned Beef	2 oz	80	3.5	20	1.5	0	35	520	0	1	13	2 lean meat

Lean Beef Salami	2 oz	90	5	50	3	0	25	480	0	1	9	1 med-fat meat
Pastrami	2 oz	80	3	25	1	0	30	520	0	1	11	2 lean meat
Hebrew National Franks												
97% Fat Free Beef Franks	1	40	1	10	0	0	10	520	3	0	6	1 lean meat
Beef Franks	1	150	14	130	6	0.5	25	460	1	0	6	1 high-fat meat, 1 fat
Jumbo Beef Franks	1	270	25	230	10	0	45	810	2	0	10	1 high-fat meat, 3 fat
Reduced Fat Beef Franks	1	110	9	80	3.5	0	20	490	2	0	5	1 high-fat meat
Hillshire Farm Deli Select												
Baked Ham	2 oz	60	1.5	15	0.5	0	30	730	0	1	9	1 lean meat
Brown Sugar Baked Ham	2 oz	60	1.5	15	0.5	0	25	600	0	2	10	1 lean meat
Honey Ham	2 oz	70	1.5	15	0.5	0	30	720	0	3	9	1 lean meat
Honey Roasted Turkey Breast	2 oz	50	0.5	5	0	0	25	580	0	2	9	1 lean meat

PROCESSED MEAT, BREAKFAST MEAT, LUNCH MEAT

	Serving	Calories	Fat (g)	Cal. from Fat	Sat. Fat (g)	Trans Fat (g)	Chol. (mg)	Sod. (mg)	Carb. (g)	Fiber (g)	Prot. (g)	Servings/Exchanges
Oven Roasted Chicken Breast	2 oz	60	0.5	5	0	0	25	620	0	2	11	2 lean meat
Oven Roasted Turkey Breast	2 oz	50	0.5	5	0	0	25	610	0	1	10	1 lean meat
Pastrami	2 oz	60	1	10	0.5	0	30	600	0	0	11	2 lean meat
Roast Beef	2 oz	60	1	10	0.5	0	25	670	0	1	11	2 lean meat
Smoked Chicken Breast	2 oz	60	1	10	0	0	25	730	0	2	10	1 lean meat
Smoked Ham	2 oz	60	1.5	15	0.5	0	25	600	0	1	10	1 lean meat
Smoked Turkey Breast	2 oz	50	0.5	5	0	0	20	590	0	3	9	1 lean meat
Hillshire Farm Hearty Slices												
Honey Ham	1 oz	30	0.5	5	0	0	10	260	0	<1	5	1 lean meat
Honey Roasted Turkey	1 oz	25	0	0	0	0	10	260	0	1	6	1 lean meat
Oven Roasted Chicken	1 oz	25	0	0	0	0	15	280	0	<1	5	1 lean meat

Hillshire Farm Ultra Thin

Hard Salami	1 oz	110	10	90	4	0	30	500	0	0	6	1 high-fat meat
Honey Ham	2 oz	60	1.5	15	0.5	0	25	500	0	2	10	1 lean meat
Oven Roasted Turkey Breast	2 oz	50	0.5	5	0	0	20	620	0	2	9	1 lean meat
Roast Beef	2 oz	60	3	25	1	0	25	450	0	0	9	1 med-fat meat
Smoked Ham	2 oz	60	1.5	15	0.5	0	30	620	0	1	9	1 lean meat

Hormel Natural Choice

Deli Roast Beef	2 oz	70	2.5	25	1	0	25	500	0	0	11	2 lean meat
Honey Deli Ham 97% Fat Free	2 oz	70	1.5	15	0.5	0	25	520	0	3	10	1 lean meat

Land O'Frost

DeliShaved

Chicken	2 oz	90	6	50	1.5	0	30	760	0	0	10	1 med-fat meat
Honey Ham	2 oz	80	5	45	2	0	30	540	0	4	10	1 med-fat meat
Oven Roasted Turkey	2 oz	90	6	50	1.5	0	35	540	0	0	9	1 med-fat meat

PROCESSED MEAT, BREAKFAST MEAT, LUNCH MEAT

	Serving	Calories	Fat (g)	Cal. from Fat	Sat. Fat (g)	Trans Fat (g)	Chol. (mg)	Sod. (mg)	Carb. (g)	Fiber (g)	Prot. (g)	Servings/Exchanges
Smoked Turkey	2 oz	90	6	50	2	0	40	740	0	0	9	1 med-fat meat
Premium												
Chicken Breast	2 oz	80	5	45	1	0	35	650	0	2	7	1 med-fat meat
Honey Ham	1.8 oz	70	3	25	1	0	25	530	0	2	9	1 lean meat
Smoked Ham	1.8 oz	60	3	25	1	0	25	560	0	1	9	1 lean meat
Select												
Honey Smoked White Turkey	3 oz	110	4.5	40	1	0	35	1080	0	6	12	1 med-fat meat
Oven Roasted White Turkey	1.9 oz	70	3.5	35	1	0	25	630	0	1	8	1 med-fat meat
Smoked Ham	3 oz	100	5	45	1.5	0	45	1060	0	1	14	2 lean meat
Taste Escapes												
Hickory Smoked Black Pepper Ham	2 oz	70	2.5	20	1	0	30	690	0	2	10	1 lean meat

Hickory Smoked Maple Ham	2 oz	70	2	15	0.5	0	30	640	0	3	10	1 lean meat
Peppered Beef	2 oz	70	2	20	1	0	20	680	0	2	10	1 lean meat
Traditional												
Chicken	2 oz	90	5	45	1.5	0	35	800	0	0	9	1 med-fat meat
Ham	2 oz	90	5	45	2	0	30	690	0	1	9	1 med-fat meat
Honey Ham	2 oz	90	4.5	40	1.5	0	30	610	0	3	9	1 med-fat meat
Honey Turkey	2 oz	90	5	45	1.5	0	35	780	3	0	9	1 med-fat meat
Turkey	2 oz	90	6	50	2	0	40	790	0	0	9	1 med-fat meat
Oscar Mayer												
Baked Ham	2.25 oz	60	2	20	1	0	30	760	0	1	10	1 lean meat
Beef Bologna	1 oz	90	8	70	3.5	0	20	310	0	1	3	1 high-fat meat
Beef Cotto Salami	1 oz	60	4.5	40	2	0	20	360	0	1	4	1 med-fat meat
Beef Salami, Deli Thin	1.8 oz	150	13	120	6	1	40	640	0	1	8	1 high-fat meat
Boiled Ham	2.25 oz	60	2	20	1	0	30	820	0	1	10	1 lean meat
Bologna	1 oz	90	8	80	3	0	30	300	0	1	3	1 high-fat meat

PROCESSED MEAT, BREAKFAST MEAT, LUNCH MEAT

	Serving	Calories	Fat (g)	Cal. from Fat	Sat. Fat (g)	Trans Fat (g)	Chol. (mg)	Sod. (mg)	Carb. (g)	Fiber (g)	Prot. (g)	Servings/Exchanges
Bologna, 98% Fat Free	1 oz	25	0	0.5	0	0	10	240	0	3	3	1 lean meat
Braunschweiger Liver Sausage	2 oz	190	17	155	6	0	90	630	0	1	8	1 high-fat meat, 1 fat
Chopped Ham	1 oz	50	3	30	1.5	0	15	340	0	1	4	1 lean meat
Cotto Salami	1 oz	70	6	50	2	0	25	280	0	1	4	1 med-fat meat
Fat Free Bologna	1 oz	20	0	0	0	0	10	250	0	2	3	1 lean meat
Ham & Cheese Loaf	1 oz	60	4.5	40	2.5	0	20	350	0	1	4	1 med-fat meat
Hard Salami	1 oz	100	8	70	3	0	25	510	0	1	7	1 high-fat meat
Honey Ham	2.25 oz	70	2	20	1	0	30	770	0	2	11	2 lean meat
Honey Ham, 98% Fat Free	2.25 oz	70	2	20	1	0	30	770	0	2	11	2 lean meat
Light Beef Bologna	1 oz	60	4	35	1.5	0	15	310	0	2	3	1 med-fat meat
Liver Cheese	1.5 oz	120	10	90	3.5	0	80	420	0	1	6	1 high-fat meat
Olive Loaf	1 oz	70	6	55	2	0	20	360	0	2	3	1 med-fat meat

Oven Roasted White Turkey	1 oz	25	1	10	0	0	10	340	0	1	6	1 lean meat
Pickle & Pimiento Loaf	1 oz	80	6	55	2	0	20	360	0	2	3	1 med-fat meat
Sandwich Spread	2 oz	130	9	80	4	0	25	460	0	9	4	1 high-fat meat
Turkey Bologna	1 oz	50	4	35	1	0	20	270	0	1	3	1 med-fat meat
Turkey Bologna, 50% Less Fat	1 oz	50	4	35	1	0	20	270	0	1	3	1 med-fat meat
Turkey Cotto Salami	1 oz	45	3	25	1	0	20	310	0	0	4	1 lean meat
Turkey Cotto Salami, 50% Less Fat	1 oz	45	3	25	1	0	20	310	0	0	4	1 lean meat
Turkey Ham	1 oz	35	1.5	10	0	0	20	350	0	1	5	1 lean meat
Turkey, Smoked, White, 95% Fat Free	1 oz	30	1	10	0	0	10	320	0	1	4	1 lean meat
Turkey, White, Smoked	1 oz	30	1	10	0	0	10	320	0	1	4	1 lean meat
Deli Fresh Meats												
Brown Sugar Ham, Shaved	1.8 oz	60	1.5	10	0	0	25	740	0	3	9	1 lean meat

PROCESSED MEAT, BREAKFAST MEAT, LUNCH MEAT

	Serving	Calories	Fat (g)	Cal. from Fat	Sat. Fat (g)	Trans Fat (g)	Chol. (mg)	Sod. (mg)	Carb. (g)	Fiber (g)	Prot. (g)	Servings/Exchanges
Chicken Breast, Rotisserie Style, Shaved	1.8 oz	50	1	10	0	0	25	480	0	2	9	1 lean meat
Honey Ham–Shaved	1.8 oz	50	1	10	0.5	0	25	650	0	2	9	1 lean meat
Roast Beef Slow Roasted, Shaved	1.8 oz	60	2.5	20	1	0	30	520	0	0	10	1 lean meat
Smoked Ham, Shaved	1.8 oz	45	1	10	0	0	25	640	0	0	9	1 lean meat
Smoked Turkey Breast	2.25 oz	60	0.5	5	0	0	25	760	0	0	13	2 lean meat
Oscar Mayer Hot Dogs												
Jumbo Beef Franks	1	300	27	240	11	1.5	55	1090	2	0	10	1 high-fat meat, 3 fat
Jumbo Wieners	1	290	27	240	10	0	60	930	2	0	10	1 high-fat meat, 3 fat
Quarter Pound Beef Franks	1	370	34	310	14	1.5	70	1370	3	0	13	2 high-fat meat, 3 fat
Regular Beef Franks	1	180	17	150	7	1	35	680	1	0	7	1 high-fat meat, 1 fat

Food	Serving											Exchanges
Turkey Franks	1	100	8	70	2.5	0	30	510	2	0	5	1 high-fat meat
Wieners	1	140	13	120	5	0	30	460	<1	0	5	1 high-fat meat, 1 fat
Trader Joe's												
Black Forest Ham	2 oz	70	1	10	0	0	35	730	0	2	12	1 lean meat
Oven Roasted Turkey Breast	2 oz	50	0	0	0	0	25	630	0	2	11	2 lean meat
Pastrami	2 oz	80	2	15	0.5	0	25	270	0	<1	13	2 lean meat
Roast Beef	2 oz	80	2	20	0.5	0	30	460	0	0	15	2 lean meat
Smoked Turkey Breast	2 oz	50	0	0	0	0	25	630	0	2	11	2 lean meat

CANNED MEAT

Fish/Seafood

Food	Serving											Exchanges
Anchovies in Oil, Canned, Drained	5	42	2	18	<1	0	17	734	0	0	8	1 lean meat
Clams, Canned, Drained Solids	1 oz	42	<1	5	<1	0	19	32	1	0	7	1 lean meat
Clams, Smoked, Canned in Oil, Small	5	88	6	54	1	0	19	161	1	0	7	1 med-fat meat

PROCESSED MEAT, BREAKFAST MEAT, LUNCH MEAT

	Serving	Calories	Fat (g)	Cal. from Fat	Sat. Fat (g)	Trans Fat (g)	Chol. (mg)	Sod. (mg)	Carb. (g)	Fiber (g)	Prot. (g)	Servings/Exchanges
Crab, Canned, Drained Solids	1 oz	28	<1	5	<1	0	26	95	0	0	6	1 lean meat
Salmon, Canned in Water	1 oz	40	2	18	<1	0	11	139	0	0	6	1 lean meat
Sardines, Oil-Packed, Drained	2	50	3	27	<1	0	34	121	0	0	6	1 lean meat
Shrimp, Canned, Drained Solids	1 oz	34	<1	0	<1	0	50	48	<1	0	7	1 lean meat
Squid, Pickled	1 oz	26	<1	0	<1	0	64	397	1	0	4	1 lean meat
Tuna, Canned in Oil, Drained	1 oz	56	2	9	<1	0	5	100	0	0	8	1 lean meat
Tuna, Canned, Water Packed, Solids Only	1 oz	33	<1	0	<1	0	9	96	0	0	7	1 lean meat
Beef												
Liver Pate, Canned	2 Tbsp	52	3	27	1	0	66	100	2	0	4	1 lean meat

Pickled Beef Trip	1 oz	18	<1	0	<1	0	19	13	0	0	3	1 lean meat
Pork												
Ham, Canned	1 oz	48	2	18	<1	0	12	304	<1	0	6	1 lean meat
Sausage, Vienna, Canned	1 oz	79	7	63	3	0	15	270	<1	0	3	1 high-fat meat
Canned Fish												
Bumble Bee												
Blueback Salmon	2.2 oz	110	7	60	1.5	0	40	270	0	0	13	2 lean meat
Chunk Light Tuna in Oil	2 oz	70	3	25	0.5	0	25	180	0	0	13	2 lean meat
Chunk Light Tuna in Water	2 oz	50	0.5	5	0	0	3	180	0	0	13	2 lean meat
Chunk White Albacore Tuna, Very Low Sodium, in Water	2 oz	60	1	10	0	0	25	35	0	0	15	2 lean meat
Fancy Whole Baby Clams	2 oz	50	1	10	0.5	0	40	270	2	0	9	1 lean meat

PROCESSED MEAT, BREAKFAST MEAT, LUNCH MEAT

	Serving	Calories	Fat (g)	Cal. from Fat	Sat. Fat (g)	Trans Fat (g)	Chol. (mg)	Sod. (mg)	Carb. (g)	Fiber (g)	Prot. (g)	Servings/Exchanges
Jumbo Shrimp	2 oz	40	0	0	0	0	115	430	0	0	10	1 lean meat
Keta Salmon	2.2 oz	90	4	35	1	0	40	270	0	0	13	2 lean meat
Medium Red Salmon (Alaska Coho)	2.2 oz	90	5	45	1	0	40	270	0	0	12	2 lean meat
Medium Shrimp	2 oz	40	0	0	0	0	115	430	0	0	10	1 lean meat
Minced Clams	2 oz	25	0	0	0	0	10	320	2	0	4	1 lean meat
Pink Crabmeat	2 oz	35	0.5	5	0	0	50	300	0	0	7	1 lean meat
Pink Salmon	2.2 oz	90	5	45	1	0	40	270	0	0	12	2 lean meat
Premium Light Tuna in Water Pouch	2 oz	60	0.5	5	0	0	30	180	0	0	13	2 lean meat
Prime Fillet Albacore Steak Entrées, Mesquite Grilled	4 oz	150	1.5	10	0	0	40	370	0	0	35	5 lean meat
Prime Fillet Atlantic Salmon	2 oz	80	3	30	1.5	0	10	170	0	0	12	2 lean meat

Prime Fillet Salmon Steaks	4 oz	160	3	25	0.5	0	45	690	8	0	24	3 lean meat
Prime Fillet Solid Light Tuna, Tonno in Oil	2 oz	110	5	50	1	0	30	220	0	0	15	2 lean meat
Prime Fillet Solid White Albacore in Water	2 oz	70	1	10	0	0	25	180	0	0	16	2 lean meat
Red Salmon (Sockeye)	2.2 oz	110	7	60	1.5	0	40	270	0	0	13	2 lean meat
Sardines in Oil	2.7-oz can	130	9	80	2	0	35	340	0	0	13	2 med-fat meat
Sardines in Water	2.7-oz can	120	7	70	2	0	35	340	0	0	13	2 lean meat
Sensations Easy Peel Bowls, Spicy Thai Chili	3 oz	110	3	30	0.5	0	25	350	2	0	18	2 lean meat
Sensations Easy Peel Tuna Bowls, Lemon & Cracked Pepper	3 oz	110	4	35	1	0	25	300	2	0	16	2 lean meat

PROCESSED MEAT, BREAKFAST MEAT, LUNCH MEAT

	Serving	Calories	Fat (g)	Cal. from Fat	Sat. Fat (g)	Trans Fat (g)	Chol. (mg)	Sod. (mg)	Carb. (g)	Fiber (g)	Prot. (g)	Servings/Exchanges
Skinless Boneless Pink Salmon	2 oz	70	1.5	10	0	0	30	240	0	0	12	2 lean meat
Small Shrimp	2 oz	40	0	0	0	0	115	430	0	0	10	1 lean meat
Smoked Clams	2 oz	130	8	80	2	0	40	460	1	0	11	2 med-fat meat
Smoked Oysters	2 oz	120	7	60	1.5	0	35	210	6	0	10	1 med-fat meat
Smoked Salmon Fillets in Oil	3 oz	150	9	80	2	0	55	400	0	0	16	2 med-fat meat
Solid White Albacore Tuna in Oil	2 oz	80	3	25	0.5	0	25	180	0	0	14	2 lean meat
Solid White Albacore Tuna in Water	2 oz	60	1	10	0	0	25	180	0	0	13	2 lean meat
White Crabmeat	2 oz	40	1	10	0	0	50	300	0	0	8	1 lean meat
Whole Oysters	2 oz	70	3	30	0.5	0	45	140	3	0	7	1 lean meat

Chicken of the Sea

Chunk Light Tuna in Oil	2 oz	100	6	50	1	0	25	250	0	0	10	1 med-fat meat
Chunk Light Tuna in Water	2 oz	50	0.5	50	0	0	25	250	0	0	11	2 lean meat
Chunk Light Tuna in Water Low Sodium	2 oz	50	0.5	50	0	0	25	90	0	0	11	2 lean meat
Chunk Light Tuna, 50% Less Sodium	2 oz	50	0.5	5	0	0	25	125	0	0	11	2 lean meat
Chunk White Albacore Low Sodium	3 oz	80	1	10	0	0	35	50	0	0	18	3 lean meat
Chunk White Albacore Tuna	2 oz	50	1	10	0	0	25	250	0	0	11	2 lean meat
Fancy Crabmeat	2 oz	40	0	0	0	0	50	400	2	0	7	1 lean meat
Genova Skinless Boneless Salmon in Water	2 oz	60	2	20	1	0	20	280	0	0	10	1 lean meat
Genova Solid White Albacore Tuna in Oil	2 oz	110	6	50	1	0	25	250	0	0	13	2 lean meat

PROCESSED MEAT, BREAKFAST MEAT, LUNCH MEAT

	Serving	Calories	Fat (g)	Cal. from Fat	Sat. Fat (g)	Trans Fat (g)	Chol. (mg)	Sod. (mg)	Carb. (g)	Fiber (g)	Prot. (g)	Servings/Exchanges
Genova Tonno Tuna in Olive Oil	2 oz	120	8	70	2	0	25	250	0	0	13	2 med-fat meat
Medium or Small Shrimp	2 oz	45	0.5	5	0	0	145	400	1	0	10	1 lean meat
Minced Clams	1/4 cup	30	0	0	0	0	12	370	2	0	5	1 lean meat
Pink Crabmeat	2 oz	30	0	0	0	0	50	400	0	0	7	1 lean meat
Sardines in Water	3.75-oz can	100	4	40	2	0	45	430	2	0	13	2 lean meat
Skinless & Boneless Pink Salmon	2 oz	60	2	20	0.5	0	20	280	0	0	10	1 lean meat
Smoked Oysters in Oil	3.75 oz	170	8	70	2	0	45	280	8	0	10	1 high-fat meat
Smoked Oysters in Water	3.75 oz	120	3	30	1	0	55	400	10	0	12	2 lean meat
Smoked Sardines in Oil	3.75-oz can	190	14	130	6	0	45	430	2	0	12	2 med-fat meat, 1 fat

Solid White Albacore Tuna in Oil	2 oz	90	4	40	0	0	25	250	0	0	13	2 lean meat
Solid White Albacore Tuna in Water	2 oz	80	4	40	0	0	25	250	0	0	11	2 lean meat
Traditional Pink Salmon	1/4 cup	90	5	45	1	0	40	270	0	0	12	2 lean meat
Very Low Sodium Chunk White Albacore Tuna	2 oz	50	0.5	5	0	0	25	35	0	0	12	2 lean meat
Whole Baby Clams	1/4 cup	30	0	0	0	0	10	290	1	0	6	1 lean meat
Whole Oysters	2 oz	80	3	30	1	0	35	220	6	0	7	1 lean meat
Starkist												
Chunk Light Tuna in Water	2 oz	50	1	0	0	0	25	180	<1	<1	11	2 lean meat
Hickory Smoked Tuna Creations	2 oz	80	2.5	0	0	0	30	NA	<1	0	14	2 lean meat
Low Sodium Albacore	2 oz	50	0.5	0	0	0	20	125	0	0	12	2 lean meat

PROCESSED MEAT, BREAKFAST MEAT, LUNCH MEAT

	Serving	Calories	Fat (g)	Cal. from Fat	Sat. Fat (g)	Trans Fat (g)	Chol. (mg)	Sod. (mg)	Carb. (g)	Fiber (g)	Prot. (g)	Servings/Exchanges
Low Sodium Chunk Light Tuna	2 oz	50	0.5	0	0	0	20	125	0	0	12	2 lean meat
Solid White Albacore Tuna in Water	2 oz	70	2	0	0.5	0	25	200	0	0	13	2 lean meat
Canned Chicken												
Swanson												
Premium White Chunk Chicken Breast in Water	2 oz	50	1	10	0	0	25	260	1	0	9	1 lean meat
Tyson												
Premium Chunk Chicken	2 oz	60	2	20	0	0	30	200	0	0	10	1 lean meat
Premium Chunk Chicken Pouch (97% Fat Free)	2 oz	70	1	15	0	0	45	210	0	0	14	2 lean meat

RICE, RICE MIXES

	Serving	Calories	Fat (g)	Cal. from Fat	Sat. Fat (g)	Trans Fat (g)	Chol. (mg)	Sod. (mg)	Carb. (g)	Fiber (g)	Prot. (g)	Servings/Exchanges
Brown Rice, Long Grain, Cooked	1/2 cup	108	<1	0	<1	0	0	5	22	2	3	1 1/2 starch
Brown Rice, Medium Grain, Cooked	1/2 cup	109	<1	0	<1	0	0	1	23	2	2	1 1/2 starch
White Rice, Glutinous, Cooked	1/2 cup	85	<1	0	0	0	0	5	19	<1	2	1 starch
White Rice, Long Grain, Cooked	1/2 cup	103	<1	0	<1	0	0	1	22	<1	2	2 starch
White Rice, Long Grain, Instant, Cooked	1/2 cup	97	<1	0	<1	0	0	4	21	<1	2	1 starch
White Rice, Long Grain, Parboiled, Cooked	1/2 cup	97	<1	0	<1	0	0	2	21	<1	2	1/2 starch
White Rice, Medium Grain, Cooked	1/2 cup	121	<1	0	<1	0	0	0	27	<1	2	2 starch

RICE, RICE MIXES

	Serving	Calories	Fat (g)	Cal. from Fat	Sat. Fat (g)	Trans Fat (g)	Chol. (mg)	Sod. (mg)	Carb. (g)	Fiber (g)	Prot. (g)	Servings/Exchanges
White Rice, Short Grain, Cooked	1/2 cup	121	<1	0	<1	0	0	0	27	<1	2	2 starch
Wild Rice, Cooked	1/2 cup	83	<1	0	<1	0	0	3	18	2	3	1 starch
Brands												
Knorr/Lipton												
Cheddar Broccoli	1 cup	260	6	55	1	0	<5	900	47	2	6	3 starch, 1 fat
Chicken Fried Rice	1 cup	270	8	75	1	0	<5	750	46	2	6	3 starch, 2 fat
Spanish Rice	1 cup	290	7	65	1	0	0	860	50	2	6	3 starch, 1 fat
Mahatma												
Authenic Spanish Rice	2/3 cup	180	0	5	0	0	0	650	42	1	4	3 starch
Brown Rice	3/4 cup	150	1	10	0	0	0	0	32	1	3	2 starch
Classic Pilaf	2/3 cup	190	0.5	5	0	0	0	790	43	1	5	3 starch
Gold Rice, Parboiled	1 cup	160	0	0	0	0	0	0	37	1	3	2 1/2 starch
Thai Jasmine Rice	3/4 cup	160	0	0	0	0	0	0	36	0	3	2 1/2 starch

Minute Rice

Boil-In-Bag Rice	1 cup	180	0	0	0	0	0	10	42	<1	4	3 starch
Brown Rice, Instant	2/3 cup	150	1.5	0	15	0	0	10	34	2	3	2 starch
White Rice, Instant	1 cup	200	0	0	0	0	0	5	45	<1	5	3 starch

Near East

Long Grain & Wild Rice

Garlic & Herb	1 cup	220	4	2	35	0	10	720	43	2	5	3 starch, 1 fat
Original	1 cup	220	4	2	35	0	10	830	43	2	5	3 starch, 1 fat

Rice Pilaf

Garlic & Herb	1 cup	220	4	0.5	30	0	0	680	44	1	5	3 starch, 1 fat
Original	1 cup	220	4	2	30	0	10	820	44	1	5	3 starch, 1 fat
Roasted Chicken & Garlic	1 cup	220	3	1.5	25	0	5	600	44	2	5	3 starch, 1 fat
Spanish Rice	1 cup	310	8	5	70	0	0	1090	54	2	5	3 1/2 starch, 2 fat
Sundried Tomato & Basil	1 cup	290	7	1	60	0	0	1030	54	2	6	3 1/2 starch, 1 fat

RICE, RICE MIXES

	Serving	Calories	Fat (g)	Cal. from Fat	Sat. Fat (g)	Trans Fat (g)	Chol. (mg)	Sod. (mg)	Carb. (g)	Fiber (g)	Prot. (g)	Servings/Exchanges
Toasted Almond	1 cup	230	6	50	0	0	10	670	40	2	5	2 1/2 starch, 1 fat
Wild Mushroom & Herb	1 cup	220	4	30	2	0	10	570	43	1	5	3 starch, 1 fat
Rice-A-Roni												
Beef	1 cup	310	9	80	1.5	1.5	0	1100	51	2	7	3 1/2 starch, 2 fat
Chicken & Garlic	1 cup	260	8	70	1.5	1.5	0	820	41	1	5	2 1/2 starch, 2 fat
Chicken & Broccoli	1 cup	220	5	45	1	1	0	1020	40	2	6	2 1/2 starch, 1 fat
Country Cheddar	1 cup	370	17	150	5	2	10	1080	49	2	6	3 starch, 3 fat
Creamy Four Cheese	1 cup	280	12	110	4	1.5	5	810	37	1	6	2 1/2 starch, 2 fat
Long Grain & Wild Rice	1 cup	240	6	50	1	1	0	910	42	2	5	3 starch, 1 fat
Mexican Style	1 cup	250	8	70	1.5	1	0	820	40	2	6	2 1/2 starch, 2 fat
Parmesan Chicken	1 cup	370	15	140	4.5	2	5	1360	51	3	8	3 1/2 starch, 3 fat
Spanish	1 cup	260	7	60	1.5	1	0	1340	44	2	6	3 starch, 1 fat
Rice-A-Roni Savory Whole Grain Blends												
Chicken Herb Classico	1 cup	260	8	70	1	0	0	760	41	4	6	2 1/2 starch, 2 fat

Roasted Garlic Italiano	1 cup	270	9	80	1.5	0	0	760	41	3	6	2 1/2 starch, 2 fat
Spanish	1 cup	250	8	60	1	0	0	760	42	3	5	3 starch, 2 fat

Uncle Ben's

Country Inn Rice Dishes

Broccoli Rice Au Gratin	1 cup	200	2	20	1	0	5	790	43	1	4	3 starch
Chicken & Broccoli	1 cup	190	1	10	0	0	0	910	42	1	5	3 starch
Chicken & Vegetable	1 cup	200	1.5	15	0.5	0	0	720	41	1	5	2 1/2 starch
Chicken & Wild Rice	1 cup	200	1	5	0.5	0	0	800	42	1	5	3 starch
Chicken Flavored	1 cup	200	1	10	0	0	0	940	41	1	6	2 1/2 starch
Mexican Fiesta	1 cup	200	1	5	0	0	0	680	42	1	5	3 starch
Oriental Fried Rice	1 cup	200	1	20	0	0	0	580	42	1	6	3 starch
Rice Pilaf	1 cup	200	0.5	5	0	0	0	640	43	1	5	3 starch

Long Grain & Wild Rice

Butter & Herb	1 cup	190	1	10	0	0	0	810	40	1	5	2 1/2 starch
Fast Cook Recipe	1 cup	190	0.5	5	0	0	0	680	41	1	5	2 1/2 starch
Original Recipe	1 cup	200	0	0	0	0	0	670	44	1	6	3 starch

RICE, RICE MIXES

	Serving	Calories	Fat (g)	Cal. from Fat	Sat. Fat (g)	Trans Fat (g)	Chol. (mg)	Sod. (mg)	Carb. (g)	Fiber (g)	Prot. (g)	Servings/Exchanges
Roasted Garlic & Olive Oil	1 cup	180	1	10	0	0	0	590	39	3	5	2 1/2 starch
Vegetable Pilaf	1 cup	180	1	10	0	0	0	610	40	3	5	2 1/2 starch
Whole Grain & Wild Rice with Mushroom	1 cup	200	1.5	10	1.5	0	0	570	42	3	6	3 starch
Ready Rice												
Long Grain & Wild	1 cup	220	3	25	0	0	0	900	43	2	5	3 starch, 1 fat
Original Long Grain	1 cup	200	2.5	25	0	0	0	10	40	1	4	2 1/2 starch, 1 fat
Rice Pilaf	1 cup	220	3.5	35	0.5	0	0	970	42	2	6	2 1/2 starch, 1 fat
Roasted Chicken	1 cup	220	3.5	30	0	0	0	1020	41	2	5	2 1/2 starch
Spanish Style	1 cup	200	2.5	30	0	0	0	680	41	3	4	2 1/2 starch, 1 fat
Teriyaki Style	1 cup	220	3	25	0	0	5	870	42	3	6	3 starch, 1 fat
Ready Whole Grain Medley												
Brown & Wild	1 cup	220	3.5	30	0	0	0	730	42	3	6	3 starch, 1 fat

Santa Fe	1 cup	220	3	25	0	0	0	700	42	5	7	3 starch, 1 fat
Vegetable Harvest	1 cup	220	3	25	0	0	0	780	44	5	5	3 starch, 1 fat
White Rice											
Boil-In-Bag	1 cup	190	0.5	5	0	0	0	0	44	1	4	3 starch
Instant	1 cup	190	0.5	5	0	0	0	15	43	1	3	3 starch
Original Converted Rice	1 cup	170	0	0	0	0	0	0	37	0	4	2 1/2 starch
Whole Grain Brown Rice											
Fast & Natural Instant Brown Rice	1 cup	170	1	10	0	0	0	20	36	2	4	2 1/2 starch
Natural Whole Grain Brown Rice	1 cup	170	1.5	10	0	0	0	0	35	2	5	2 starch

SALAD DRESSING

	Serving	Calories	Fat. (g)	Cal. from Fat	Sat. Fat (g)	Trans Fat (g)	Chol. (mg)	Sod. (mg)	Carb. (g)	Fiber (g)	Prot. (g)	Servings/Exchanges
Mayonnaise	1 tsp	33	4	35	<1	0	2	26	0	0	0	1 fat
Mayonnaise, Fat-Free	1 Tbsp	13	<1	0	0	0	1	126	2	0	0	free
Mayonnaise, Light/ Reduced Fat	1 Tbsp	45	5	45	<1	0	4	120	1	0	0	1 fat
Oil & Vinegar	2 Tbsp	144	16	145	3	0	0	<1	<1	0	0	3 fat
Salad Dressing, Fat-Free	1 Tbsp	20	0	0	0	0	0	145	5	0	0	free
Salad Dressing, Reduced Fat, Cream Based	2 Tbsp	70	4	35	<1	0	0	241	8	0	0	1/2 carb, 1 fat
Salad Dressing, Regular	1 Tbsp	69	7	65	<1	0	0	125	2	0	0	1 fat
Brands												
Bernstein's												
Balsamic Italian	2 Tbsp	110	11	100	0.5	0	0	270	2	0	0	2 fat

Food	Serving											
Basil Parmesan	2 Tbsp	100	10	90	1	0	5	400	2	0	1	2 fat
Cheese & Garlic Italian	2 Tbsp	110	11	100	1	0	0	340	2	0	1	2 fat
Cheese Fantastico	2 Tbsp	100	10	90	1	0	5	400	2	0	1	2 fat
Creamy Caesar	2 Tbsp	120	13	115	1	0	15	200	1	0	0	3 fat
Herb Garden French	2 Tbsp	130	12	110	1	0	0	260	6	0	0	1/2 carb, 2 fat
Light Fantastic Cheese Fantastico	2 Tbsp	25	1.5	15	0.5	0	0	370	2	0	1	free
Light Fantastic Parmesan Garlic Ranch	2 Tbsp	50	2.5	25	0.5	0	5	330	6	0	1	1/2 carb, 1 fat

Best Foods

Food	Serving											
Canola Cholesterol Free Mayonnaise	1 Tbsp	45	4.5	40	0	0	0	90	<1	0	0	1 fat
Light Mayonnaise	1 Tbsp	35	3.5	30	0	0	<5	120	1	0	0	1 fat
Low Fat Mayonnaise Dressing	1 Tbsp	15	1	10	0	0	0	130	2	0	0	free

SALAD DRESSING

	Serving	Calories	Fat (g)	Cal. from Fat	Sat. Fat (g)	Trans Fat (g)	Chol. (mg)	Sod. (mg)	Carb. (g)	Fiber (g)	Prot. (g)	Servings/Exchanges
Mayonnaise Dressing with Olive Oil	1 Tbsp	50	5	45	0.5	0	5	120	<1	0	0	1 fat
Real Mayonnaise	1 Tbsp	90	10	90	1.5	0	5	85	0	0	0	2 fat
Cardini's												
Balsamic Vinaigrette	2 Tbsp	100	8	80	1.5	0	0	250	5	0	0	2 fat
Fat Free Caesar	2 Tbsp	40	0	0	0	0	0	510	9	0	0	1/2 carb
Honey Mustard	2 Tbsp	140	13	120	2	0	0	220	5	0	0	3 fat
Italian	2 Tbsp	100	8	70	1	0	0	310	7	0	0	1/2 carb, 3 fat
Light Caesar	2 Tbsp	60	5	45	1	0	0	450	2	0	1	1 fat
Original Caesar	2 Tbsp	160	17	150	2.5	0	30	240	10	0	1	1/2 carb, 3 fat
Pear Vinaigrette	2 Tbsp	100	9	80	1.5	0	0	150	6	0	0	1/2 carb, 2 fat
Roasted Asian Sesame	2 Tbsp	120	10	90	1.5	0	0	360	7	0	0	1/2 carb, 2 fat
Dorothy Lynch												
Fat Free Dressing	2 Tbsp	60	0	0	0	0	0	160	14	0	0	1 carb

Home Style Dressing	2 Tbsp	110	6	55	1	0	0	170	12	0	0	1 carb, 1 fat
Girard's												
Balsamic Basil	2 Tbsp	90	9	80	1.5	0	0	330	3	0	0	2 fat
Blue Cheese Vinaigrette	2 Tbsp	100	10	90	2	0	5	500	3	0	1	2 fat
Caesar	2 Tbsp	140	15	130	2.5	0	10	350	1	0	1	3 fat
Chinese Chicken Salad	2 Tbsp	120	11	100	1.5	0	0	350	6	0	0	1/2 carb, 2 fat
Greek Feta Vinaigrette	2 Tbsp	100	11	100	1.5	0	0	300	2	0	0	2 fat
Light Caesar	2 Tbsp	90	8	70	1.5	0	10	370	5	0	1	2 fat
Romano Cheese	2 Tbsp	130	13	120	2	0	0	500	2	0	1	3 fat
Spinach Salad	2 Tbsp	70	2	15	0	0	0	250	14	0	1	1 carb
Girard's Fat Free												
Balsamic Vinaigrette	2 Tbsp	25	0	0	0	0	0	390	6	0	0	1/2 carb
Raspberry	2 Tbsp	60	0	0	0	0	0	210	14	0	0	1 carb
Fat Free Caesar	2 Tbsp	40	0	0	0	0	0	510	9	0	0	1/2 carb
Hidden Valley												
Buttermilk Ranch Light	2 Tbsp	70	5	50	1	0	5	310	3	0	1	1 fat

SALAD DRESSING

	Serving	Calories	Fat (g)	Cal. from Fat	Sat. Fat (g)	Trans Fat (g)	Chol. (mg)	Sod. (mg)	Carb. (g)	Fiber (g)	Prot. (g)	Servings/Exchanges
Coleslaw Dressing	2 Tbsp	150	15	130	2.5	0	15	170	5	0	0	3 fat
Old-Fashioned Buttermilk Ranch	2 Tbsp	140	14	130	2	0	10	340	2	0	0	3 fat
Original Ranch	2 Tbsp	140	14	130	2.5	0	10	260	2	0	1	3 fat
Original Ranch Fat Free	2 Tbsp	30	0	0	0	0	0	310	6	0	0	1/2 carb
Original Ranch Light	2 Tbsp	80	7	70	1	0	5	290	3	0	1	1 fat
Ken's Steak House												
Buttermilk Ranch	2 Tbsp	180	20	180	3	0	5	280	1	0	0	4 fat
Country French	2 Tbsp	130	12	110	1.5	0	0	150	9	0	0	1/2 carb, 2 fat
Lite Caesar	2 Tbsp	70	6	60	1	0	0	620	3	0	1	1 fat
Lite Country French	2 Tbsp	100	6	50	1	0	0	230	11	0	0	1 carb, 1 fat
Lite Olive Oil Vinaigrette	2 Tbsp	60	6	50	1	0	0	240	3	0	0	1 fat
Kraft												
Catalina	2 Tbsp	130	11	100	1.5	0	0	380	7	0	0	1/2 carb, 2 fat

	Serving	Cal	Fat	Fat Cal	Sat Fat		Chol	Sod	Carb	Fiber	Sugar	Exchanges
Classic Caesar	2 Tbsp	130	12	110	2.5	0	15	380	2	0	2	2 fat
Honey Dijon Vinaigrette	2 Tbsp	90	7	60	0.5	0	0	340	6	0	<1	1/2 carb, 1 fat
Ranch	2 Tbsp	120	12	110	2	0	5	370	3	0	0	2 fat
Roka Blue Cheese	2 Tbsp	120	13	120	2	0	5	380	1	0	0	3 fat
Thousand Island	2 Tbsp	110	10	90	1.5	0	0	330	5	0	0	2 fat
Three Cheese Ranch	2 Tbsp	120	12	110	2	0	0	360	3	0	0	2 fat
Zesty Italian	2 Tbsp	70	6	50	1	0	0	370	3	0	0	1 fat
Kraft Free (Fat Free)												
Catalina	2 Tbsp	50	0	0	0	0	0	350	11	0	0	1 carb
French	2 Tbsp	45	0	0	0	0	0	290	11	0	0	1 carb
Honey Dijon	2 Tbsp	50	0	0	0	0	0	330	12	0	0	1 carb
Ranch	2 Tbsp	50	0	0	0	0	0	330	11	0	0	1 carb
Kraft Light												
Caesar	2 Tbsp	60	4.5	40	1	0	10	320	3	0	0	1 fat
Ranch	2 Tbsp	80	6	60	1	0	10	440	7	0	0	1/2 carb, 1 fat
Red Wine Vinaigrette	2 Tbsp	45	4	35	0	0	0	310	3	0	0	1 fat

SALAD DRESSING

	Serving	Calories	Fat (g)	Cal. from Fat	Sat. Fat (g)	Trans Fat (g)	Chol. (mg)	Sod. (mg)	Carb. (g)	Fiber (g)	Prot. (g)	Servings/Exchanges
Thousand Island	2 Tbsp	60	3	20	0	0	10	340	11	0	0	1 carb
Three Cheese Ranch	2 Tbsp	70	8	70	1.5	0	0	450	2	0	0	2 fat
Kraft Miracle Whip, Mayonnaise												
Mayonnaise	1 Tbsp	90	10	90	1.5	0	5	70	0	0	0	2 fat
Mayonnaise, Fat Free	1 Tbsp	10	0	0	0	0	0	120	2	0	0	free
Mayonnaise, Light	1 Tbsp	45	4	35	0.5	0	5	95	2	0	0	1 fat
Mayonnaise, Reduced Fat with Olive Oil	1 Tbsp	45	4	35	0	0	0	95	2	0	0	1 fat
Miracle Whip	1 Tbsp	40	3.5	35	0.5	0	5	105	2	0	0	1 fat
Miracle Whip, Fat Free	1 Tbsp	15	0	0	0	0	0	125	3	0	0	free
Miracle Whip, Light	1 Tbsp	25	1.5	15	0	0	5	140	3	0	0	free
Litehouse												
Big Bleu	2 Tbsp	160	17	150	2	0	15	230	1	0	1	3 fat
Coleslaw	2 Tbsp	100	8	70	0.5	0	5	120	8	0	0	1/2 carb, 2 fat

Creamy Asian	2 Tbsp	130	13	110	1	0	10	170	4	0	0	3 fat
Creamy Cilantro	2 Tbsp	110	10	90	1	0	10	230	3	0	1	2 fat
Lite Bleu Cheese	2 Tbsp	70	6	60	0.5	0	5	240	2	0	1	1 fat
Lite Ranch	2 Tbsp	60	6	50	0.5	0	10	230	3	0	1	1 fat
Original Bleu Cheese	2 Tbsp	150	16	140	1.5	0	15	220	1	0	1	3 fat
Parmesan Caesar	2 Tbsp	100	10	90	1	0	5	220	3	0	1	2 fat
Ranch	2 Tbsp	120	12	110	1	0	10	220	2	0	1	2 fat
Sesame Ginger, Fat Free	2 Tbsp	35	0	0	0	0	0	230	8	0	0	1/2 carb
Spinach Salad	2 Tbsp	50	0	0	0	0	0	260	11	0	1	1 carb
Sweet & Sour	2 Tbsp	70	3.5	30	0	0	5	240	9	0	0	1/2 carb, 1 fat
Tangy Orange Citrus, Fat Free	2 Tbsp	50	0	0	0	0	0	190	13	0	0	1 carb
Thai Peanut	2 Tbsp	60	3	30	0	0	0	280	6	1	1	1/2 carb, 1 fat
Maple Grove Farms of Vermont												
Fat Free Balsamic Vinaigrette	2 Tbsp	5	0	0	0	0	0	160	1	0	0	free

SALAD DRESSING

	Serving	Calories	Fat (g)	Cal. from Fat	Sat. Fat (g)	Trans Fat (g)	Chol. (mg)	Sod. (mg)	Carb. (g)	Fiber (g)	Prot. (g)	Servings/Exchanges
Fat Free Cranberry Balsamic	2 Tbsp	20	0	0	0	0	0	180	7	0	0	1/2 carb
Fat Free Honey Dijon	2 Tbsp	40	0	0	0	0	0	200	10	<1	0	1 carb
Honey Mustard	2 Tbsp	100	8	70	0.5	0	0	260	8	0	<1	1/2 carb, 2 fat
Light Caesar	2 Tbsp	60	4.5	40	1	0	5	270	4	0	0	1 fat
Light Romano	2 Tbsp	40	3.5	30	0	0	0	260	1	0	<1	1 fat
Parmesan & Cracked Pepper	2 Tbsp	120	11	100	1	0	0	360	3	0	<1	2 fat
Marie's												
Balsamic Vinaigrette	2 Tbsp	50	4.5	40	0.5	0	0	220	3	0	0	1 fat
Caesar	2 Tbsp	170	19	170	3.5	0	15	170	1	0	1	4 fat
Chunky Blue Cheese	2 Tbsp	160	17	150	3.5	0	15	170	0	0	1	3 fat
Coleslaw	2 Tbsp	150	13	120	2	0	10	170	8	0	0	1/2 carb, 3 fat
Creamy Ranch	2 Tbsp	170	19	170	3	0	15	150	1	0	1	4 fat

	Serving										Exchanges
Italian Vinaigrette	2 Tbsp	80	8	70	1.5	0	0	350	3	0	0	2 fat
Lite Chunky Blue Cheese	2 Tbsp	80	6	60	1.5	0	5	280	7	4	1	1/2 carb, 1 fat
Lite Creamy Ranch	2 Tbsp	90	6	60	1	0	5	240	6	0	1	1/2 carb, 1 fat
Poppy Seed	2 Tbsp	150	13	120	2	0	10	170	8	0	0	1/2 carb, 3 fat
Premium Spinach Salad	2 Tbsp	70	1.5	15	0	0	0	330	13	0	1	1 carb
Raspberry Vinaigrette	2 Tbsp	40	0.5	5	0	0	0	60	8	0	0	1/2 carb
Red Wine Vinaigrette	2 Tbsp	60	4.5	40	0.5	0	0	210	6	0	0	1/2 carb, 1 fat
Thousand Island	2 Tbsp	150	15	140	2.5	0	15	210	4	0	0	3 fat
Yogurt Feta Cheese	2 Tbsp	70	7	60	1.5	0	15	190	2	0	1	1 fat

Newman's Own

	Serving										Exchanges
Balsamic Vinaigrette	2 Tbsp	90	9	80	1	0	0	350	3	0	0	2 fat
Caesar	2 Tbsp	150	16	140	1.5	0	0	420	1	0	1	3 fat
Family Recipe Italian	2 Tbsp	120	13	120	1	0	0	400	1	0	1	3 fat
Olive Oil & Vinegar	2 Tbsp	150	16	150	2.5	0	0	150	1	0	0	3 fat
Ranch	2 Tbsp	140	15	130	2	0	10	250	2	0	0	3 fat

SALAD DRESSING

	Serving	Calories	Fat (g)	Cal. from Fat	Sat. Fat (g)	Trans Fat (g)	Chol. (mg)	Sod. (mg)	Carb. (g)	Fiber (g)	Prot. (g)	Servings/Exchanges
Newman's Own Lighten Up												
Balsamic Vinaigrette	2 Tbsp	45	4	40	0.5	0	0	470	2	0	0	1 fat
Caesar	2 Tbsp	70	6	50	1	0	5	520	3	0	1	1 fat
Honey Mustard	2 Tbsp	70	4	35	0.5	0	0	290	7	0	0	1 fat
Italian	2 Tbsp	60	6	50	1	0	0	260	0	0	0	1 fat
Raspberry & Walnut	2 Tbsp	70	5	45	0.5	0	0	120	7	0	0	1/2 carb, 1 fat
Rao's Homemade												
8 Star Balsamic	2 Tbsp	140	14	130	1.5	0	0	240	2	0	0	3 fat
Caesar Salad	2 Tbsp	80	8	70	1	0	0	310	2	0	1	2 fat
Italian Herb	2 Tbsp	80	8	70	0.5	0	0	370	2	0	0	2 fat
Roasted Garlic Vinaigrette	2 Tbsp	140	16	140	1.5	0	0	180	1	0	0	3 fat
Seven Seas												
Creamy Italian	2 Tbsp	110	12	110	2	0	0	510	2	0	0	2 fat

Green Goddess	2 Tbsp	130	13	120	2	0	0	260	2	0	0	3 fat
Red Wine Vinaigrette	2 Tbsp	90	9	80	1	0	0	470	2	0	0	2 fat
Viva Italian Fat Free	2 Tbsp	15	0	0	0	0	0	480	2	0	0	free
Viva Italian Reduced Fat	2 Tbsp	45	4	35	0.5	0	0	370	2	0	0	1 fat
Viva Robust Italian	2 Tbsp	90	9	80	0.5	0	0	380	2	0	0	2 fat
South Beach												
Italian with Extra Virgin Olive Oil	2 Tbsp	50	4.5	40	0	0	0	300	3	0	0	1 fat
Ranch	2 Tbsp	70	7	60	1	0	0	300	2	0	1	1 fat
Trader Joe's												
Balsamic Vinaigrette	2 Tbsp	80	6	60	0	0	0	60	5	0	0	1 fat
Fat Free Balsamic Vinaigrette	2 Tbsp	25	0	0	0	0	0	170	6	0	0	1/2 carb
Goddess	2 Tbsp	130	13	120	1	0	0	320	1	0	1	3 fat
Organic Red Wine & Olive Oil Vinaigrette	2 Tbsp	140	15	140	2	0	0	190	0	0	0	3 fat

SALAD DRESSING

	Serving	Calories	Fat (g)	Cal. from Fat	Sat. Fat (g)	Trans Fat (g)	Chol. (mg)	Sod. (mg)	Carb. (g)	Fiber (g)	Prot. (g)	Servings/Exchanges
Raspberry Vinaigrette	2 Tbsp	35	1.5	15	0	0	0	75	5	0	0	1 fat
Romano Caesar	2 Tbsp	180	20	180	1.5	0	1	150	<1	0	<1	4 fat
Sesame Soy Ginger Vinaigrette	2 Tbsp	35	0	0	0	0	0	230	9	0	0	1/2 carb
Sweet Poppyseed	2 Tbsp	90	5	45	0.5	0	0	45	11	0	0	1 carb, 1 fat
Tuscan Italian	2 Tbsp	80	7	60	0.5	0	0	240	5	0	0	1 fat
Vidalia												
Creamy Vidalia	2 Tbsp	60	4.5	40	0	0	0	160	7	0	0	1/2 carb, 1 fat
Honey Mustard	2 Tbsp	60	3.5	35	3.5	0	0	95	6	0	0	1/2 carb, 1 fat
Raspberry Vinaigrette	2 Tbsp	35	0	0	0	0	0	25	9	0	0	1/2 carb
Sun Dried Tomato	2 Tbsp	90	8	70	1	0	0	330	4	0	0	2 fat
Wish-Bone												
Blue Cheese with Gorgonzola	2 Tbsp	140	15	140	2.5	0	<5	300	1	0	0	3 fat

Chunky Blue Cheese	2 Tbsp	150	15	140	2.5	0	5	260	2	0	0	3 fat
Creamy Caesar	2 Tbsp	170	18	160	3	0	10	300	1	0	<1	4 fat
Creamy Italian	2 Tbsp	110	10	90	1.5	0	0	240	4	0	<1	2 fat
Deluxe French	2 Tbsp	120	11	100	1.5	0	0	170	5	0	<1	2 fat
Fat Free Western	2 Tbsp	50	0	0	0	0	0	280	12	0	0	1 carb
House Italian	2 Tbsp	100	10	90	1.5	0	5	260	3	0	0	2 fat
Italian	2 Tbsp	80	7	60	1	0	0	510	3	0	0	2 fat
Olive Oil Vinaigrette	2 Tbsp	60	5	45	0.5	0	0	250	4	0	0	1 fat
Ranch	2 Tbsp	120	13	120	2	0	5	250	2	0	0	3 fat
Raspberry Hazelnut Vinaigrette	2 Tbsp	80	5	45	0.5	0	0	260	9	0	0	1/2 carb, 1 fat
Red Wine Vinaigrette	2 Tbsp	80	5	45	1	0	0	240	9	0	0	1/2 carb, 1 fat
Russian	2 Tbsp	120	6	50	1	0	0	360	14	0	0	1 carb, 1 fat
Sweet & Spicy French	2 Tbsp	130	12	110	1.5	0	0	330	6	0	0	1/2 carb, 2 fat
Thousand Island	2 Tbsp	130	12	110	2	0	10	300	6	0	0	1/2 carb, 2 fat
Western	2 Tbsp	160	12	110	1.5	0	0	230	11	0	0	1 carb, 2 fat

SALAD DRESSING

	Serving	Calories	Fat (g)	Cal. from Fat	Sat. Fat (g)	Trans Fat (g)	Chol. (mg)	Sod. (mg)	Carb. (g)	Fiber (g)	Prot. (g)	Servings/Exchanges
Wish-Bone Fat Free												
Chunky Blue Cheese	2 Tbsp	35	0	0	0	0	0	270	7	<1	<1	1/2 carb
Italian	2 Tbsp	20	0	0	0	0	0	350	4	0	0	free
Ranch	2 Tbsp	30	0	0	0	0	0	280	7	<1	0	1/2 carb
Red Wine Vinaigrette	2 Tbsp	30	0	0	0	0	0	230	7	0	0	1/2 carb

SAUCES, GRAVIES, CONDIMENTS, RELISHES

	Serving	Calories	Fat (g)	Cal. from Fat	Sat. Fat (g)	Trans Fat (g)	Chol. (mg)	Sod. (mg)	Carb. (g)	Fiber (g)	Prot. (g)	Servings/Exchanges
Apple Butter	2 Tbsp	65	<1	0	<1	0	0	0	17	<1	<1	1 carb
Catsup/Ketchup	1 Tbsp	16	<1	0	<1	0	0	182	4	<1	<1	free
Catsup/Ketchup, Low Sodium	1 Tbsp	16	<1	0	<1	0	0	3	4	<1	<1	free
Chutney	1 Tbsp	26	<1	0	<1	0	0	38	7	<1	<1	1/2 carb
Gravy, Au Jus, Canned	1/2 cup	19	<1	0	<1	NA	0	60	3	0	1	free
Gravy, Beef, Canned	1/2 cup	62	3	27	1	NA	4	652	6	<1	4	1/2 carb, 1 fat
Gravy, Beef, Homemade	1/2 cup	89	5	45	2	0	3	767	7	<1	4	1/2 carb, 1 fat
Gravy, Brown, Dry Mix with Water	1/2 cup	38	<1	0	<1	0	1	538	7	<1	1	1/2 carb
Gravy, Chicken Giblet, Homemade	1/2 cup	97	5	45	1	0	55	683	6	<1	6	1/2 carb, 1 fat
Gravy, Chicken, Canned	1/2 cup	94	7	63	2	NA	2	687	7	<1	2	1/2 carb, 1 fat

SAUCES, GRAVIES, CONDIMENTS, RELISHES

	Serving	Calories	Fat (g)	Cal. from Fat	Sat. Fat (g)	Trans Fat (g)	Chol. (mg)	Sod. (mg)	Carb. (g)	Fiber (g)	Prot. (g)	Servings/Exchanges
Gravy, Mushroom, Canned	1/2 cup	60	6	54	<1	NA	0	678	7	<1	2	1/2 carb, 1 fat
Gravy, Sausage	1/2 cup	206	16	144	6	NA	33	408	8	<1	8	1/2 carb, 3 fat
Gravy, Turkey, Canned	1/2 cup	61	3	27	<1	NA	2	687	6	<1	3	1/2 starch, 1 fat
Guacamole with Tomatoes	1 Tbsp	17	2	17	<1	0	0	27	1	<1	<1	free
Honey	1 Tbsp	64	0	0	0	0	0	<1	17	<1	<1	1 carb
Horseradish, Prepared	1 Tbsp	7	<1	0	<1	0	0	47	2	<1	<1	free
Jam, Cherry/Strawberry	1 Tbsp	54	<1	0	0	0	0	2	14	<1	<1	1 carb
Jam/Marmalade, Artifically Sweetened	1 Tbsp	2	<1	0	<1	0	0	0	11	<1	<1	free
Jam/Marmalade, Reduced Sugar	1 Tbsp	36	<1	0	<1	0	0	5	9	<1	<1	1/2 carb
Jam/Preserves	1 Tbsp	48	<1	0	<1	0	0	8	13	<1	<1	1 carb

Food	Serving									
Jelly	1 Tbsp	52	<1	0	0	7	14	<1	<1	1 carb
Jelly, Blackberry	1 Tbsp	50	0	0	0	10	13	0	0	1 carb
Jelly, Dietetic	1 Tbsp	6	0	0	0	<1	11	<1	<1	free
Jelly, Reduced Sugar	1 Tbsp	34	<1	<1	0	<1	9	<1	<1	1/2 carb
Marmalade, Orange	1 Tbsp	49	0	0	0	11	13	<1	<1	1 carb
Mustard, Dijon	1 Tbsp	19	1	9	<1	379	2	<1	<1	free
Mustard, Honey	1 Tbsp	50	3	27	<1	91	7	<1	<1	1/2 carb
Mustard, Prepared	1 Tbsp	12	<1	0	<1	196	1	<1	<1	free
Olives, Green, Pitted	10	45	5	45	<1	936	<1	<1	<1	1 fat
Olives, Small Ripe	10	37	3	27	<1	279	2	1	<1	1 fat
Olives, Stuffed Green	10	41	5	41	<1	827	<1	<1	<1	1 fat
Peppers, Pickled Hot Jalapeño	2	8	<1	0	<1	121	2	<1	<1	free
Pickle Slices, Dill	10	11	<1	0	0	769	3	<1	<1	free
Pickle Slices, Dill, Low Sodium	10	11	<1	0	0	11	3	<1	<1	free

SAUCES, GRAVIES, CONDIMENTS, RELISHES

	Serving	Calories	Fat (g)	Cal. from Fat	Sat. Fat (g)	Trans Fat (g)	Chol. (mg)	Sod. (mg)	Carb. (g)	Fiber (g)	Prot. (g)	Servings/Exchanges
Pickle Slices, Fresh Pack	4	22	<1	0	0	0	0	202	5	<1	<1	free
Pickle Slices, Sour	10	8	<1	0	<1	0	0	846	2	<1	<1	free
Pickle, Dill	1	12	<1	0	<1	0	0	833	3	<1	<1	free
Pickle, Dill, Low Sodium	1	12	<1	0	<1	0	0	12	3	<1	<1	free
Pickle, Sour	1	4	<1	0	<1	0	0	423	<1	<1	<1	free
Pickle, Sweet	1 medium	41	<1	0	<1	0	0	329	11	<1	<1	1/2 carb
Relish, Hot Dog	1 Tbsp	14	<1	0	<1	0	0	167	4	<1	<1	free
Relish, Sweet Pickle	1 Tbsp	20	<1	0	<1	0	0	124	5	<1	<1	free
Sauce, Bearnaise, Homemade	1/2 cup	321	34	306	20	0	237	444	1	<1	2	7 fat
Sauce, Black Bean	1/2 cup	129	6	54	1	0	0	1322	14	2	3	1 starch, 1 fat
Sauce, Cheese	1/2 cup	221	16	144	10	0	36	515	9	<1	10	1/2 carb, 1 med-fat meat, 2 fat

Food	Serving											
Sauce, Curry	1/2 cup	74	6	54	1	0	0	392	3	<1	3	1 fat
Sauce, Hollandaise, Dry Mix & Water	1/2 cup	119	10	90	6	0	26	783	7	<1	2	1/2 carb, 2 fat
Sauce, Hot Chili/Red Pepper	2 Tbsp	7	<1	0	<1	0	0	8	1	<1	<1	free
Sauce, Hot Green Chili	1 Tbsp	6	<1	0	0	0	0	4	2	<1	<1	free
Sauce, Salsa/Mexican, Homemade	1/2 cup	23	<1	0	<1	0	0	468	5	1	<1	1 vegetable
Sauce, Soy	1 Tbsp	10	<1	0	0	0	0	1028	2	0	<1	free
Sauce, Spanish-Style Tomato	1/2 cup	40	<1	0	<1	0	0	576	9	2	2	1/2 carb
Sauce, Tartar	1 Tbsp	74	8	72	2	0	7	99	<1	<1	<1	2 fat
Sauce, Teriyaki	1 Tbsp	15	0	0	0	0	0	690	3	<1	1	free
Sauce, White, Homemade	1/2 cup	178	14	126	4	0	14	185	10	<1	4	1/2 starch, 3 fat
Sauce, Worcestershire	1 Tbsp	11	0	0	0	0	0	167	3	0	0	free

SAUCES, GRAVIES, CONDIMENTS, RELISHES

	Serving	Calories	Fat (g)	Cal. from Fat	Sat. Fat (g)	Trans Fat (g)	Chol. (mg)	Sod. (mg)	Carb. (g)	Fiber (g)	Prot. (g)	Servings/Exchanges
Syrup, Maple	1 Tbsp	52	<1	0	0	0	0	2	13	0	0	1 carb
Syrup, Pancake	1 Tbsp	57	0	0	0	0	0	17	15	0	0	1 carb
Brands												
A1 Steakhouse												
Marinade, Carb Well	1 Tbsp	5	0	0	0	0	0	230	1	0	0	free
Marinade, Chicago Steakhouse	1 Tbsp	20	1	10	0	0	0	270	3	0	0	free
Marinade, Ginger Teriyaki	1 Tbsp	25	0	0	0	0	0	490	5	0	0	free
Marinade, Jamaican Jerk	1 Tbsp	25	0.5	5	0	0	0	190	5	0	0	free
Marinade, New Orleans Cajun	1 Tbsp	25	0	0	0	0	0	180	5	0	0	free
Marinade, Texas Mesquite	1 Tbsp	15	0	0	0	0	0	400	4	0	0	free

Steak Sauce	1 Tbsp	15	0	0	0	0	280	3	0	0	free

Aunt Jemima

Butter Lite Syrup	1/4 cup	100	0	0	0	0	210	26	1	0	2 carb
Butter Rich Syrup	1/4 cup	210	0	0	0	0	210	53	0	0	3 1/2 carb
Country Rich Lite Syrup	1/4 cup	100	0	0	0	0	180	26	1	0	2 carb
Country Rich Syrup	1/4 cup	210	0	0	0	0	120	53	0	0	3 1/2 carb
Lite Syrup	1/4 cup	100	0	0	0	0	190	26	0	0	2 carb
Original Syrup	1/4 cup	210	0	0	0	0	120	52	0	0	3 1/2 carb

Betty Crocker

Bac-Os Bits or Chips	1 1/2 Tbsp	30	1.5	10	0	0	120	2	0	3	1 fat

Braswell's

Pear Preserves	1 Tbsp	30	0	0	0	0	0	7	0	0	1/2 carb
Red Pepper Jelly	1 Tbsp	35	0	0	0	0	0	9	0	0	1/2 carb

Campbell's

Gravy, Beef	1/4 cup	25	3	25	1	5	270	3	0	1	1 fat

SAUCES, GRAVIES, CONDIMENTS, RELISHES

	Serving	Calories	Fat (g)	Cal. from Fat	Sat. Fat (g)	Trans Fat (g)	Chol. (mg)	Sod. (mg)	Carb. (g)	Fiber (g)	Prot. (g)	Servings/Exchanges
Gravy, Chicken	1/4 cup	40	3	25	1	0	5	260	3	0	0	1 fat
Gravy, Country Style Cream Gravy	1/4 cup	45	3	25	1	0	5	190	3	0	1	1 fat
Gravy, Cream Style Sausage Gravy	1/4 cup	70	5	45	1.5	0	5	270	4	0	2	1 fat
Gravy, Turkey	1/4 cup	25	1	10	0.5	0	0	270	3	0	1	free
Cary's												
Syrup, Maple	1/4 cup	210	0	0	0	0	0	5	53	0	0	3 1/2 carb
Syrup, Sugar Free	1/4 cup	30	0	0	0	0	0	115	12	0	0	1 carb
Claussen												
Pickle Relish, Sweet	1 Tbsp	14	<1	0	<1	0	0	90	3	NA	<1	free
Pickles, Bread 'n Butter	1 oz	20	0	0	0	0	0	180	4	0	0	free
Pickles, Kosher Dill, Halves	1	5	0	0	0	0	0	270	1	0	0	free

Pickles, Kosher Dill Mini Dills	1	5	0	0	0	0	290	<1	<1	<1	free
Pickles, Kosher Dill Sandwich Slices	1	5	0	0	0	0	420	1	0	0	free
Pickles, Kosher Dill Spears	1	5	0	0	0	0	312	<1	0	0	free
Dynasty											
Bead Molasses	1 Tbsp	60	0	0	0	0	45	16	0	0	1 carb
Chinese Brown Gravy Sauce	1 Tbsp	60	0	0	0	0	65	14	0	0	1 carb
Hoisin Sauce	2 Tbsp	50	1	0	0	10	410	9	0	0	1/2 carb
Hot Chili Oil	1 tsp	40	4	0.5	40	0	0	0	0		1 fat
Spicy Hot Kung Pao Sauce	2 Tbsp	45	1.5	0	15	0	590	7	0	1	1/2 carb
Emeril's											
BAM! B-Q Sauce, Kicked Up	2 Tbsp	40	0	0	0	0	360	11	0	0	1 carb

SAUCES, GRAVIES, CONDIMENTS, RELISHES

	Serving	Calories	Fat (g)	Cal. from Fat	Sat. Fat (g)	Trans Fat (g)	Chol. (mg)	Sod. (mg)	Carb. (g)	Fiber (g)	Prot. (g)	Servings/Exchanges
BAM! B-Q Sauce, Sweet	2 Tbsp	45	0	0	0	0	0	390	12	0	0	1 carb
Dijon Mustard	1 Tbsp	5	0	0	0	0	0	120	1	0	0	free
Famous Dave's												
BBQ Sauce, Devil's Spit	2 Tbsp	50	0	0	0	0	0	350	12	<1	0	1 carb
BBQ Sauce, Rich & Sassy	2 Tbsp	60	0	0	0	0	0	350	15	<1	0	1 carb
BBQ Sauce, Sweet & Zesty	2 Tbsp	70	0	0	0	0	0	320	17	0	0	1 carb
Fifty50												
Sugar Free, Low Calorie, Strawberry Spread	1 Tbsp	5	0	0	0	0	0	25	3	0	0	free
Franco-American												
Gravy, Slow Roast Beef	1/4 cup	25	0.5	5	0	0	5	310	3	0	1	free

Gravy, Slow Roast Chicken	1/4 cup	20	0.5	5	0	0	<5	240	3	0	1	free
Gravy, Slow Roast Turkey	1/4 cup	25	0	0	0	0	<5	320	4	0	1	free
Grey Poupon											
Country Dijon Mustard	1 tsp	5	0	0	0	0	0	120	0	0	0	free
Heinz											
57 Sauce	1 Tbsp	20	0	0	0	0	0	190	4	0	0	free
Chili Sauce	1 Tbsp	20	0	0	0	0	0	230	5	0	0	free
Cocktail Sauce	1/4 cup	60	0	0	0	0	0	690	15	0	1	1 carb
Gravy, Home Style Classic Chicken	1/4 cup	30	2	20	0.5	0	<5	250	3	0	0	1 fat
Gravy, Home Style Rich Mushroom	1/4 cup	20	0.5	5	0	0	0	320	3	0	<1	free
Gravy, Home Style Roasted Turkey	1/4 cup	25	1	0	0	0	<5	290	3	0	1	free

SAUCES, GRAVIES, CONDIMENTS, RELISHES

	Serving	Calories	Fat (g)	Cal. from Fat	Sat. Fat (g)	Trans Fat (g)	Chol. (mg)	Sod. (mg)	Carb. (g)	Fiber (g)	Prot. (g)	Servings/Exchanges
Gravy, Home Style Savory Beef	1/4 cup	30	1	10	0.5	0	<5	390	4	0	1	1 fat
Worcestershire Sauce	1 tsp	0	0	0	0	0	0	60	0	0	0	free
Hormel												
Real Bacon Bits	1 Tbsp	25	1.5	15	1	0	5	240	0	0	3	1 fat
Real Bacon Pieces	1 Tbsp	25	1.5	15	0.5	0	5	200	0	0	3	1 fat
Hunt's												
BBQ Sauce, Hickory & Brown Sugar	2 Tbsp	70	0	0	0	0	0	390	18	<1	0	1 carb
BBQ Sauce, Honey Hickory	2 Tbsp	50	0	0	0	0	0	420	13	<1	0	1 carb
BBQ Sauce, Original	2 Tbsp	60	0	0	0	0	0	280	15	<1	0	1 carb
Jack Daniels												
Barbecue Sauce, Hickory Brown Sugar	2 Tbsp	50	0	0	0	0	0	290	13	0	0	1 carb

	Serving									
Barbecue Sauce, Honey Smokehouse	2 Tbsp	50	0	0	0	290	12	0	0	1 carb
Steak Sauce, Original	1 Tbsp	50	0	0	0	290	12	0	0	1 carb
Karo										
Dark Corn Syrup	2 Tbsp	120	0	0	0	45	31	0	0	2 carb
Light Corn Syrup	2 Tbsp	120	0	0	0	35	30	0	0	2 carb
Lite Syrup	2 Tbsp	80	0	0	0	80	20	0	0	1 carb
Pancake Syrup	4 Tbsp	240	0	0	0	85	63	0	0	4 carb
KC Masterpiece										
Barbecue Sauce, Hickory Brown Sugar	2 Tbsp	60	0	0	0	320	15	0	0	1 carb
Barbecue Sauce, Mesquite	2 Tbsp	60	0	0	0	260	14	0	0	1 carb
Barbecue Sauce, Original	2 Tbsp	60	0	0	0	240	15	0	0	1 carb
Marinade, Caribbean Jerk	1 Tbsp	25	0	0	0	320	6	0	0	1/2 carb

SAUCES, GRAVIES, CONDIMENTS, RELISHES

	Serving	Calories	Fat (g)	Cal. from Fat	Sat. Fat (g)	Trans Fat (g)	Chol. (mg)	Sod. (mg)	Carb. (g)	Fiber (g)	Prot. (g)	Servings/Exchanges
Marinade, Garlic & Herb	1 Tbsp	30	1	10	0	0	0	220	5	0	0	1/2 carb
Marinade, Honey Teriyaki	1 Tbsp	40	0.5	5	0	0	0	360	9	0	<1	1/2 carb
Marinade, Lemon Pepper	1 Tbsp	40	1.5	15	0	0	0	310	7	0	0	1/2 carb
Marinade, Roasted Garlic Balsamic	1 Tbsp	15	0	0	0	0	0	220	4	0	0	free
Kitchen Bouquet												
Browning & Seasoning Sauce	1 tsp	15	0	0	0	0	0	10	3	0	0	free
Knott's Berry Farm												
Apple Cinnamon Jelly	1 Tbsp	50	0	0	0	0	0	0	13	0	0	1 carb
Apricot Preserves	1 Tbsp	50	0	0	0	0	0	0	13	0	0	1 carb
Bing Cherry Preserves	1 Tbsp	50	0	0	0	0	0	0	13	0	0	1 carb

Boysenberry Light Preserves	1 Tbsp	20	0	0	0	0	0	5	0	0	free
Boysenberry Preserves	1 Tbsp	50	0	0	0	0	0	13	0	0	1 carb
California Plum Jam	1 Tbsp	50	0	0	0	0	0	13	0	0	1 carb
Jalapeño Jelly	1 Tbsp	50	0	0	0	0	0	13	0	0	1 carb
Mint Flavored Apple Jelly	1 Tbsp	50	0	0	0	0	0	13	0	0	1 carb
Red Currant Jelly	1 Tbsp	50	0	0	0	0	10	13	0	0	1 carb
Seedless Blackberry Jam	1 Tbsp	50	0	0	0	0	0	13	0	0	1 carb
Seedless Red Raspberry Jam	1 Tbsp	50	0	0	0	0	0	13	0	0	1 carb
Strawberry Preserves	1 Tbsp	50	0	0	0	0	0	13	0	0	1 carb
Kraft											
Barbecue Sauce, Hickory Smoke	2 Tbsp	60	0	0	0	0	430	13	0	0	1 carb
Barbecue Sauce, Honey	2 Tbsp	50	0	0	0	0	360	13	0	0	1 carb

SAUCES, GRAVIES, CONDIMENTS, RELISHES

	Serving	Calories	Fat (g)	Cal. from Fat	Sat. Fat (g)	Trans Fat (g)	Chol. (mg)	Sod. (mg)	Carb. (g)	Fiber (g)	Prot. (g)	Servings/Exchanges
Barbecue Sauce, Honey Hickory Smoke	2 Tbsp	70	0	0	0	0	0	460	16	0	0	1 carb
Barbecue Sauce, Honey Roasted Garlic	2 Tbsp	50	0	0	0	0	0	350	12	0	0	1 carb
Barbecue Sauce, Light Original	2 Tbsp	20	0	0	0	0	0	340	5	0	0	free
Barbecue Sauce, Mesquite Smoke	2 Tbsp	50	0	0	0	0	0	450	12	0	0	1 carb
Barbecue Sauce, Original	2 Tbsp	50	0	0	0	0	0	440	12	0	0	1 carb
Sauce, Cocktail	1/4 cup	60	0.5	5	0	0	0	880	11	1	1	1 carb
Sauce, Coleslaw Maker	1/4 cup	110	9	80	1.5	10	0	230	7	0	0	1/2 carb, 2 fat
Sauce, Horseradish	1 tsp	15	1.5	15	0	0	0	40	1	0	0	free
Sauce, Sweet & Sour	2 Tbsp	60	0	0	0	0	0	130	13	0	0	1 carb
Sauce, Tartar	2 Tbsp	60	4.5	40	0.5	0	5	230	4	0	0	1 fat

Sauce, Tartar, Fat Free	2 Tbsp	25	0	0	0	200	5	0	0	free
Sauce, Tartar, Lemon & Herb	2 Tbsp	150	16	2.5	15	170	1	0	0	3 fat
La Choy										
Marinade & Sauce, Teriyaki	1 Tbsp	40	0	0	0	570	10	0	<1	1/2 carb
Sauce, Soy	1 Tbsp	10	0	0	0	1160	1	0	1	free
Sauce, Soy, Lite	1 Tbsp	15	0	0	0	550	2	0	1	free
Sauce, Sweet & Sour	1 Tbsp	60	0	0	0	110	14	0	0	1 carb
La Victoria										
Enchilada Sauce, Green	1/4 cup	15	0	0	0	310	3	0	0	free
Enchilada Sauce, Red	1/4 cup	15	2	0	0	310	2	0	0	free
Taco Sauce, Green	1 Tbsp	0	0	0	0	70	<1	0	0	free
Taco Sauce, Red	1 Tbsp	5	0	0	0	90	1	0	0	free
Las Palmas										
Enchilada Sauce, Green	1/4 cup	25	1.5	0	0	340	1	0	0	free

SAUCES, GRAVIES, CONDIMENTS, RELISHES

	Serving	Calories	Fat (g)	Cal. from Fat	Sat. Fat (g)	Trans Fat (g)	Chol. (mg)	Sod. (mg)	Carb. (g)	Fiber (g)	Prot. (g)	Servings/Exchanges
Enchilada Sauce, Original Style	1/4 cup	15	0.5	5	0	0	0	330	2	1	0	free
Sauce, Red Chile	1/4 cup	15	0	0	0	0	0	330	2	1	0	free
Lawry's												
Marinade, Baja Chipotle	1 Tbsp	15	0	0	0	0	0	390	4	0	0	free
Marinade, Herb & Garlic	1 Tbsp	10	0	0	0	0	0	420	2	0	0	free
Marinade, Lemon Pepper	1 Tbsp	10	0	0	0	0	0	390	2	0	0	free
Marinade, Mesquite	1 Tbsp	5	0	0	0	0	0	350	1	0	0	free
Marinade, Sesame Ginger	1 Tbsp	30	0	0	0	0	0	580	7	0	0	1/2 carb
Marinade, Tequila Lime	1 Tbsp	15	0	0	0	0	0	490	4	0	0	free
Marinade, Teriyaki	1 Tbsp	20	0	0	0	0	0	560	5	0	0	free
Log Cabin												
Original Syrup	1/4 cup	210	0	0	0	0	0	105	52	0	0	3 1/2 carb

Sugar Free Syrup	1/4 cup	30	0	0	0	0	110	11	0	0	1 carb

Maple Grove Farms Cozy Cottage

Blueberry Syrup	1/4 cup	210	0	0	0	0	120	52	0	0	3 1/2 carb
Maple Syrup	1/4 cup	200	0	0	0	0	5	53	0	0	3 1/2 carb

McCormick

Bac'n Pieces, Bits	1 Tbsp	30	1	10	0	0	180	2	0	3	1 fat
Salad Toppins	1 1/3 Tbsp	35	1.5	15	0	0	70	3	0	2	1 fat

Mezzetta

Cocktail Onions	8 pieces	5	0	0	0	0	300	1	0	0	free
Garlic Olives	1	10	1	10	0	0	140	0	0	0	free
Grape Leaves	1 leaf	5	0	0	0	0	100	1	0	0	free
Jalapeño Stuffed Olives	1	10	1	10	0	0	140	1	0	0	free
Martini Olives	1	10	1	10	0	0	170	1	0	0	free
Roasted Bell Peppers	1 1/2 Tbsp	10	0	0	0	0	110	1	0	0	free

SAUCES, GRAVIES, CONDIMENTS, RELISHES

	Serving	Calories	Fat (g)	Cal. from Fat	Sat. Fat (g)	Trans Fat (g)	Chol. (mg)	Sod. (mg)	Carb. (g)	Fiber (g)	Prot. (g)	Servings/Exchanges
Sliced Jalapeño Peppers	1/4 cup	5	0	0	0	0	0	380	1	0	0	free
Spanish Queen Olives	1	10	1	10	0	0	0	170	1	1	0	free
Sweet Banana Peppers	3	10	0	0	0	0	0	320	1	0	0	free
Sweet Cherry Peppers Relish	3 pieces	15	0.5	5	0	0	0	340	2	1	1	free
Mrs. Butterworth's												
Original Syrup	1/4 cup	210	0	0	0	0	0	115	53	0	0	3 1/2 carb
Mrs. Dash												
10 Minute Marinade, Lemon Herb Peppercorn	1 Tbsp	25	2	20	0	0	0	0	2	0	0	free
10 Minute Marinade, Mesquite Grille	1 Tbsp	25	1.5	15	0	0	0	0	2	0	0	free

10 Minute Marinade, Southwest Chipotle	1 Tbsp	20	1.5	15	0	0	0	2	0	0	free
10 Minute Marinade, Zesty Garlic Herb	1 Tbsp	25	2	20	0	0	0	3	0	0	free
Musselman's										
Apple Butter	1 Tbsp	30	0	0	0	0	0	8	0	0	1/2 carb
Old El Paso										
Enchilada Sauce, Green Chile Mild	1/4 cup	25	1.5	15	0	0	280	4	0	0	free
Enchilada Sauce, Mild	1/4 cup	20	0	0	0	0	360	3	0	0	free
Taco Sauce, Hot	1 Tbsp	5	0	0	0	0	90	1	0	0	free
Taco Sauce, Medium	1 Tbsp	5	0	0	0	0	90	1	0	0	free
Taco Sauce, Mild	1 Tbsp	5	0	0	0	0	90	1	0	0	free
Ortega										
Enchilada Sauce	1/4 cup	10	0.5	5	0	0	340	4	<1	<1	free
Sauce Picante, Mild	1/4 cup	10	0	0	0	0	220	2	0	1	free

SAUCES, GRAVIES, CONDIMENTS, RELISHES

	Serving	Calories	Fat (g)	Cal. from Fat	Sat. Fat (g)	Trans Fat (g)	Chol. (mg)	Sod. (mg)	Carb. (g)	Fiber (g)	Prot. (g)	Servings/Exchanges
Taco Sauce, Original	1 Tbsp	10	0	0	0	0	0	60	1	0	0	free
Oscar Mayer												
Bacon Bits	1 Tbsp	25	1.5	15	0.5	0	5	170	0	0	2	free
Polaner												
All Fruit Strawberry Spread	1 Tbsp	40	0	0	0	0	0	0	10	0	0	1/2 carb
Strawberry Preserves	1 Tbsp	50	0	0	0	0	0	0	13	0	0	1 carb
Sugar Free Strawberry Preserves	1 Tbsp	10	0	0	0	0	0	0	5	0	0	free
Progresso												
Artichoke Hearts, Marinated	2 pieces	60	5	45	1	0.5	0	110	2	0	0	1 fat
Sauce, Lobster	1/2 cup	100	7	60	1	0	5	430	6	2	3	1/2 carb, 1 fat
Sauce, Red Clam with Tomato & Basil	1/2 cup	60	1	10	0	0	10	350	8	1	4	1 carb

Sauce, White Clam, Deluxe	1/2 cup	150	10	90	1.5	0	20	710	5	0	9	1 med-fat meat, 1 fat

Regina

Cooking Wine, Red	1/4 cup	20	1	9	0	0	0	365	1	0	1	free
Cooking Wine, Sherry	1/4 cup	20	0	0	0	0	0	70	5	0	1	free
Vinegar, Red Wine	1 oz	4	0	0	0	0	0	0	0	0	0	free
Vinegar, White Wine	1 oz	4	0	0	0	0	0	0	1	0	0	free

Smucker's

Apricot Preserves	1 Tbsp	50	0	0	0	0	0	0	13	0	0	1 carb
Apricot-Pineapple Preserves	1 Tbsp	50	0	0	0	0	0	0	13	0	0	1 carb
Blueberry Syrup	1/4 cup	210	0	0	0	0	0	0	52	0	0	3 1/2 carb
Boysenberry Preserves	1 Tbsp	50	0	0	0	0	0	0	13	0	0	1 carb
Boysenberry Syrup	1/4 cup	210	0	0	0	0	0	0	52	0	0	3 1/2 carb
Cider Apple Butter	1 Tbsp	45	0	0	0	0	0	10	11	0	0	1 carb
Concord Grape Jam	1 Tbsp	50	0	0	0	0	0	0	13	0	0	1 carb

SAUCES, GRAVIES, CONDIMENTS, RELISHES

	Serving	Calories	Fat (g)	Cal. from Fat	Sat. Fat (g)	Trans Fat (g)	Chol. (mg)	Sod. (mg)	Carb. (g)	Fiber (g)	Prot. (g)	Servings/Exchanges
Currant Jelly	1 Tbsp	50	0	0	0	0	0	0	13	0	0	1 carb
Low Sugar Apricot	1 Tbsp	25	0	0	0	0	0	0	6	0	0	1/2 carb
Low Sugar Apricot Preserves	1 Tbsp	25	0	0	0	0	0	0	6	0	0	1/2 carb
Low Sugar Concord Grape Jelly	1 Tbsp	25	0	0	0	0	0	0	6	0	0	1/2 carb
Low Sugar Strawberry Preserves	1 Tbsp	25	0	0	0	0	0	0	6	0	0	1/2 carb
Red Raspberry Preserves	1 Tbsp	50	0	0	0	0	0	0	13	0	0	1 carb
Reduced Sugar Sweet Orange Marmalade	1 Tbsp	25	0	0	0	0	0	0	6	0	0	1/2 carb
Seedless Strawberry Jam	1 Tbsp	50	0	0	0	0	0	0	13	0	0	1 carb

Simply Fruit Spreadable Fruit, Strawberry	1 Tbsp	40	0	0	0	0	0	10	0	1/2 carb
Squeeze Grape Jelly	1 Tbsp	50	0	0	0	5	0	13	0	1 carb
Squeeze Strawberry Fruit Spread	1 Tbsp	50	0	0	0	0	0	13	0	1 carb
Strawberry Preserves	1 Tbsp	50	0	0	0	0	0	13	0	1 carb
Sugar Free Blackberry with Splenda	1 Tbsp	10	0	0	0	0	0	5	0	free
Sugar Free Strawberry with Nutra Sweet	1 Tbsp	10	0	0	0	0	0	5	0	free
Sweet Orange Marmalade Preserves	1 Tbsp	50	0	0	0	0	0	13	0	1 carb
Tabasco										
Sauce, Green Pepper	1 tsp	0	0	0	0	150	0	0	0	free
Sauce, Pepper	1 tsp	0	0	0	0	35	0	0	0	free
Trappey's Red Devil										
Cayenne Pepper Sauce	1 tsp	0	0	0	0	150	0	0	0	free

SAUCES, GRAVIES, CONDIMENTS, RELISHES

	Serving	Calories	Fat (g)	Cal. from Fat	Sat. Fat (g)	Trans Fat (g)	Chol. (mg)	Sod. (mg)	Carb. (g)	Fiber (g)	Prot. (g)	Servings/Exchanges
Vermont												
Sugar Free Low Calorie Syrup	1/4 cup	25	0	0	0	0	0	110	7	0	0	1/2 carb
Vlasic												
Sweet Gherkins	1 oz	35	0	0	0	0	0	170	9	0	0	1/2 carb
Sweet Relish	1 Tbsp	15	0	0	0	0	0	140	4	0	0	free
Welch's												
Concord Grape Jam	1 Tbsp	50	0	0	0	0	0	10	13	0	0	1 carb
Concord Grape Jelly	1 Tbsp	50	0	0	0	0	0	10	13	0	0	1 carb
Squeezable Concord Grape Jelly	1 Tbsp	50	0	0	0	0	0	10	13	0	0	1 carb
Squeezable Strawberry Spread	1 Tbsp	50	0	0	0	0	0	10	13	0	0	1 carb
Strawberry Spread	1 Tbsp	50	0	0	0	0	0	10	13	0	0	1 carb

SNACKS, CRACKERS, CHIPS, POPCORN, SNACK BARS

	Serving	Calories	Fat (g)	Cal. from Fat	Sat. Fat (g)	Trans Fat (g)	Chol. (mg)	Sod. (mg)	Carb. (g)	Fiber (g)	Prot. (g)	Servings/Exchanges
Chips, Bagel	5	298	7	63	1	0	0	419	52	6	6	3 1/2 starch, 1 fat
Chips, Potato	3/4 oz	114	7	65	2	0	0	171	11	<1	2	1 starch, 1 fat
Chips, Potato, Baked	3/4 oz	82	1	10	0	0	0	112	17	1.5	2	1 starch
Chips, Potato, Fat Free	3/4 oz	56	0	0	0	0	0	150	14	<1	2	1 starch
Crackers, Animal	8	89	3	25	0.5	0	0	79	15	0	1	1 starch
Crackers, Graham	3 squares	99	2	20	<1	0	0	142	18	<1	2	1 starch
Crackers, Matzoh, Plain	3/4 oz	83	<1	0	<1	0	0	0	18	<1	2	1 starch
Crackers, Oyster	20	86	2	20	<1	0	0	214	14	<1	2	1 starch
Crackers, Round Butter Type	6	90	5	45	0.5	0	0	152	11	<1	1	1 starch, 1 fat
Crackers, Saltines	6	77	2	20	<1	0	0	193	13	0.5	2	1 starch
Crackers, Whole Wheat, Baked	5	89	3.5	30	<1	0	0	132	14	2	2	1 starch, 1 fat

SNACKS, CRACKERS, CHIPS, POPCORN

	Serving	Calories	Fat (g)	Cal. from Fat	Sat. Fat (g)	Trans Fat (g)	Chol. (mg)	Sod. (mg)	Carb. (g)	Fiber (g)	Prot. (g)	Servings/Exchanges
Crackers, Whole Wheat, Reduced Fat	5	80	2	20	<1	0	0	110	15	2.5	2	1 starch
Crispbread	2 slices	73	<1	0	0	0	0	53	16	3	2	1 starch
Granola Bar	1	134	6	55	1	0	0	83	18	1.5	3	1 starch, 1 fat
Granola Bar, Chewy, Low Fat	1	109	2	20	0.5	0	0	70	22	1	1	1 1/2 starch
Meal Replacement Bar, Small	1 1/3 oz bar	140	4	35	2	0	2	75	22	4	6	1 1/2 starch, 1 fat
Meal Replacement Bar, Medium	2 oz bar	202	5	45	3	0	2	130	27	2	12	2 carb, 1 med-fat meat
Melba Toast	4 pieces	78	<1	0	0	0	0	166	15	1	2	1 starch
Oriental Snack Mix	1 oz	155	12	108	5	0	0	235	9	4	5	1/2 starch, 2 fat
Pita Chips	3/4 oz	86	3	25	1	0	0	246	12	<1	2	1 starch, 1 fat
Popcorn, Microwave, 94% Fat Free	3 cups	65	1	10	<1	0	0	155	14	2.5	2	1 starch

	Serving Size	Cal.	Fat (g)	% Cal. Fat	Sat. Fat (g)	Chol. (mg)	Sod. (mg)	Carb. (g)	Fiber (g)	Prot. (g)	Exchanges/Choices
Popcorn, Microwave, Butter	3 cups	96	6	55	3	0	216	11	2	2	1 starch, 1 fat
Popcorn, No Salt Added	3 cup	93	1	10	0	0	2	19	3.5	3	1 starch
Pretzels, Sticks or Rings	3/4 oz	80	<1	0	0	0	360	17	<1	2	1 starch
Rice Cakes	2	70	<1	0	0	0	59	15	<1	2	1 starch
Sandwich Crackers, Cheese Filled	3	100	4	35	1	0	294	13	<1	2	1 starch, 1 fat
Sandwich Crackers, Peanut Butter	3	102	5	45	1	0	198	12	<1	2	1 starch, 1 fat
Tortilla Chips	3/4 oz	106	6	55	1	0	131	13	<1	2	1 starch, 1 fat
Tortilla Chips, Fat Free	3/4 oz	82	<1	0	0	0	111	18	3	2	1 starch
Trail Mix, Fruit Based	1 oz	115	5	45	2	0	3	19	2	2	1 starch, 1 fat

Brands

Act II Microwave Popcorn

	Serving Size	Cal.	Fat (g)	% Cal. Fat	Sat. Fat (g)	Chol. (mg)	Sod. (mg)	Carb. (g)	Fiber (g)	Prot. (g)	Exchanges/Choices
94% Fat Free Butter Popcorn	3 Tbsp	130	2.5	20	0.5	0	310	28	5	4	2 starch, 1 fat

SNACKS, CRACKERS, CHIPS, POPCORN

	Serving	Calories	Fat (g)	Cal. from Fat	Sat. Fat (g)	Trans Fat (g)	Chol. (mg)	Sod. (mg)	Carb. (g)	Fiber (g)	Prot. (g)	Servings/Exchanges
94% Fat Free Kettle Corn	3 Tbsp	130	2.5	20	1	0	0	370	28	5	4	2 starch, 1 fat
Light Butter Popcorn	2 Tbsp	110	4.5	40	2	0	0	400	19	3	3	1 starch, 1 fat
Movie Theatre Pop 'n Serve Tub	2 Tbsp	160	10	90	2	4.5	0	300	18	3	3	1 starch, 2 fat
Austin												
Cheese Crackers with Cheddar Cheese	1 pkg	190	10	90	2.5	0	0	350	23	<1	3	1 1/2 starch, 2 fat
Cheese Crackers with Peanut Butter	1 pkg	190	10	90	1.5	0	0	330	23	1	4	1 1/2 starch, 2 fat
Toasty Crackers with Peanut Butter	1 pkg	130	6	50	1	0	0	200	16	<1	3	1 starch, 1 fat
Barbara's Bakery												
Crunchy Organic Granola Bar, Oats & Honey	2 bars	190	8	70	1	0	0	60	27	3	4	2 carb, 2 fat

Fruit & Yogurt Bar, Strawberry Apple	1 bar	150	3	25	0	0	125	28	1	3	2 carb, 1 fat
Nature's Choice Multigrain Cereal Bar, Apple Cinnamon	1 bar	140	2	20	0	0	80	28	1	2	2 carb
Betty Crocker											
Fruit By The Foot	1 roll	80	1	10	0	0	45	17	0	0	1 carb
Fruit Gushers	1 pouch	90	1	10	0	0	45	20	0	0	1 carb
Fruit Roll-Ups	1	50	1	5	0	0	55	12	0	0	1 carb
Fruit-Flavored Shapes, Batman	1 pouch	80	0	0	0	0	30	21	0	0	1 1/2 carb
Cracker Jack											
Original	1/2 cup	120	2	15	0	0	70	23	1	2	1 1/2 carb
Entenmann's											
Apple Cinnamon Cereal Bar	1 bar	140	3	25	1.5	0	105	28	1	1	2 carb, 1 fat

SNACKS, CRACKERS, CHIPS, POPCORN

	Serving	Calories	Fat (g)	Cal. from Fat	Sat. Fat (g)	Trans Fat (g)	Chol. (mg)	Sod. (mg)	Carb. (g)	Fiber (g)	Prot. (g)	Servings/Exchanges
Chewy Chocolate Chip Cereal Bar	1 bar	150	6	50	2.53	0	5	110	25	2	2	1 1/2 carb, 1 fat
Strawberry Cereal Bar	1 bar	140	3	25	1.5	0	0	105	28	1	1	2 carb, 1 fat
Extend Bar												
Peanut Butter Chocolate Delight	1 bar	150	3	30	1	0	0	180	21	5	11	1 1/2 carb, 1 lean meat
Franklin												
Crunch 'n Munch, Buttery Toffee	2/3 cup	140	5	45	1.5	0	<5	160	23	1	2	1 1/2 carb, 1 fat
Crunch 'n Munch, Caramel	2/3 cup	150	6	50	2.5	0	10	100	23	<1	2	1 1/2 carb, 1 fat
Frito-Lay												
Baken-ets Fried Pork Skins, Traditional	8	90	6	55	2	0	15	550	<1	<1	7	1 med-fat meat

Cheetos, Baked	1 oz	130	5	45	1	0	0	240	19	0	2	1 starch, 1 fat
Cheetos, Baked! 100 Calorie Mini Bites	1 pkg	100	4	35	0.5	0	0	180	14	0	2	1 starch, 1 fat
Cheetos, Crunchy	1 oz	160	10	90	2	0	<5	290	15	<1	2	1 starch, 2 fat
Cheetos, Flamin' Hot	1 oz	170	11	100	1.5	0	0	250	15	<1	2	1 starch, 2 fat
Cheetos, Natural White Cheddar Puffs	1 oz	150	9	80	1.5	0	0	290	16	<1	2	1 starch, 2 fat
Cheetos, Puffs	1 oz	160	10	90	1.5	0	0	370	15	<1	2	1 starch, 2 fat
Chester's Butter Popcorn	1 oz	160	11	100	1.5	0	0	300	12	<1	1	1 starch 2 fat
Chester's Cheddar Cheese Popcorn	1 oz	150	10	90	1.5	0	0	200	15	3	2	1 starch, 2 fat
Crackers, Peanut Butter on Toast	1 pkg	200	10	90	2.5	1	0	310	23	2	4	1 1/2 starch, 2 fat
Crackers, Peanut Butter Sandwich Crackers	1 pkg	190	9	80	2.5	1	0	370	23	2	5	1 1/2 starch, 2 fat

SNACKS, CRACKERS, CHIPS, POPCORN

	Serving	Calories	Fat (g)	Cal. from Fat	Sat. Fat (g)	Trans Fat (g)	Chol. (mg)	Sod. (mg)	Carb. (g)	Fiber (g)	Prot. (g)	Servings/Exchanges
Doritos, 100 Calorie Mini Bites, Nacho Cheese	1 pkg	100	6	60	1	0	0	140	12	0	2	1 starch, 1 fat
Doritos, Cooler Ranch	1 oz	150	8	70	1	0	0	180	18	2	2	1 starch, 2 fat
Doritos, Diablo	1 oz	150	8	70	1	0	0	310	17	2	2	1 starch, 2 fat
Doritos, Last Call Jalapeño Popper	1 oz	150	8	70	1.5	0	0	230	17	2	2	1 starch, 2 fat
Doritos, Nacho Cheese	1 oz	150	8	70	1.5	0	0	180	17	1	2	1 starch, 2 fat
Doritos, Reduced Fat Nacho Cheese	1 pkg	130	5	45	1	0	0	220	19	1	2	1 starch, 1 fat
Doritos, Reduced Fat, Cool Ranch	1 pkg	130	5	45	1	0	0	160	19	2	2	1 starch, 1 fat
Doritos, Salsa Verde	1 oz	140	7	70	1	0	0	210	19	1	2	1 starch, 1 fat
Doritos, Spicy Nacho	1 oz	140	7	60	1	0	0	210	18	1	2	1 starch, 1 fat
Doritos, Toasted Corn	1 oz	140	7	60	1	0	0	120	18	1	2	1 starch, 1 fat

Food	Serving											Exchanges
Fritos, BBQ	1 oz	150	10	90	1.5	0	0	280	16	1	2	1 starch, 2 fat
Fritos, Chili Cheese	1 oz	160	10	90	1.5	0	0	260	15	1	2	1 starch, 2 fat
Fritos, Flamin' Hot	1 oz	160	10	90	1.5	0	0	160	15	1	2	1 starch, 2 fat
Fritos, Flavor Twists, Honey BBQ	1 oz	160	10	90	1.5	0	0	210	16	1	2	1 starch, 2 fat
Fritos, Original	1 oz	160	10	90	1.5	0	0	170	15	1	2	1 starch, 2 fat
Fritos, Scoops	1 oz	160	10	90	1.5	0	0	110	16	1	2	1 starch, 2 fat
Funyuns Onion Flavored Rings	1 oz	140	7	60	1	0	0	270	18	<1	2	1 starch, 1 fat
Lay's, Baked BBQ Potato Chips	1 oz	120	3	30	0.5	0	0	210	22	2	2	1 1/2 starch, 1 fat
Lay's, Baked Original Potato Chips	1 oz	120	2	15	0	0	0	180	23	2	2	1 1/2 starch
Lay's, Baked Sour Cream & Onion Potato Chips	1 oz	120	3	25	0.5	0	0	210	21	2	2	1 1/2 starch, 1 fat

SNACKS, CRACKERS, CHIPS, POPCORN

	Serving	Calories	Fat (g)	Cal. from Fat	Sat. Fat (g)	Trans Fat (g)	Chol. (mg)	Sod. (mg)	Carb. (g)	Fiber (g)	Prot. (g)	Servings/Exchanges
Lay's, BBQ Potato Chips	1 oz	150	10	90	1	0	0	200	15	1	2	1 starch, 2 fat
Lay's, Classic Potato Chips	1 oz	150	10	90	1	0	0	180	15	1	2	1 starch, 2 fat
Lay's, Kettle Cooked, Original	1 oz	150	8	80	1	0	0	110	18	1	2	1 starch, 2 fat
Lay's, Light Original	1 oz	75	0	0	0	0	0	200	17	1	2	1 starch
Lay's, Natural Sea Salt & Vinegar	1 oz	140	7	60	1	0	0	260	17	1	2	1 starch, 1 fat
Lay's, Salt & Vinegar Potato Chips	1 oz	150	10	90	1	0	0	380	15	1	2	1 starch, 2 fat
Lay's, Stax, Original Potato Crisps	1 oz	150	9	80	1	0	0	160	16	1	2	1 starch, 2 fat
Lay's, Wavy Au Gratin Potato Chips	1 oz	150	10	90	1.5	0	<5	200	14	1	2	1 starch, 2 fat

Lay's, Wavy Original Potato Chips	1 oz	150	10	90	1	0	0	180	15	1	2	1 starch, 2 fat
Lay's, Wavy Ranch Potato Chips	1 oz	150	10	80	1.5	0	0	200	16	1	2	1 starch, 2 fat
Munchies, Flamin' Hot Snack Mix	3/4 cup	140	7	60	1	0	0	200	18	1	2	1 starch, 1 fat
Munchos Potato Crisps	1 oz	160	10	90	1.5	0	0	230	16	1	1	1 starch, 2 fat
Rold Gold, Cheddar Cheese Tiny Twists Pretzels	1 oz	110	1	10	0	0	0	370	22	1	3	1 1/2 starch
Rold Gold, Classic Style Tiny Twists Pretzels	1 oz	110	1	10	0	0	0	450	23	1	3	1 1/2 starch
Rold Gold, Fat Free Tiny Twists Pretzels	1 oz	100	0	0	0	0	0	420	23	1	3	1 1/2 starch
Rold Gold, Honey Mustard Tiny Twists Pretzels	1 oz	110	1	10	0	0	0	430	23	1	3	1 1/2 starch

SNACKS, CRACKERS, CHIPS, POPCORN

	Serving	Calories	Fat (g)	Cal. from Fat	Sat. Fat (g)	Trans Fat (g)	Chol. (mg)	Sod. (mg)	Carb. (g)	Fiber (g)	Prot. (g)	Servings/Exchanges
Rold Gold, Pretzel Sticks	1 oz	100	0	0	0	0	0	580	23	1	2	1 1/2 starch
Ruffles, Authentic Barbecue Flavored	1 oz	150	10	90	1	0	0	190	16	1	2	1 starch, 2 fat
Ruffles, Baked, Cheddar & Sour Cream	1 oz	120	3.5	30	0.5	0	0	270	21	2	2	1 1/2 starch, 1 fat
Ruffles, Baked, Original	1 oz	120	3	30	0	0	0	200	21	2	2	1 1/2 starch, 1 fat
Ruffles, Cheddar & Sour Cream	1 oz	160	11	90	1.5	0	0	230	14	1	2	1 starch, 2 fat
Ruffles, Light Original	1 oz	70	0	0	0	0	0	190	17	1	2	1 starch
Ruffles, Original	1oz	160	10	90	1	0	0	160	14	1	2	1 starch, 2 fat
Ruffles, Sour Cream & Onion	1 oz	160	11	90	1.5	0	0	190	14	1	2	1 starch, 2 fat
Santitas White Corn Tortilla Chips	1 oz	130	6	50	1	0	0	110	19	1	2	1 starch, 1 fat

Santitas Yellow Corn Tortilla Chips	1 oz	140	6	50	1	0	0	110	19	2	2	1 starch, 1 fat
Smartfood White Cheddar Cheese Popcorn	1 pkg	100	6	60	1.5	0	<5	180	9	1	2	1/2 starch, 1 fat
Smartfood White Cheddar Cheese Popcorn, Reduced Fat	3 cups	140	6	50	1.5	0	<5	280	19	3	4	1 starch, 1 fat
Sunchips, French Onion	1 oz	140	6	60	1	0	0	130	18	2	2	1 starch, 1 fat
Sunchips, Harvest Cheddar	1 oz	140	6	50	1	0	0	160	19	2	2	1 starch, 1 fat
Sunchips, Original	1 oz	140	6	50	1	0	0	120	19	2	2	1 starch, 1 fat
Tostitos, Baked Scoops	1 oz	120	3	25	0.5	0	0	125	22	2	1	1 1/2 starch, 1 fat
Tostitos, Bite Size Rounds	1 oz	140	8	70	1	0	0	110	18	1	2	1 starch, 2 fat
Tostitos, Crispy Rounds	1 oz	140	7	70	1	0	0	120	18	1	2	1 starch, 1 fat

SNACKS, CRACKERS, CHIPS, POPCORN

	Serving	Calories	Fat (g)	Cal. from Fat	Sat. Fat (g)	Trans Fat (g)	Chol. (mg)	Sod. (mg)	Carb. (g)	Fiber (g)	Prot. (g)	Servings/Exchanges
Tostitos, Restaurant Style	1 oz	140	7	60	1	0	0	115	19	2	2	1 starch, 1 fat
Tostitos, Restaurant Style, Hint of Lime	1 oz	150	8	70	1	0	0	160	18	1	2	1 starch, 2 fat
Gardetto's												
Snack Mix, Original	1/2 cup	150	6	60	1	1	0	270	20	1	3	1 starch, 1 fat
Snack Mix, Reduced Fat Original	1/2 cup	130	4	35	1	0.5	0	330	20	1	3	1 starch, 1 fat
General Mills												
Bugles, Original	1 1/3 cup	160	9	80	8	0	0	310	18	<1	1	1 starch, 2 fat
Cheerios Snack Mix, Cheddar	2/3 cup	120	3	30	0.5	0	0	310	21	1	3	1 1/2 carb, 1 fat
Cheerios Snack Mix, Original	2/3 cup	130	3.5	30	0.5	0	0	290	22	1	3	1 1/2 carb, 1 fat

Chex Mix Bar, Chocolate Chunk	1 bar	140	3	30	0	0	0	135	26	2	2	2 carb, 1 fat
Chex Mix Select, Chocolate Turtle	1/2 cup	130	4.5	40	2	0	<5	130	20	<1	2	1 starch, 1 fat
Chex Mix Sweet 'n Salty, Trail Mix	1/2 cup	140	5	45	1.5	0	0	140	23	1	2	1 1/2 starch, 1 fat
Chex Mix, Bold Party Blend	1/2 cup	120	4.5	40	1	0.5	0	260	18	<1	2	1 starch, 1 fat
Chex Mix, Cheddar	1/2 cup	120	3.5	30	0.5	0	0	210	20	1	2	1 starch, 1 fat
Chex Mix, Peanut Lovers	1/2 cup	140	5	50	1	0	0	270	20	1	3	1 starch, 1 fat
Chex Mix, Traditional	1/2 cup	110	3	30	0.5	0	0	240	19	<1	2	1 starch, 1 fat
Fiber One Chewy Bar, Oats & Caramel	1 bar	140	3.5	30	1.5	0	0	105	30	9	2	2 carb, 1 fat
Fiber One Chewy Bar, Oats & Peanut Butter	1 bar	150	4.5	40	2	0	0	105	28	9	3	2 carb, 1 fat

SNACKS, CRACKERS, CHIPS, POPCORN

	Serving	Calories	Fat (g)	Cal. from Fat	Sat. Fat (g)	Trans Fat (g)	Chol. (mg)	Sod. (mg)	Carb. (g)	Fiber (g)	Prot. (g)	Servings/Exchanges
Health Valley Organic												
Cereal Bar, Strawberry Cobbler	1 bar	130	2.5	20	0	0	0	85	26	1	2	2 carb, 1 fat
Crackers, Sesame	4	70	3	30	0	0	0	200	10	<1	1	1/2 starch, 1 fat
Crackers, Stoned Wheat	4	70	3	30	0	0	0	170	10	<1	1	1/2 starch, 1 fat
Graham Crackers, Amaranth Bran	6	120	3	25	0	0	0	80	22	3	3	1 1/2 starch, 1 fat
Graham Crackers, Oat Bran	6	120	3	25	0	0	0	80	22	3	3	1 1/2 carb, 1 fat
Granola Bar, Chocolate Chewy	1 bar	110	2	20	1	0	0	10	22	<1	1	1 1/2 carb
Jolly Time												
Blast O Butter Popcorn	3 1/2 cups	150	12	110	3	4	0	340	19	9	3	1 starch, 2 fat

Healthy Pop Popcorn, 94% Fat Free	5 cups	90	2	20	0	0	0	210	23	9	3	1 1/2 starch
Mallow Magic Popcorn	2 1/2 cups	170	12	110	2	3	0	170	16	3	1	1 starch, 2 fat
The Big Cheez Popcorn	3 1/2 cups	160	11	100	2.5	4	0	340	17	6	2	1 starch, 2 fat
Kashi												
TLC Fruit & Grain Bar, Dark Chocolate Coconut	1 bar	120	3.5	30	1.5	0	0	50	21	4	4	1 1/2 carb, 1 fat
TLC Fruit & Grain Bar, Raspberry Chocolate	1 bar	120	3	30	0.5	0	0	50	21	4	4	1 1/2 carb, 1 fat
Kay's Naturals												
Better Balance Pretzel Sticks, Jalapeño Honey Mustard	1 oz	120	6	60	1.5	0	0	150	9	2	10	1/2 carb, 1 med-fat meat
Better Balance Pretzel Sticks, Wasabi	1 oz	120	6	60	1.5	0	0	200	9	2	10	1/2 carb, 1 med-fat meat

SNACKS, CRACKERS, CHIPS, POPCORN

	Serving	Calories	Fat (g)	Cal. from Fat	Sat. Fat (g)	Trans Fat (g)	Chol. (mg)	Sod. (mg)	Carb. (g)	Fiber (g)	Prot. (g)	Servings/Exchanges
Keebler												
Crackers, Club, Multi-Grain	4	70	3	25	0	0	0	120	9	<1	1	1/2 starch, 1 fat
Crackers, Club, Original	4	70	3	25	0.5	0	0	125	9	<1	<1	1/2 starch, 1 fat
Crackers, Club, Reduced Fat	5	70	2	20	0	0	0	150	12	<1	1	1 starch
Crackers, Graham, Cinnamon	8	130	3.5	35	1	0	0	140	23	1	2	1 1/2 starch, 1 fat
Crackers, Graham, Cinnamon, Low-Fat	8	110	1.5	15	0	0	0	140	23	1	2	1 1/2 starch
Crackers, Graham, Original	8	120	1	30	1	0	0	160	22	1	2	1 1/2 starch
Crackers, Honey Graham	8	140	4	35	1	0	0	150	23	<1	2	1 1/2 starch, 1 fat

Crackers, Honey Graham, Bug Bites	13	130	4	35	1.5	0	0	125	22	<1	2	1 1/2 starch, 1 fat
Crackers, Krispy Soup & Oyster	16	60	1.5	15	0	0	0	230	11	<1	1	1 starch
Crackers, Toasteds, Buttercrisps	5	80	4	35	0.5	0	0	150	10	<1	<1	1/2 starch, 1 fat
Crackers, Toasteds, Onion	5	80	3	35	0.5	0	0	150	10	<1	<1	1/2 starch, 1 fat
Crackers, Toasteds, Sesame	5	80	4	35	0.5	0	0	140	10	<1	1	1/2 starch, 1 fat
Crackers, Toasteds, Wheat	5	80	3.5	30	0.5	0	0	150	10	<1	1	1/2 starch, 1 fat
Crackers, Town House Original	5	80	4.5	40	1	0	0	130	10	<1	<1	1/2 starch, 1 fat
Crackers, Town House, Reduced Fat	6	60	1.5	15	0	0	0	160	11	<1	1	1 starch
Crackers, Wheatables, Original Golden Wheat	17	140	6	50	1.5	0	0	340	20	1	2	1 starch, 1 fat

SNACKS, CRACKERS, CHIPS, POPCORN

	Serving	Calories	Fat (g)	Cal. from Fat	Sat. Fat (g)	Trans Fat (g)	Chol. (mg)	Sod. (mg)	Carb. (g)	Fiber (g)	Prot. (g)	Servings/Exchanges
Crackers, Wheatables, Reduced Fat	19	140	4	35	1	0	0	320	22	1	2	1 1/2 starch, 1 fat
Crackers, Zesta Saltines, Original	5	60	1.5	15	0	0	0	150	11	<1	1	1 starch
Crackers, Zesta Saltines, Whole Wheat	5	60	1.5	15	0	0	0	230	11	<1	1	1 starch
Kellogg's												
FiberPlus Antioxidants Bar, Chocolate Chip	1 bar	120	4	40	2	0	0	55	26	9	2	2 carb, 1 fat
Nutri-Grain Cereal Bars (All Varieties)	1 bar	130	3	30	0.5	0	0	120	24	2	2	1 1/2 carb, 1 fat
Nutri-Grain Yogurt Bar, Strawberry	1 bar	140	3.5	30	0.5	0	0	110	25	2	2	1 1/2 carb, 1 fat
Rice Krispies Treats, Original	1	90	2.5	20	1	0	0	105	17	0	1	1 starch, 1 fat

	Serving	Cal.	Fat (g)	% Cal. Fat	Sat. Fat (g)	Trans Fat (g)	Chol. (mg)	Sod. (mg)	Carb. (g)	Fiber (g)	Prot. (g)	Exchanges/Choices
Special K Bars	1 bar	90	1.5	15	1	0	0	95	18	<1	1	1 carb
Kraft/Nabisco												
Barnum's Animal Crackers	10	120	4	35	<1	0	0	140	22	0	0	1 1/2 starch, 1 fat
Better Cheddars, Baked Snack Crackers	22	160	8	70	1.5	0	5	360	18	<1	3	1 starch, 2 fat
Chicken-In-A-Biskit Crackers	12	160	8	70	1.5	0	0	310	19	1	2	1 starch, 2 fat
Handi-Snacks, Premium Breadsticks 'n Cheez	1 pkg	110	4.5	40	1	0	5	350	14	0	3	1 starch, 1 fat
Handi-Snacks, Ritz Crackers 'n Cheez	1 pkg	100	6	50	1.5	0	<5	330	11	0	2	1 starch, 1 fat
Honey Maid Grahams, Cinnamon	8	130	2.5	25	0.5	0	0	170	25	1	2	1 1/2 starch, 1 fat
Honey Maid Grahams, Cinnamon, Low Fat	8	120	1.5	15	0	0	0	180	26	1	2	2 starch
Honey Maid Grahams, Honey	8	130	3	25	0.5	0	0	190	24	1	2	1 1/2 starch, 1 fat

SNACKS, CRACKERS, CHIPS, POPCORN

	Serving	Calories	Fat (g)	Cal. from Fat	Sat. Fat (g)	Trans Fat (g)	Chol. (mg)	Sod. (mg)	Carb. (g)	Fiber (g)	Prot. (g)	Servings/Exchanges
Honey Maid Grahams, Honey, Low Fat	8	120	2	15	0	0	0	190	25	1	2	1 1/2 starch
Premium Saltine Crackers	5	60	1.5	10	0	0	0	190	11	0	1	1 starch
Premium Saltine Crackers, Hint of Salt	5	60	1.5	10	0	0	0	30	12	0	1	1 starch
Ritz Bits, Cheese	13	150	9	80	3	0	0	250	17	0	2	1 starch, 2 fat
Ritz Bits, Peanut Butter	12	140	8	70	1.5	0	0	240	16	1	3	1 starch, 2 fat
Ritz Crackers	5	80	4.5	40	1	0	10	135	10	0	1	1 starch, 1 fat
Ritz Crackers, Hint of Salt	5	80	4	35	1	0	0	35	10	0	1	1/2 starch, 1 fat
Ritz Crackers, Reduced Fat	5	70	2	20	0	0	0	160	11	0	1	1 starch
Ritz Crackers, Whole Wheat	5	70	2.5	25	0.5	0	0	120	11	<1	1	1 starch, 1 fat

Sociables	5	70	3.5	30	0.5	0	0	140	9	0	1	1/2 starch, 1 fat
Triscuit Thin Crisps, Parmesan Garlic	15	140	5	40	1	0	0	180	22	3	3	1 1/2 starch, 1 fat
Triscuits	6	120	4.5	40	1	0	0	180	19	3	3	1 starch, 1 fat
Triscuits, Reduced Fat	7	120	3	25	0.5	0	0	160	21	3	3	1 1/2 starch, 1 fat
Vegetable Thins, Baked Snack Crackers	21	150	7	60	2	0	0	320	19	1	2	1 starch, 1 fat
Wheat Thins Toasted Chips, Multi-Grain	14	120	4	35	0.5	0	0	240	20	1	2	1 starch, 1 fat
Wheat Thins, Multi-Grain	15	140	4.5	40	0.5	0	0	230	22	2	2	1 1/2 starch, 1 fat
Wheat Thins, Original	16	140	5	45	1	0	0	230	22	2	2	1 1/2 starch, 1 fat
Wheat Thins, Reduced Fat	16	130	3.5	35	0.5	0	0	260	21	1	2	1 1/2 starch, 1 fat,

Orville Redenbacher's Gourmet Popping Corn

Butter	4 1/2 cups	170	12	110	6	0	0	260	17	3	2	1 starch, 2 fat

SNACKS, CRACKERS, CHIPS, POPCORN

	Serving	Calories	Fat (g)	Cal. from Fat	Sat. Fat (g)	Trans Fat (g)	Chol. (mg)	Sod. (mg)	Carb. (g)	Fiber (g)	Prot. (g)	Servings/Exchanges
Kettle Korn	5 cups	170	13	110	7	0	<5	130	16	3	2	1 starch, 3 fat
Light Butter	5 1/2 cups	120	5	45	2.5	0	0	190	19	4	3	1 starch, 1 fat
Movie Theatre Butter	4 1/2 cups	170	12	110	6	0	0	360	16	3	2	1 starch, 2 fat
Smart Pop! 94% Fat Free Butter	6 1/2 cups	110	2	20	0.5	0	0	220	24	4	3	1 1/2 starch
Tender White	3 1/2 cups	170	12	110	6	0	0	250	15	2	3	1 starch, 2 fat
Ultimate Butter	5 cups	170	12	110	6	0	0	380	16	3	2	1 starch, 2 fat
Pepperidge Farm												
Crackers, Cheese Crisps, Four Cheese	20	140	6	55	1	0	<5	270	19	1	3	1 starch, 1 fat
Crackers, Golden Butter	4	70	2.5	25	1	0	<5	100	11	0	1	1 starch, 1 fat

Food											
Crackers, Harvest Wheat	3	80	3.5	30	0.5	0	0	125	11	<1	1	1 starch, 1 fat
Goldfish Crackers, Chocolate Grahams	50	130	4	35	1	0	0	125	22	2	2	1 1/2 starch, 1 fat
Goldfish Crackers, Honey Graham	50	140	4.5	40	1	0	0	150	23	1	2	1 1/2 starch, 1 fat
Goldfish Crackers, Original	55	140	5	45	1	0	<5	250	20	<1	4	1 starch, 1 fat
Goldfish Crackers, Parmesan	60	130	4	35	1	0	0	280	20	<1	4	1 starch, 1 fat
Goldfish Crackers, Pizza Flavor	55	140	5	45	1	0	0	230	20	<1	3	1 starch, 1 fat
Goldfish Crackers, Pretzel	43	130	2.5	25	0.5	0	0	430	24	<1	3	1 1/2 starch, 1 fat
Goldfish Crackers, Whole Grain	55	140	5	45	1	0	<5	250	19	2	4	1 starch, 1 fat

SNACKS, CRACKERS, CHIPS, POPCORN

	Serving	Calories	Fat (g)	Cal. from Fat	Sat. Fat (g)	Trans Fat (g)	Chol. (mg)	Sod. (mg)	Carb. (g)	Fiber (g)	Prot. (g)	Servings/Exchanges
Snack Sticks, Toasted Sesame	12	140	5	45	1	0	0	290	20	2	4	1 starch, 1 fat
Planters												
Double Peanut Bar	1	220	13	110	3	0	0	160	22	3	7	1 1/2 carb, 3 fat
Fiddle Faddle	3/4 cup	150	7	63	3	0	10	180	20	1	2	1 carb, 1 fat
Fiddle Faddle, Fat-Free	1 cup	110	0	0	0	0	0	210	28	0	2	2 carb
Poore Brothers												
Chips, Original	1 oz	140	9	80	2.5	0	0	180	15	1	2	1 starch, 2 fat
Chips, Salt & Vinegar	1 oz	150	9	80	2.5	0	0	470	15	1	2	1 starch, 2 fat
Pop-Secret Microwave Popcorn												
94% Fat Free Butter	6 cups	120	2	20	0.5	0	0	400	26	4	4	2 starch
Butter	4 cups	180	11	100	2.5	5	0	330	17	3	3	1 starch, 2 fat
Homestyle	4 cups	180	11	100	1.5	5	0	410	18	3	3	1 starch, 2 fat
Kettle Corn	4 cups	180	13	120	3	6	0	150	15	3	2	1 starch, 3 fat

Movie Theater Butter	4 cups	180	12	100	2.5	5	0	300	18	3	2	1 starch, 2 fat
Power Bar												
Performance Energy Bar, Chocolate	1	240	3	30	1	0	0	200	45	3	8	3 carb, 1 fat
Performance Energy Bar, Vanilla Crisp	1	240	3.5	35	0.5	0	0	200	45	1	8	3 carb, 1 fat
Pringles												
Chips, Original	1 oz	150	9	90	2.5	0	0	150	15	1	1	1 starch, 2 fat
Chips, Original, Light	1 oz	70	0	0	0	0	0	160	15	0	1	1 starch
Chips, Sour Cream & Onion	1 oz	150	9	80	2.5	0	0	170	15	1	1	1 starch, 2 fat
Chips, Sour Cream & Onion, Light	1 oz	70	0	0	0	0	0	190	15	1	2	1 starch
Quaker												
Cheesy Nacho Tortillaz	1 oz	130	5	45	0.5	0	0	230	20	1	2	1 carb, 1 fat
Chewy 25% Less Sugar Bar, Baked Apple	1 bar	100	3.5	30	1	0	0	75	17	3	1	1 carb, 1 fat

SNACKS, CRACKERS, CHIPS, POPCORN

	Serving	Calories	Fat (g)	Cal. from Fat	Sat. Fat (g)	Trans Fat (g)	Chol. (mg)	Sod. (mg)	Carb. (g)	Fiber (g)	Prot. (g)	Servings/Exchanges
Chewy Granola Bar, Chocolate Chip	1 bar	100	3	20	0.5	0	15	80	19	1	1	1 carb
Fiber & Omega-3 Bar, Peanut Butter Chocolate	1 bar	150	5	45	2	0	0	35	25	9	3	1 1/2 carb, 1 fat
Granola Bites	1 bag	90	3.5	30	2	0	0	30	14	2	2	1 carb, 1 fat
Mini Rice Cakes, Apple Cinnamon	8	60	0	0	0	0	0	50	15	0	1	1 carb
Mini Rice Cakes, Caramel Corn	7	60	0	0	0	0	0	150	13	0	1	1 carb
Rice Cakes, Apple Cinnamon	1	50	0	0	0	0	0	0	11	0	1	1 carb
Rice Cakes, Butter Popped Corn	1	35	0	0	0	0	0	45	8	0	1	1/2 carb
Rice Cakes, Caramel Corn	1	50	0	0	0	0	0	30	11	0	1	1 carb

Food	Serving	Calories	Fat (g)	Cal. from Fat	Sat. Fat (g)	Chol. (mg)	Sodium (mg)	Carb. (g)	Fiber (g)	Prot. (g)	Exchanges
Rice Cakes, Peanut Butter Chocolate Chip	1	60	1	10	0	0	70	12	0	1	1 carb
Rice Cakes, Salt Free	1	35	0	0	0	0	0	7	0	1	1 carb
Ross											
Chewy Glucerna Meal Bar, Oatmeal Raisin	1 bar	220	6	50	3.5	<5	105	35	2	10	2 carb, 1 med-fat meat
Ry Krisp											
Crackers, Seasoned, Fat Free	2	60	1	10	0	0	80	11	3	1	1 starch
Crackers, Sesame Rye	2	60	1.5	15	0	0	80	10	3	1	1/2 starch
Snyder's of Hanover											
Butter Snaps	24	120	1	10	0	0	270	25	1	3	1 1/2 starch
Honey Mustard & Onion Nibblers	13	130	3	25	1.5	0	95	23	<1	3	1 1/2 starch, 1 fat
Hot Buffalo Wing Pieces	1/3 cup	140	7	60	3	0	380	17	<1	2	1 starch, 1 fat
Mini Pretzels	20	110	0	0	0	0	250	25	<1	3	1 1/2 starch
Rods	3	120	1	10	0	0	290	24	1	3	1 1/2 starch

SNACKS, CRACKERS, CHIPS, POPCORN

	Serving	Calories	Fat (g)	Cal. from Fat	Sat. Fat (g)	Trans Fat (g)	Chol. (mg)	Sod. (mg)	Carb. (g)	Fiber (g)	Prot. (g)	Servings/Exchanges
South Beach Living												
High Protein Cereal Bar, Peanut Butter	1	140	5	50	2	0	0	160	15	3	10	1 carb, 1 med-fat meat
Stacy's												
Pita Chips, Multigrain	1 oz	140	5	50	0.5	0	0	270	19	2	3	1 starch, 1 fat
Pita Chips, Simply Naked	1 oz	130	5	45	0.5	0	0	270	19	1	3	1 starch, 1 fat
Sunshine												
Cheez-It, Original	27	150	8	70	3	0	0	250	17	<1	3	1 starch, 2 fat
Cheez-It, Party Mix	1/2 cup	130	4.5	40	1	0	0	370	20	1	3	1 starch, 1 fat
Cheez-It, Reduced Fat	29	130	4.5	45	1	0	0	320	20	<1	4	1 starch, 1 fat
Cheez-It, White Cheddar	25	130	4	35	1	0	0	240	22	<1	3	1 1/2 starch, 1 fat
Krispy Saltine Crackers	5	60	1.5	15	0	0	0	150	11	<1	1	1 starch
Krispy Saltine Crackers, Wheat	5	60	1.5	15	0	0	0	230	11	<1	1	1 starch

SOUPS, STEW, CHILI

READY-TO-SERVE CANNED SOUP

Brands

Campbell's Chunky

	Serving	Calories	Fat (g)	Cal. from Fat	Sat. Fat (g)	Trans Fat (g)	Chol. (mg)	Sod. (mg)	Carb. (g)	Fiber (g)	Prot. (g)	Servings/Exchanges
Baked Potato with Cheddar & Bacon Bits	1 cup	190	9	80	3	0	10	790	23	3	5	1 1/2 carb, 2 fat
Beef & Dumplings with Hearty Vegetables	1 cup	130	2	20	0.5	0	25	800	20	2	8	1 carb, 1 lean meat
Beef with Country Vegetables	1 cup	130	3	25	1	0	15	920	18	4	8	1 carb, 1 lean meat
Beef with White & Wild Rice	1 cup	140	1.5	15	0.5	0	10	890	24	2	8	1 1/2 carb, 1 lean meat
Chicken & Dumplings	1 cup	180	8	70	2	0	30	890	19	3	8	1 carb, 1 med-fat meat, 1 fat

SOUPS, STEW, CHILI

	Serving	Calories	Fat (g)	Cal. from Fat	Sat. Fat (g)	Trans Fat (g)	Chol. (mg)	Sod. (mg)	Carb. (g)	Fiber (g)	Prot. (g)	Servings/Exchanges
Chicken Broccoli Cheese & Potato	1 cup	210	11	100	4	0	20	880	20	3	7	1 carb, 1 med-fat meat, 1 fat
Classic Chicken Noodle	1 cup	120	3	25	1	0	25	790	14	2	8	1 carb, 1 lean meat
Grilled Chicken & Sausage Gumbo	1 cup	140	3	25	1.5	0	20	850	21	2	7	1 1/2 carb, 1 lean meat
Hearty Bean 'N' Ham	1 cup	180	2	20	0.5	0	10	780	30	5	11	2 carb, 1 lean meat
Hearty Chicken & Vegetable	1 cup	110	2	20	0.5	0	15	710	17	3	6	1 carb, 1 lean meat
Manhattan Clam Chowder	1 cup	130	3.5	30	1	0	5	830	19	3	5	1 carb, 1 fat
New England Clam Chowder	1 cup	230	13	115	2	0	10	890	20	3	7	1 carb, 1 med-fat meat, 2 fat
Old Fashioned Vegetable Beef	1 cup	120	2.5	20	1	0	15	890	17	4	8	1 carb, 1 lean meat
Roasted Beef Tips with Vegetables	1 cup	130	1.5	15	0.5	0	15	800	20	2	8	1 carb, 1 lean meat

Salisbury Steak Mushrooms & Onions	1 cup	140	4.5	40	2.5	0	15	800	19	2	7	1 carb, 1 med-fat meat
Sirloin Burger with Country Vegetables	1 cup	130	2.5	20	1	0	15	800	18	4	10	1 carb, 1 lean meat
Split Pea & Ham	1 cup	190	2.5	20	1	0	10	780	30	5	12	2 carb, 1 lean meat
Steak & Potato	1 cup	120	2	20	0.5	0	15	920	18	3	8	1 carb, 1 lean meat

Campbell's Chunky Fully Loaded

Creamy Chicken Alfredo	1 cup	230	12	110	5	0	30	780	18	2	12	1 carb, 1 med-fat meat, 1 fat
Rigatoni & Meatball	1 cup	210	7	65	3	0	20	800	25	8	11	1 1/2 carb, 1 med-fat meat
Turkey Pot Pie	1 cup	200	8	70	1.5	0	35	800	21	4	11	1 1/2 carb, 1 med-fat meat, 1 fat
Campbell's Chunky Healthy Request	1 cup	140	3.5	32	1.5	0	10	730	24	2	3	1 1/2 carb, 1 fat
Chicken Corn Chowder	1 cup	140	3	25	1	0	10	410	22	2	7	1 1/2 carb, 1 lean meat
Chicken Noodle	1 cup	120	2.5	20	1	0	10	410	17	2	8	1 carb, 1 lean meat

SOUPS, STEW, CHILI

	Serving	Calories	Fat (g)	Cal. from Fat	Sat. Fat (g)	Trans Fat (g)	Chol. (mg)	Sod. (mg)	Carb. (g)	Fiber (g)	Prot. (g)	Servings/Exchanges
New England Clam Chowder	1 cup	130	3	25	1	0	10	410	20	2	5	1 carb, 1 fat
Old Fashioned Vegetable Beef	1 cup	120	2	20	1	0	10	410	19	3	7	1 carb, 1 lean meat
Sirloin Burger	1 cup	130	2	20	1	0	15	410	19	3	9	1 carb, 1 lean meat
Vegetable	1 cup	120	1	10	0.5	0	0	410	24	4	4	1 1/2 carb
Campbell's Low Sodium												
Chicken Broth	1 can	25	0.5	5	0.5	0	5	140	1	0	4	free
Chicken with Noodles	1 can	160	4.5	40	1.5	0	30	140	17	2	12	1 carb, 1 med-fat meat
Chunky Vegetable Beef	1 can	170	4.5	40	1.5	0	30	50	18	6	14	1 carb, 2 lean meat
Cream of Mushroom	1 can	160	8	70	2.5	0	10	60	19	3	4	1 carb, 2 fat
Split Pea	1 can	240	4	35	1.5	0	5	30	38	6	12	2 1/2 carb, 1 med-fat meat
Tomato with Tomato Pieces	1 can	150	4	45	1.5	0	10	90	25	4	4	1 1/2 carb, 1 fat

Campbell's Select Harvest

Light Italian-Style Vegetable	1 cup	50	0	0	0	0	480	14	4	3	1 carb
Light Minestrone with Whole Grain Pasta	1 cup	80	0.5	0	0	0	480	14	4	4	1 carb
Light Roasted Chicken with Italian Herbs	1 cup	80	2.5	0.5	25	10	480	8	3	6	1/2 carb, 1 lean meat
Light Vegetable & Pasta	1 cup	60	0	0	0	0	480	13	4	3	1 carb

Health Valley Organic (Fat Free)

Black Bean, No Added Salt	1 cup	130	1	0	0	0	25	25	5	7	1 1/2 carb
Chicken Noodle	1 cup	80	2	0	20	10	480	11	1	4	1 carb, 1 lean meat
Italian Minestrone, 40% Less Sodium	1 cup	110	0	0	0	0	470	26	7	6	2 carb
Lentil, No Added Salt	1 cup	100	1	0	0	0	25	21	8	8	1 1/2 carb
Minestrone, No Added Salt	1 cup	70	0	0	0	0	45	17	3	3	1 carb

SOUPS, STEW, CHILI

	Serving	Calories	Fat (g)	Cal. from Fat	Sat. Fat (g)	Trans Fat (g)	Chol. (mg)	Sod. (mg)	Carb. (g)	Fiber (g)	Prot. (g)	Servings/Exchanges
Split Pea, No Added Salt	1 cup	110	0	0	0	0	0	115	23	8	10	1 1/2 carb, 1 very lean meat
Tomato Vegetable, 40% Less Sodium	1 cup	70	0	0	0	0	0	470	17	5	3	1 carb
Tomato, No Added Salt	1 cup	80	0	0	0	0	0	35	18	1	3	1 carb
Vegetable Barley, 40% Less Sodium	1 cup	80	0	0	0	0	0	480	19	4	3	1 carb
Vegetable, No Added Salt	1 cup	90	0	0	0	0	0	70	16	4	3	1 carb
Healthy Choice												
Bean & Ham	1 cup	180	2	20	1	0	5	480	29	10	11	2 carb, 1 lean meat
Chicken & Dumplings	1 cup	140	2.5	20	0.5	0	20	480	21	3	9	1 1/2 carb, 1 lean meat
Chicken with Rice	1 cup	110	1.5	15	0	0	10	480	17	3	7	1 carb, 1 lean meat
Country Vegetable	1 cup	110	1	10	0	0	0	480	19	4	5	1 carb
Fiesta Chicken	1 cup	120	2	20	0.5	0	15	480	20	3	6	1 carb, 1 lean meat

Garden Vegetable	1 cup	120	0.5	5	0	0	5	480	24	4	5	1 1/2 carb
Hearty Chicken	1 cup	130	2	15	0.5	0	20	480	20	3	9	1 carb, 1 lean meat
New England Clam Chowder	1 cup	110	1	10	0.5	0	10	480	19	2	5	1 carb
Old Fashioned Chicken Noodle	1 cup	100	1.5	15	0	0	15	480	13	2	9	1 carb, 1 lean meat
Split Pea & Ham	1 cup	170	2	15	0.5	0	5	480	22	3	9	1 1/2 carb, 1 lean meat
Vegetable Beef	1 cup	130	1	10	0	0	15	480	22	4	9	1 1/2 carb, 1 lean meat
Zesty Gumbo	1 cup	100	2	15	0.5	0	20	480	16	4	6	1 carb
Progresso (99% Fat Free)											
Beef Barley	1 cup	120	1.5	15	0.5	0	10	720	20	4	7	1 carb, 1 lean meat
Chicken Noodle	1 cup	90	2	20	0.5	0	20	670	12	1	6	1 carb, 1 lean meat
Lentil	1 cup	140	1.5	15	0	0	0	500	25	3	8	1 1/2 carb, 1 lean meat
Minestrone	1 cup	100	1	10	0	0	0	600	19	5	5	1 carb
New England Clam Chowder	1 cup	110	1.5	15	0	0	5	810	21	2	4	1 1/2 carb

SOUPS, STEW, CHILI

	Serving	Calories	Fat (g)	Cal. from Fat	Sat. Fat (g)	Trans Fat (g)	Chol. (mg)	Sod. (mg)	Carb. (g)	Fiber (g)	Prot. (g)	Servings/Exchanges
Progresso												
Beef & Vegetable	1 cup	120	2	15	1	0	15	690	18	2	8	1 carb, 1 lean meat
Chickarina w/Meatballs	1 cup	130	5	45	2	0	20	690	14	1	8	1 carb, 1 med-fat meat
Chicken & Wild Rice	1 cup	100	1.5	15	0.5	0	15	650	15	1	6	1 carb, 1 lean meat
Chicken Noodle	1 cup	100	2.5	20	0.5	0	20	690	12	1	7	1 carb, 1 lean meat
Creamy Mushroom	1 cup	120	8	70	2	0	5	890	9	1	2	1/2 carb, 2 fat
Creamy Tomato Basil	1 cup	130	4	35	1	0	5	690	26	7	3	2 carb, 1 fat
French Onion	1 cup	50	1	10	0	0	0	690	9	1	2	1/2 carb
Green Split Pea	1 cup	160	2	20	0.5	0	0	690	28	4	9	2 carb, 1 lean meat
Hearty Black Bean	1 cup	160	1	10	0.5	0	<5	690	29	8	8	2 carb
Hearty Penne in Chicken Broth	1 cup	80	1	10	0	0	0	710	14	1	3	1 carb
Hearty Tomato	1 cup	110	0.5	5	0	0	0	690	24	3	3	1 1/2 carb
Lentil	1 cup	160	2	20	0.5	0	0	810	30	5	9	2 carb, 1 lean meat

Macaroni & Bean	1 cup	160	3.5	30	1	0	0	690	25	6	8	1 1/2 carb, 1 lean meat
Manhattan Clam Chowder	1 cup	100	2	20	0	0	5	690	17	2	3	1 carb
Minestrone	1 cup	100	2	20	0.5	0	0	690	20	4	4	1 carb
Potato Broccoli & Cheese Chowder	1 cup	210	12	110	3.5	0	15	860	20	2	5	1 carb, 2 fat
Roasted Chicken Rotini	1 cup	80	2	15	0.5	0	10	670	10	<1	5	1/2 carb, 1 lean meat
Southwestern Style Corn Chowder	1 cup	120	2	15	0.5	0	10	740	18	2	6	1 carb, 1 lean meat
Split Pea with Ham	1 cup	140	1	10	0	0	5	690	24	4	9	1 1/2 carb, 1 lean meat
Tomato Basil	1 cup	150	3	30	0.5	0	0	680	29	2	3	2 carb, 1 fat
Tomato Rotini	1 cup	130	0.5	5	0	0	0	690	28	4	4	2 carb
Turkey Noodle	1 cup	80	1	10	0	0	15	690	12	1	5	1 carb, 1 lean meat
Vegetable	1 cup	80	0	0	0	0	0	660	15	3	5	1 carb
Vegetarian Vegetable with Barley	1 cup	80	0	0	0	0	0	670	18	3	3	1 carb

SOUPS, STEW, CHILI

	Serving	Calories	Fat (g)	Cal. from Fat	Sat. Fat (g)	Trans Fat (g)	Chol. (mg)	Sod. (mg)	Carb. (g)	Fiber (g)	Prot. (g)	Servings/Exchanges
CONDENSED CANNED SOUP												
Brands												
Campbell's Condensed												
Bean with Bacon	1/2 cup	160	3	30	1.5	0	5	860	25	8	8	1 1/2 carb, 1 lean meat
Beef Broth	1/2 cup	10	0	0	0	0	0	860	1	0	2	free
Beef Consommé	1/2 cup	20	0	0	0	0	0	810	1	0	4	free
Beef Noodle	1/2 cup	70	2	20	0.5	0	10	820	8	<1	4	1/2 carb, 1 lean meat
Beefy Mushroom	1/2 cup	50	2	20	0.5	0	5	890	6	0	3	1/2 carb
Broccoli Cheese	1/2 cup	100	4.5	40	2	0	5	820	12	0	2	1 carb, 1 fat
Chicken & Dumplings	1/2 cup	70	2.5	20	1	0	10	760	10	1	3	1/2 carb, 1 fat
Chicken & Stars	1/2 cup	70	2	20	0.5	0	5	480	11	1	3	1 carb
Chicken Alphabet	1/2 cup	70	1.5	20	0.5	0	5	480	12	1	3	1 carb
Chicken Broth	1/2 cup	20	1	10	0	0	<5	770	1	0	1	free
Chicken Gumbo	1/2 cup	70	1	10	0.5	0	5	870	12	1	2	1 carb

Chicken Noodle	1/2 cup	60	2	20	0.5	0	15	890	8	1	3	1/2 carb
Chicken Won Ton	1/2 cup	60	1	10	0.5	0	10	870	8	0	4	1/2 carb
Cream of Asparagus	1/2 cup	110	9	80	2	0	5	830	9	3	2	1/2 carb, 2 fat
Cream of Broccoli	1/2 cup	90	3.5	30	1	0	5	750	12	1	2	1 carb, 1 fat
Cream of Celery	1/2 cup	90	6	55	0.5	0	5	860	9	3	1	1/2 carb, 1 fat
Cream of Chicken	1/2 cup	120	8	70	2.5	0	10	870	10	2	3	1/2 carb, 2 fat
Cream of Mushroom	1/2 cup	100	7	65	1.5	0	5	870	9	2	1	1/2 carb, 1 fat
French Onion	1/2 cup	45	1.5	15	1	0	<5	900	6	1	2	1/2 carb
Golden Mushroom	1/2 cup	80	3.5	30	1	0	5	890	10	1	2	1/2 carb, 1 fat
Green Pea	1/2 cup	180	3	25	1	0	0	870	28	4	9	2 carb, 1 lean meat
Lentil	1/2 cup	140	1	10	0.5	0	0	800	24	6	9	1 1/2 carb, 1 lean meat
Manhattan Clam Chowder	1/2 cup	60	0.5	5	0.5	0	0	880	12	2	2	1 carb
Minestrone	1/2 cup	90	1	10	0.5	0	5	960	17	3	4	1 carb
New England Clam Chowder	1/2 cup	90	2.5	20	0.5	0	5	880	13	1	4	1 carb, 1 fat

SOUPS, STEW, CHILI

	Serving	Calories	Fat (g)	Cal. from Fat	Sat. Fat (g)	Trans Fat (g)	Chol. (mg)	Sod. (mg)	Carb. (g)	Fiber (g)	Prot. (g)	Servings/Exchanges
Pepper Pot	1/2 cup	90	4	35	1.5	0	25	980	9	1	5	1/2 carb, 1 fat
Split Pea with Ham & Bacon	1/2 cup	180	3.5	30	2	0	5	850	27	5	10	2 carb, 1 med-fat meat
Tomato	1/2 cup	90	0	0	0	0	0	480	20	1	2	1 carb
Tomato Bisque	1/2 cup	130	3.5	30	1.5	0	5	880	23	1	2	1 1/2 carb, 1 fat
Vegetable	1/2 cup	100	0.5	5	0.5	0	5	890	20	3	4	1 carb
Campbell's Condensed Light												
Chicken Gumbo	1/2 cup	70	1	10	0.5	0	5	870	12	1	2	1 carb
Italian-Style Wedding	1/2 cup	80	2	20	1	0	5	790	12	2	4	1 carb
Campbell's Healthy Request Condensed												
Chicken Noodle	1/2 cup	60	2	20	0.5	0	10	410	8	1	3	1/2 carb
Chicken Rice	1/2 cup	70	1.5	15	0.5	0	5	410	13	1	2	1 carb
Cream of Celery	1/2 cup	70	2	20	0.5	0	<5	410	12	1	1	1 carb
Cream of Chicken	1/2 cup	80	2.5	20	1	0	5	410	12	1	2	1 carb

Cream of Mushroom	1/2 cup	70	2	20	0.5	0	5	410	10	1	2	1/2 carb, 1 fat
Homestyle Chicken Noodle	1/2 cup	70	2	20	0.5	0	10	410	10	1	3	1/2 carb, 1 fat
Minestrone	1/2 cup	80	0.5	5	0	0	0	410	15	3	3	1 carb
Tomato	1/2 cup	90	1.5	15	0.5	0	0	410	17	1	2	1 carb
Vegetable	1/2 cup	100	1	9	10	0	0	410	20	3	4	1 carb

READY-TO-SERVE SINGLE-SERVING CANNED SOUP

Brands

Campbell's Soup at Hand

Chicken & Stars	1 Container	70	2	20	0.5	0	5	960	10	1	3	1 carb
Classic Tomato	1 Container	120	0.5	5	0	0	0	890	25	2	3	1 1/2 carb
Cream of Broccoli	1 Container	150	7	65	2	0	5	890	17	7	3	1 carb, 1 fat
Creamy Chicken	1 Container	150	8	70	2.5	0	10	880	9	2	3	1/2 carb, 2 fat

SOUPS, STEW, CHILI

	Serving	Calories	Fat (g)	Cal. from Fat	Sat. Fat (g)	Trans Fat (g)	Chol. (mg)	Sod. (mg)	Carb. (g)	Fiber (g)	Prot. (g)	Servings/Exchanges
Creamy Tomato	1 Container	180	4	35	1	0	5	940	32	2	4	2 carb, 1 fat
Creamy Tomato Parmesan Bisque	1 Container	220	7	65	2	0	10	810	35	2	5	2 carb, 1 fat
New England Clam Chowder	1 Container	160	10	90	2	0	5	890	13	5	4	1 carb, 2 fat
Vegetable Beef	1 Container	70	1	10	0.5	0	5	930	11	1	3	1 carb
Vegetable with Mini Round Noodles	1 Container	100	0.5	5	0	0	5	650	21	1	2	1 1/2 carb
Campbell's Microwavable Classic Bowls												
Chicken Noodle	1 cup	70	2	20	0.5	0	15	870	10	<1	4	1/2 carb, 1 lean meat
Tomato	1 cup	110	0	0	0	0	0	790	24	3	3	1 1/2 carb
Vegetable Beef	1 cup	80	0.5	5	0.5	0	10	880	15	3	5	1 carb

Healthy Choice Microwavable Bowls

Beef Pot Roast	1 cup	110	1	10	0	0	0	480	18	5	7	1 carb, 1 lean meat
Chicken with Rice	1 cup	90	1.5	15	0.5	0	15	440	13	2	6	1 carb, 1 lean meat
Country Vegetable	1 cup	100	0.5	5	0	0	0	480	21	5	4	1 1/2 carb

Knorr Ready to Serve

Broccoli with Boursin Cheese	1 cup	140	9	80	5	0	15	810	12	1	2	1 carb, 2 fat
Classic Tomato with Real Cream	1 cup	140	3	25	1.5	0	0	650	25	3	3	1 1/2 carb, 1 fat
Red Soup	1 cup	120	2.5	25	0.5	0	0	650	20	3	3	1 carb, 1 fat
Rustic Vegetable & Potato	1 cup	80	1.5	15	1	0	5	730	14	2	2	1 carb

MULTI-SERVE SOUP MIX

Brands

Bear Creek

Creamy Potato	1 cup	150	3.5	35	2	0	0	860	27	0	2	2 carb, 1 fat

SOUPS, STEW, CHILI

	Serving	Calories	Fat (g)	Cal. from Fat	Sat. Fat (g)	Trans Fat (g)	Chol. (mg)	Sod. (mg)	Carb. (g)	Fiber (g)	Prot. (g)	Servings/Exchanges
Minestrone	1 cup	110	0	0	0	0	0	870	23	2	4	1 1/2 carb
Tortilla	1 cup	90	0.5	5	0	0	0	830	22	5	3	1 1/2 carb
Vegetable Beef	1 cup	115	0.5	5	0	0	0	740	25	3	5	1 1/2 carb
Fantastic Foods Simmer Soups												
Blarneystone Creamy Potato	1 cup	110	2	15	1	0	5	760	28	3	9	2 carb
Dutch Split Pea	1 cup	120	1	10	1	0	0	590	21	5	8	1 1/2 carb
Vegetarian Chicken Noodle	1 cup	90	1	10	0	0	0	700	14	1	7	1 carb, 1 lean meat
SINGLE-SERVING SOUP MIX												
Brands												
Health Valley (Fat Free Soup Cups)												
Chicken Flavored Noodles w/Vegetable	1/2 cup	110	0	0	0	0	0	390	24	3	5	1 1/2 carb

Creamy Potato with Broccoli	1/3 cup	80	0	0	0	0	0	390	17	3	4	1 carb
Lentil with Couscous	1/3 cup	130	0	0	0	0	0	310	28	5	7	2 carb
Spicy Black Bean with Couscous	1/3 cup	130	0	0	0	0	0	290	29	5	6	2 carb

Lipton Cup-a-Soup

Chicken Noodle	1 envelope	45	1	0	0	0	10	540	8	0	2	1/2 carb

Maruchan Noodle Cups

Chicken	1 container	290	12	110	6	0	0	1200	38	2	7	2 1/2 carb, 2 fat

Maruchan Ramen Noodle Soup

Chicken	1/2 pkg	190	7	70	3.5	0	0	830	26	1	5	2 carb, 1 fat

Nissin Noodle Cup

Chicken	1 container	300	13	120	7	0	<5	1060	38	2	6	2 1/2 carb, 3 fat

SOUPS, STEW, CHILI

	Serving	Calories	Fat (g)	Cal. from Fat	Sat. Fat (g)	Trans Fat (g)	Chol. (mg)	Sod. (mg)	Carb. (g)	Fiber (g)	Prot. (g)	Servings/Exchanges
Nissin Top Ramen Noodle Soup												
Chicken	1/2 pkg	190	7	60	3.5	0	0	910	26	2	5	2 carb, 1 fat
CHILI & STEW												
Brands												
Amy's Organic												
Black Bean Chili	1 cup	200	3	30	0	0	0	680	31	13	13	2 carb, 1 lean meat
Medium Chili	1 cup	280	9	80	1	0	0	680	35	7	15	2 carb, 2 med-fat meat
Medium Chili with Vegetables	1 cup	190	6	50	0.5	0	0	590	29	8	7	2 carb, 1 fat
Southwestern Black Bean Chili	1 cup	240	4	35	0.5	0	0	680	40	10	12	2 1/2 carb, 1 med-fat meat
Spicy Chili	1 cup	250	9	80	1	0	0	340	30	7	13	2 carb, 1 med-fat meat, 1 fat
Campbell's												

Chunky Hot & Spicy Beef & Bean Chili	1 cup	230	8	70	3.5	0.5	30	870	25	8	15	1 1/2 carb, 2 med-fat meat
Chunky Grilled Steak Chili with Beans	1 cup	200	3	25	1	0	15	870	27	7	16	2 carb, 1 lean meat
Chunky Hold the Beans Chili	1 cup	240	10	90	4	0.5	35	770	20	5	18	1 carb, 2 med-fat meat
Chunky Roadhouse Beef & Bean Chili	1 cup	230	8	70	3.5	0.5	30	870	25	8	15	1 1/2 carb, 2 med-fat meat
Dennison's											
Chunky Chili Con Carne with Beans	1 cup	300	10	90	4.5	0.5	40	1020	32	9	20	2 carb, 2 med-fat meat
Hot Chili Con Carne with Beans	1 cup	350	14	130	6	1	40	930	36	11	21	2 1/2 carb, 2 med-fat meat, 1 fat
Original Chili Con Carne with Beans	1 cup	360	14	130	6	1	40	1030	38	11	20	2 1/2 carb, 2 med-fat meat, 1 fat
Dinty Moore											
Beef Stew	1 cup	210	10	90	4	0	30	970	19	1	11	1 carb, 1 med-fat meat, 1 fat

SOUPS, STEW, CHILI

	Serving	Calories	Fat (g)	Cal. from Fat	Sat. Fat (g)	Trans Fat (g)	Chol. (mg)	Sod. (mg)	Carb. (g)	Fiber (g)	Prot. (g)	Servings/Exchanges
Health Valley Chunky Chili												
Vegetarian, Mild	1 cup	150	1	0	0	0	0	480	31	10	9	2 carb, 1 lean meat
Vegetarian, Mild, Black Bean Mole	1 cup	150	1	0	0	0	0	480	32	8	10	2 carb, 1 lean meat
Vegetarian, Mild, No Salt Added	1 cup	150	1	0	0	0	0	75	31	10	9	2 carb, 1 lean meat
Vegetarian, Mild, Three Bean Chipotle	1 cup	150	1	0	0	0	0	480	32	10	10	2 carb, 1 lean meat
Vegetarian, Spicy	1 cup	150	1	0	0	0	0	480	31	10	9	2 carb, 1 lean meat
Vegetarian, Spicy, Black Bean Mango	1 cup	150	1	0	0	0	0	480	32	8	10	2 carb, 1 lean meat
Hormel Chili												
Chili No Beans	1 cup	220	9	80	4	0	40	970	18	3	16	1 carb, 2 med-fat meat
Chili with Beans	1 cup	260	7	60	3	0	30	1200	33	7	16	2 carb, 1 med-fat meat

Chunky Chili No Beans	1 cup	210	8	70	3.5	0	40	1130	19	4	16	1 carb, 2 med-fat meat
Chunky Chili with Beans	1 cup	260	7	60	3	0	30	1160	32	7	17	2 carb, 2 lean meat
Hot Chili No Beans	1 cup	220	9	80	4	0	40	970	18	3	16	1 carb, 2 med-fat meat
Hot Chili with Beans	1 cup	260	7	60	3	0	30	1190	33	7	16	2 carb, 1 med-fat meat
Less Sodium Chili with Beans	1 cup	260	7	60	3	0	30	880	33	7	16	2 carb, 1 med-fat meat
Turkey Chili with Beans, 98% Fat Free	1 cup	210	3	25	1	0	45	1250	28	6	17	2 carb, 2 lean meat

Hormel Chili Master

Chipotle Chicken Chili with Beans	1 cup	240	7	65	2	0	50	970	28	7	17	2 carb, 2 lean meat
Roasted Tomato Chili with Beans	1 cup	210	6	55	2	0	25	990	25	7	14	2 carb, 2 lean meat
White Chicken Chili with Beans	1 cup	220	8	70	4	0	50	990	17	4	19	1 1/2 carb, 2 med-fat meat

SOUPS, STEW, CHILI

	Serving	Calories	Fat (g)	Cal. from Fat	Sat. Fat (g)	Trans Fat (g)	Chol. (mg)	Sod. (mg)	Carb. (g)	Fiber (g)	Prot. (g)	Servings/Exchanges
Shelton's												
Mild Turkey Chili	1 cup	220	2.5	20	0.5	0	50	1060	29	6	21	2 carb, 2 lean meat
Spicy Turkey Chili	1 cup	220	2.5	20	0.5	0	50	1060	29	6	21	2 carb, 2 lean meat
Stagg Chili												
Chunkero Chili with Beans	1 cup	320	16	140	6	0.5	40	850	28	6	16	2 carb, 1 med-fat meat, 2 fat
Classic Chili with Beans	1 cup	330	17	150	7	0.05	45	810	27	6	16	2 carb, 1 med-fat meat, 2 fat
Country Brand Chili with Beans	1 cup	330	17	150	7	1	35	1140	28	6	15	2 carb, 1 med-fat meat, 2 fat
Dynamite Hot Chili with Beans	1 cup	340	17	150	7	1	40	800	30	8	17	2 carb, 2 med-fat meat, 1 fat
Fiesta Grille Chili with Beans	1 cup	250	10	90	4	0	40	950	25	6	15	1 1/2 carb, 2 med-fat meat

Laredo Chili with Beans	1 cup	310	17	150	7	1	40	1100	25	7	15	1 1/2 carb, 2 med-fat meat, 1 fat
Ranch House Chicken Chili	1 cup	240	8	70	2	0	55	780	26	7	17	2 carb, 2 med-fat meat
Silverado Beef Chili with Beans	1 cup	250	7	60	3	0	30	860	30	6	17	2 carb, 2 lean meat
Steak House Chili No Beans	1 cup	320	22	200	10	1	65	1080	14	2	17	1 carb, 2 med-fat meat, 2 fat
Turkey Ranchero Chili with Beans	1 cup	240	3	25	1	0	35	880	31	6	22	2 carb, 2 lean meat
Vegetable Garden Four-Bean Chili	1 cup	200	1	10	0	0	0	890	37	8	10	2 1/2 carb, 1 lean meat
Trader Joe's												
99% Fat Free Beef Chili with Beans	1 cup	230	3	25	1	0	40	880	33	6	18	2 carb, 2 lean meat
Chicken Chili with Beans	1 cup	290	9	80	3	0	50	810	32	6	19	2 carb, 2 med-fat meat

SOUPS, STEWS, CHILI

	Serving	Calories	Fat (g)	Cal. from Fat	Sat. Fat (g)	Trans Fat (g)	Chol. (mg)	Sod. (mg)	Carb. (g)	Fiber (g)	Prot. (g)	Servings/Exchanges
Organic Vegetarian Chili	1 cup	190	6	60	0.5	0	0	590	26	7	8	2 carb, 1 fat
Turkey Chili with Beans	1 cup	230	3	25	1	0	40	800	30	7	21	2 carb, 2 lean meat
Wolf Brand												
Chili Hot Dog Sauce	2 Tbsp	30	1	10	0	0	0	140	4	1	1	1/2 carb
Chili No Beans	1 cup	410	28	250	12	1.5	55	1020	20	7	23	1 carb, 3 med-fat meat, 3 fat

SWEET BREADS, MUFFINS, PASTRIES, DONUTS

	Serving	Calories	Fat (g)	Cal. from Fat	Sat. Fat (g)	Trans Fat (g)	Chol. (mg)	Sod. (mg)	Carb. (g)	Fiber (g)	Prot. (g)	Servings/Exchanges
Baklava	2×2-inch piece	333	23	207	9	NA	36	291	29	2	5	2 carb, 4 fat
Bread, Banana	1 slice	178	5	45	2	NA	34	170	31	1	3	2 carb, 1 fat
Bread, Date Nut	1 slice	217	10	90	2	NA	28	140	30	<1	3	2 carb, 2 fat
Bread, Fruit, No Nuts	1 slice	150	6	54	2	NA	22	109	23	<1	2	1 1/2 carb, 1 fat
Cream Puff with Custard Filling	1	335	20	180	5	NA	174	375	30	<1	9	2 carb, 4 fat
Crepe/French Pancake	1	239	13	117	4	NA	163	274	22	<1	9	1 1/2 carb, 3 fat
Croissant, Cheese	1 medium	236	12	108	6	NA	37	316	27	2	5	2 carb, 2 fat
Danish Pastry, Cinnamon	1, 4 inches	262	15	135	4	NA	14	241	29	<1	5	2 carb, 3 fat
Danish Pastry, Fruit-Filled	1, 4 inches	263	13	115	3.5	NA	81	251	34	1	4	2 carb, 3 fat

SWEET BREADS, MUFFINS, PASTRIES, DONUTS

	Serving	Calories	Fat (g)	Cal. from Fat	Sat. Fat (g)	Trans Fat (g)	Chol. (mg)	Sod. (mg)	Carb. (g)	Fiber (g)	Prot. (g)	Servings/Exchanges
Donut Cake	1	196	11	100	3	NA	4	262	21	<1	3	1 1/2 carb, 2 fat
Donut, Cake, Sugared/Glazed	1	192	10	90	2	NA	14	181	23	<1	2	1 1/2 carb, 2 fat
Donut, Cake, with Chocolate Icing	1	194	11	100	6	NA	8	178	22	<1	2	1 1/2 carb, 2 fat
Donut, Custard-Filled with Icing	1	261	13	117	6	NA	21	125	34	1	3	2 carb, 3 fat
Donut, Yeast, Crème Filled	1	307	21	189	6	NA	20	263	26	<1	5	2 carb, 4 fat
Donut, Yeast, Glazed	1	239	12	110	3	NA	18	232	30	1	4	2 carb, 2 fat
Donut, Yeast, Jelly Filled	1	289	16	144	4	NA	22	190	33	<1	5	1 1/2 carb, 2 fat
Eclair, Chocolate with Custard Filling	1	262	16	144	4	NA	127	337	24	<1	6	1 1/2 carb, 3 fat
Muffin	1 small	133	5	45	1	NA	18	210	19	1	3	1 carb, 1 fat

Item	Serving											
Muffin, Cheese	1 small	184	8	72	3	NA	30	274	23	<1	5	1 1/2 carb, 2 fat
Muffin, Chocolate Chip	1 small	190	9	81	3	NA	25	186	27	1	4	2 carb, 2 fat
Muffin, Cranberry Nut	1 small	164	5	45	2	NA	39	326	25	<1	4	1 1/2 carb, 1 fat
Muffin, Oat Bran	1 small	175	8	70	1	NA	0	444	55	5	8	3 1/2 carb, 2 fat
Muffin, Pumpkin with Raisins & Nuts	1 small	181	4	36	<1	NA	26	154	34	1	3	2 carb, 1 fat
Muffin, Wheat Bran	1 small	161	7	63	2	NA	19	335	24	2	4	1 1/2 carb, 1 fat
Muffin, Whole Wheat	1 small	142	6	54	2	NA	21	283	20	3	4	1 carb, 1 fat
Muffin, Zucchini with Nuts	1 small	210	11	99	2	NA	37	169	26	<1	3	2 carb, 2 fat
Pannetone or Italian Sweetbread	1 slice	86	2	18	1	NA	19	96	15	<1	2	1 carb
Sweet Roll	1 roll	264	12	110	2	NA	47	272	36	2	4	2 1/2 carb, 2 fat
Sweet Roll, Cheese	1 roll	238	12	108	4	NA	40	236	29	<1	5	2 carb, 2 fat
Sweet Roll, Cinnamon Raisin	1 roll	223	10	90	2	NA	40	230	31	1	4	2 carb, 2 fat

SWEET BREADS, MUFFINS, PASTRIES, DONUTS

	Serving	Calories	Fat (g)	Cal. from Fat	Sat. Fat (g)	Trans Fat (g)	Chol. (mg)	Sod. (mg)	Carb. (g)	Fiber (g)	Prot. (g)	Servings/Exchanges
Sweet Roll, Cinnamon with Raisins & Nuts	1	196	7	63	2	NA	13	185	30	1	4	2 carb, 1 fat
Brands												
Betty Crocker												
Muffin Mix, Apple Streusel	1	230	8	70	2	0	35	280	37	<1	3	2 1/2 carb, 2 fat
Muffin Mix, Banana Nut	1	210	9	80	2	0	35	250	27	<1	2	2 carb, 2 fat
Muffin Mix, Lemon Poppy Seed	1	200	8	70	1.5	0	35	230	30	0	3	2 carb, 2 fat
Muffin Mix, Wild Blueberry	1	180	7	60	1.5	0	35	230	27	<1	3	2 carb, 1 fat
Quick Bread Mix, Banana	1 slice	170	7	60	1.5	0	35	210	25	0	3	1 1/2 carb, 1 fat
Quick Bread Mix, Cinnamon Streusel	1 slice	180	7	60	1.5	0	30	160	28	0	2	2 carb, 1 fat

	Amount	Cal.	Fat (g)	Cal. Fat	Sat. Fat (g)	Trans Fat (g)	Chol. (mg)	Sod. (mg)	Carb. (g)	Fiber (g)	Pro. (g)	Exchanges
Quick Bread Mix, Cranberry Orange	1 slice	180	6	60	1.5	0	35	180	29	<1	3	2 carb, 1 fat
Duncan Hines												
Muffin Mix, Blueberry Streusel, Whole Grain	1	210	8	70	1.5	0	35	230	32	3	3	2 carb, 2 fat
Muffin Mix, Chocolate Chip, Whole Grain	1	190	7	60	2	0	35	290	32	3	3	2 carb, 1 fat
Muffin Mix, Cinnamon Swirl, Whole Grain	1	220	8	70	1.5	0	35	230	34	3	3	2 carb, 2 fat
Eggo Bake Shop (Frozen)												
Mini Muffin Tops, Blueberry	1	140	5	45	1.5	0	15	280	21	0	2	1 1/2 carb, 1 fat
Swirlz, Strawberry	1	150	3	30	1	0	10	270	28	<1	3	2 carb, 1 fat
Twists, Apple	1	190	7	60	3.5	0	15	220	29	<1	3	2 carb, 1 fat
Entenmann's												
Apple Puffs	1	290	14	130	7	0	0	260	39	1	3	2 1/2 carb, 3 fat

SWEET BREADS, MUFFINS, PASTRIES, DONUTS

	Serving	Calories	Fat (g)	Cal. from Fat	Sat. Fat (g)	Trans Fat (g)	Chol. (mg)	Sod. (mg)	Carb. (g)	Fiber (g)	Prot. (g)	Servings/Exchanges
Cheese Topped Buns	1	320	15	140	6	0	55	320	40	1	6	2 1/2 carb, 3 fat
Cherry Cheese Danish	1/9	200	9	80	3.5	0	25	170	25	<1	3	1 1/2 carb, 2 fat
Cinnamon Swirl Rolls	1	320	14	130	5	0	45	280	44	2	5	3 carb, 3 fat
Coffee Cake, Crumb	1/10	260	13	120	4	0	15	210	34	1	3	2 carb, 3 fat
Danish Pastry Twist, Raspberry	1/8	220	11	100	4.5	0	15	170	29	<1	3	2 carb, 2 fat
Danish, Cheese Crumb	1/9	200	10	90	4	0	35	190	35	<1	3	2 carb, 2 fat
Donuts, Frosted Devil Food	1	310	18	160	12	0	10	170	36	2	3	2 1/2 carb, 4 fat
Donuts, Frosted Popettes	4	320	23	210	14	0	10	180	28	1	2	2 carb, 5 fat
Donuts, Glazed Crullers	2	210	12	210	6	0	10	140	25	0	1	1 1/2 carb, 2 fat
Donuts, Glazed Popems	4	220	10	90	5	0	0	170	30	0	2	2 carb, 2 fat
Donuts, Rich Frosted	1	300	20	180	13	0	10	190	30	1	2	2 carb, 4 fat

Food	Amount											Exchanges
Eclair	1	260	9	80	2.5	0	65	190	46	3	3	3 carb, 2 fat
Little Bites Banana Chocolate Chip Muffins	1 pkg	180	8	70	2	0	20	125	25	<1	2	1 1/2 carb, 2 fat
Little Bites Blueberry Muffins	1 pkg	180	8	70	1.5	0	25	190	25	0	2	1 1/2 carb, 2 fat
Pecan Danish Ring	1/8	240	15	140	3.5	0	20	150	24	1	3	1 1/2 carb, 3 fat
Hostess												
Donettes, Frosted	4	270	17	150	11	0	15	210	29	1	2	2 carb, 3 fat
Donettes, Powdered	4	230	11	100	5	0	20	230	31	<1	2	2 carb, 2 fat
Donuts, Powdered	1	190	9	80	4	0	10	230	25	0	2	1 1/2 carb, 2 fat
Mini Muffins, Banana Walnut	1 pkg	260	16	150	2.5	0	30	140	27	<1	3	2 carb, 3 fat
Mini Muffins, Blueberry	1 pkg	260	14	120	2.5	0	40	170	30	<1	3	2 carb, 3 fat
Jiffy												
Muffin Mix, Apple Cinnamon	1/4 cup	180	5	60	2	0	<5	320	26	0	2	2 carb, 1 fat

SWEET BREADS, MUFFINS, PASTRIES, DONUTS

	Serving	Calories	Fat (g)	Cal. from Fat	Sat. Fat (g)	Trans Fat (g)	Chol. (mg)	Sod. (mg)	Carb. (g)	Fiber (g)	Prot. (g)	Servings/Exchanges
Muffin Mix, Banana Nut	1/4 cup	170	4.5	50	2	0	<5	310	25	<1	2	1 1/2 carb, 1 fat
Muffin Mix, Blueberry	1/4 cup	180	5	60	2	0	<5	320	26	0	2	2 carb, 1 fat
Kellogg's												
Pop-Tarts Pastry, Blueberry	1	210	5	50	2	0	0	180	37	<1	2	2 1/2 carb, 1 fat
Pop-Tarts Pastry, Brown Sugar Cinnamon	1	210	8	70	2.5	0	0	190	34	1	2	2 carb, 2 fat
Pop-Tarts Pastry, Cherry, Frosted	1	200	5	45	1.5	0	0	160	38	<1	2	2 1/2 carb, 1 fat
Pop-Tarts Pastry, Chocolate Chip Cookie Dough	1	200	5	45	2	0	0	190	35	<1	2	2 carb, 1 fat
Pop-Tarts Pastry, Chocolate Fudge, Frosted	1	200	5	45	1.5	0	0	230	37	1	3	2 1/2 carb, 1 fat

Pop-Tarts Pastry, Raspberry, Frosted	1	200	5	45	1.5	0	0	160	38	<1	2	2 1/2 carb, 1 fat
Pop-Tarts Pastry, S'mores, Frosted	1	200	6	45	1.5	0	0	210	36	<1	3	2 1/2 carb, 1 fat
Pop-Tarts Pastry, Strawberry, Frosted	1	200	5	45	1.5	0	0	170	38	1	2	2 1/2 carb, 1 fat
Pop-Tarts Pastry, Whole Grain, 20% Fiber, Strawberry	1	190	5	45	1.5	0	0	150	35	5	2	2 carb, 1 fat
Kraft Bagel-fuls											
Blueberry, Bagel with Cream Cheese	1	190	4.5	40	2.5	0	10	190	30	2	6	2 carb, 1 fat
Original, Plain Bagel with Cream Cheese	1	200	5	50	3	0	15	200	31	2	6	2 carb, 1 fat
Strawberry & Cream Cheese Bagel	1	190	3	30	1.5	0	5	180	34	2	6	2 carb, 1 fat

SWEET BREADS, MUFFINS, PASTRIES, DONUTS

	Serving	Calories	Fat (g)	Cal. from Fat	Sat. Fat (g)	Trans Fat (g)	Chol. (mg)	Sod. (mg)	Carb. (g)	Fiber (g)	Prot. (g)	Servings/Exchanges
Little Debbie												
Coffee Cake, Apple Streusel	1	190	5	45	1.5	0	10	160	35	0	2	2 carb, 1 fat
Donut Stick	1	230	14	130	7	0	10	160	25	0	2	1 1/2 carb, 3 fat
Honey Bun	1	220	12	110	6	0	<5	170	26	<1	3	2 carb, 2 fat
Mini Frosted Donuts	4	290	17	150	10	0	15	230	32	1	3	2 carb, 3 fat
Mini Powdered Donuts	4	210	10	90	5	0	15	220	29	0	2	2 carb, 2 fat
Muffin, Banana Nut	1	210	9	80	1.5	0	10	170	30	<1	3	2 carb, 2 fat
Muffin, Blueberry	1	190	8	70	1.5	0	10	140	27	1	3	2 carb, 2 fat
Muffin, Chocolate Chip	1	210	9	80	2	0	20	170	28	1	3	2 carb, 2 fat
Pecan Spinwheel	1	100	4	35	1	0	<5	75	16	<1	1	1 carb, 1 fat
Pepperidge Farm Puff Pastry												
Apple Turnover	1	270	15	135	8	0	0	230	31	1	4	2 carb, 3 fat
Cherry Turnover	1	270	15	135	8	0	0	230	31	1	4	2 carb, 3 fat

Raspberry Turnover	1	280	15	135	8	0	0	230	34	2	4	2 carb, 3 fat
Pillsbury (Refrigerated)											
Cinnamon Rolls with Icing	1	140	5	45	1.5	2	0	340	23	<1	2	1 1/2 carb, 1 fat
Cinnamon Rolls with Icing, Reduced Fat	1	130	3.5	30	2.5	0	0	340	24	<1	2	1 1/2 carb, 1 fat
Flaky Supreme Cinnamon Rolls with Icing	1	370	19	170	5	5	0	650	48	1	4	3 carb, 4 fat
Flaky Twists with Icing	1	180	9	80	2.5	0	0	310	22	<1	2	1 1/2 carb, 2 fat
Orange Sweet Rolls with Icing	1	160	6	50	1.5	1.5	0	350	26	<1	2	2 carb, 1 fat
Toaster Strudel Frozen Pastries, Apple	1	190	8	80	3.5	1	5	180	26	<1	3	2 carb, 2 fat
Toaster Strudel Frozen Pastries, Strawberry	1	190	8	80	3.5	1	5	180	26	<1	3	2 carb, 2 fat

VEGETABLES, VEGETABLE JUICES

	Serving	Calories	Fat (g)	Cal. from Fat	Sat. Fat (g)	Trans Fat (g)	Chol. (mg)	Sod. (mg)	Carb. (g)	Fiber (g)	Prot. (g)	Servings/Exchanges
Alfalfa Sprouts	1 cup	10	<1	0	0	0	0	2	1	<1	1	free
Artichoke Hearts, Canned, Drained	1/2 cup	30	0	0	0	0	0	240	6	1	2	1 vegetable
Artichokes, Cooked	1/2	30	<1	0	0	0	0	57	7	<1	3	1 vegetable
Arugula, Raw	1 cup	5	0	0	0	0	0	6	<1	0	<1	free
Asparagus, Canned, Drained	1/2 cup	23	<1	0	0	0	0	347	3	2	3	1 vegetable
Asparagus, Frozen, Cooked	1/2 cup	25	<1	0	0	0	0	4	4	1	3	1 vegetable
Asparagus, Fresh, Cooked	4 spears	14	0	0	0	0	0	7	3	1	2	free
Baby Corn, Canned	1/2 cup	20	0	0	0	0	0	10	5	2	1	1 vegetable
Bamboo Shoots, Canned	1/2 cup	12	0	0	0	0	0	5	2	<1	1	free

Food	Serving										Exchanges
Bamboo Shoots, Sliced, Raw	1 cup	41	<1	0	0	0	6	8	3	4	1 vegetable
Bean Sprouts, Fresh, Cooked	1/2 cup	13	0	0	0	0	6	3	<1	1	free
Beans, Green, Canned	1/2 cup	14	0	0	0	0	178	3	1	<1	1 vegetable
Beans, Green, Fresh, Cooked	1/2 cup	22	0	0	0	0	1	5	2	1	1 vegetable
Beans, Green, Frozen	1/2 cup	19	0	0	0	0	1	4	2	<1	1 vegetable
Beets, Canned	1/2 cup	26	0	0	0	0	165	6	1	<1	1 vegetable
Beets, Harvard, Diced	1/2 cup	136	4	36	<1	0	287	25	2	<1	1 carb, 1 vegetable, 1 fat
Beets, Pickled	1/2 cup	74	<1	0	0	0	301	19	1	<1	1 carb, 1 vegetable
Bitter Melon Gourd, Cooked	1/2 cup	12	0	0	0	0	4	3	1	<1	1 vegetable
Bok Choy	1 cup	9	0	0	0	0	46	2	<1	1	free
Broccoli, Fresh, Cooked	1/2 cup	22	0	0	0	0	20	4	2	2	1 vegetable

VEGETABLES, VEGETABLE JUICES

	Serving	Calories	Fat (g)	Cal. from Fat	Sat. Fat (g)	Trans Fat (g)	Chol. (mg)	Sod. (mg)	Carb. (g)	Fiber (g)	Prot. (g)	Servings/Exchanges
Broccoli, Frozen, Cooked	1/2 cup	26	0	0	0	0	0	22	5	3	3	1 vegetable
Brussels Sprouts, Frozen, Cooked	1/2 cup	33	0	0	0	0	0	18	7	3	3	1 vegetable
Cabbage, Fresh, Cooked	1/2 cup	17	0	0	0	0	0	6	3	2	<1	1 vegetable
Cabbage, Green, Raw	1 cup	18	0	0	0	0	0	13	4	2	1	1 vegetable
Cabbage, Red, Cooked	1/2 cup	16	0	0	<1	0	0	6	4	2	<1	1 vegetable
Carrot Juice, Canned	1/2 cup	47	<1	0	<1	0	0	34	11	<1	1	2 vegetable
Carrots, Canned	1/2 cup	36	0	0	0	0	0	344	8	2	1	1 vegetable
Carrots, Fresh, Cooked	1/2 cup	35	0	0	0	0	0	51	8	3	<1	1 vegetable
Carrots, Raw	1 cup	50	0	0	0	0	0	84	12	4	1	2 vegetable
Cassava, Cooked	1/3 cup	70	0	0	0	0	0	7	17	<1	<1	1 starch
Cassava, Raw	1/4 cup	83	0	0	0	0	0	7	20	1	1	1 starch
Cauliflower, Fresh, Raw	1 cup	25	0	0	0	0	0	30	5	3	2	1 vegetable

Food	Serving									
Cauliflower, Frozen, Cooked	1/2 cup	17	0	0	0	16	3	2	1	1 vegetable
Celery, Fresh, Cooked	1/2 cup	14	0	0	0	68	3	1	<1	1 vegetable
Celery, Fresh, Raw	1 cup	17	0	0	0	99	4	2	<1	1 vegetable
Chard, Swiss, Fresh, Cooked	1/2 cup	18	0	0	0	158	4	2	2	1 vegetable
Chayote Squash, Cooked	1/2 cup	19	0	0	0	1	4	2	<1	1 vegetable
Coleslaw Mix	1/2 cup	17	0	0	0	15	3	2	0	1 vegetable
Collard Greens, Fresh, Cooked	1/2 cup	26	0	0	0	15	6	3	1	1 vegetable
Corn on the Cob, Cooked	1/2 large ear	66	<1	0	0	3	16	2	2	1 starch
Corn, Canned	1/2 cup	66	<1	0	0	175	15	2	2	1 starch
Corn, Frozen, Cooked	1/2 cup	66	<1	0	0	4	16	2	2	1 starch
Cucumber, Raw	1 cup	16	0	0	0	2	4	<1	<1	1 vegetable

VEGETABLES, VEGETABLE JUICES

	Serving	Calories	Fat (g)	Cal. from Fat	Sat. Fat (g)	Trans Fat (g)	Chol. (mg)	Sod. (mg)	Carb. (g)	Fiber (g)	Prot. (g)	Servings/Exchanges
Eggplant, Fresh, Cooked	1/2 cup	17	0	0	0	0	0	0	4	1	<1	1 vegetable
Endive/Escarole, Raw	1 cup	9	0	0	0	0	0	11	2	2	<1	1 vegetable
Green Onions, Raw	1 cup	32	0	0	0	0	0	16	7	3	2	1 vegetable
Heart of Palm, Canned	1/2 cup	20	0.5	5	0	0	0	311	3	2	2	1 vegetable
Hominy, Yellow, Canned	1/2 cup	90	1	10	0	0	0	157	18	3	2	1 starch
Jicama	1/2 cup	30	0	0	0	0	0	3	7	3	<1	1 vegetable
Kale, Fresh, Cooked	1/2 cup	18	0	0	0	0	0	15	4	1	1	1 vegetable
Kohlrabi, Cooked	1/2 cup	24	0	0	0	0	0	17	6	<1	2	1 vegetable
Leeks, Cooked	1/2 cup	16	0	0	0	0	0	5	4	<1	<1	1 vegetable
Lettuce, Butterhead, Raw	1 cup	7	0	0	0	0	0	3	1	0	0	1 vegetable
Lettuce, Iceberg, Raw	1 cup	7	<1	0	0	0	0	5	1	<1	<1	1 vegetable
Lettuce, Romaine, Chopped	1 cup	9	<1	0	<1	0	0	5	1	1	<1	free

Food	Serving										
Lettuce, Romaine, Raw	1 cup	9	<1	0	0	0	5	1	1	<1	1 vegetable
Lima Beans, Frozen, Cooked	1/2 cup	94	0	0	0	0	26	18	5	6	1 starch
Luffa, Cooked	1/2 cup	20	0	0	0	0	12	4	2	2	1 vegetable
Mixed Vegetables with Corn, Frozen, Cooked	1 cup	80	0	0	0	0	80	18	4	4	1 starch
Mixed Vegetables with Pasta, Frozen, Cooked	1 cup	80	0	0	0	0	39	15	5	3	1 starch
Mixed Vegetables, No Corn, Peas, or Pasta	1/2 cup	20	0	0	0	0	15	3	1	1	1 vegetable
Mung Bean Sprouts, Cooked	1/2 cup	13	0	0	0	0	6	3	<1	1	1 vegetable
Mushrooms, Canned	1/2 cup	20	0	0	0	0	332	4	2	1	1 vegetable
Mushrooms, Fresh	1 cup	15	0	0	0	0	4	2	<1	2	free
Mustard Greens, Fresh, Cooked	1/2 cup	10	0	0	0	0	11	2	1	2	1 vegetable

VEGETABLES, VEGETABLE JUICES

	Serving	Calories	Fat (g)	Cal. from Fat	Sat. Fat (g)	Trans Fat (g)	Chol. (mg)	Sod. (mg)	Carb. (g)	Fiber (g)	Prot. (g)	Servings/Exchanges
Okra, Frozen, Cooked	1/2 cup	34	0	0	0	0	0	3	5	3	2	1 vegetable
Onions, Fresh, Cooked	1/2 cup	46	0	0	0	0	0	3	11	2	1	2 vegetable
Onions, Fresh, Raw	1 cup	67	0	0	0	0	0	5	16	2	2	3 vegetable
Oriental Radish, Fresh	1 cup	21	0	0	0	0	0	24	5	2	<1	1 vegetable
Parsnips, Fresh, Cooked	1/2 cup	63	0	0	0	0	0	8	15	3	1	1 starch
Pea Pods, Fresh, Cooked	1/2 cup	34	0	0	0	0	0	3	6	2	3	1 vegetable
Pea Pods, Raw	1 cup	61	0	0	0	0	0	6	11	4	4	2 vegetable
Peas, Green, Canned	1/2 cup	59	0	0	0	0	0	214	11	4	4	1 starch
Peas, Green, Fresh, Cooked	1/2 cup	67	0	0	0	0	0	2	13	4	4	1 starch
Peas, Green, Frozen, Cooked	1/2 cup	62	0	0	0	0	0	70	11	4	4	1 starch
Peas, Sugar Snap, Frozen, Uncooked	1/2 cup	30	0	0	0	0	0	3	5	2	2	1 vegetable

Food	Serving										
Peppers, Green, Fresh	1 cup	18	0	0	0	0	3	4	2	<1	1 vegetable
Peppers, Hot Green Chili, Canned	1/2 cup	25	0	0	0	0	565	3	3	0	1 vegetable
Peppers, Red, Fresh, Cooked	1/2 cup	19	0	0	0	0	1	5	<1	<1	1 vegetable
Plantains, Cooked	1/3 cup	59	0	0	0	0	3	16	1	<1	1 starch
Potatoes, Baked with Skin	3 oz	79	0	0	0	0	9	18	2	2	1 starch
Potatoes, French Fried, Frozen, Baked	1 cup	98	3	25	0.5	0	18	16	2	2	1 starch, 1 fat
Potatoes, Fresh, Mashed, with Milk	1/2 cup	85	<1	0	0	0	250	19	2	2	1 starch
Potatoes, White, Cooked, Peeled	3 oz	73	0	0	0	0	4	17	2	2	1 starch
Pumpkin, canned	1 cup	83	0	0	0	0	12	20	7	3	1 starch
Radicchio, Raw	1 cup	9	0	0	0	0	9	2	0	0	1 vegetable

VEGETABLES, VEGETABLE JUICES

	Serving	Calories	Fat (g)	Cal. from Fat	Sat. Fat (g)	Trans Fat (g)	Chol. (mg)	Sod. (mg)	Carb. (g)	Fiber (g)	Prot. (g)	Servings/Exchanges
Radishes	1 cup	20	0	0	0	0	0	28	4	2	<1	1 vegetable
Rutabagas, Fresh, Cooked	1/2 cup	33	0	0	0	0	0	17	7	2	1	1 vegetable
Sauerkraut, Canned	1/2 cup	23	0	0	0	0	0	471	5	3	1	1 vegetable
Soybean Sprouts, Cooked	1/2 cup	38	2	20	0	0	0	5	3	<1	4	1 vegetable
Spinach, Canned	1/2 cup	25	0	0	0	0	0	29	4	3	3	1 vegetable
Spinach, Frozen, Cooked	1/2 cup	13	0	0	0	0	0	92	5	4	4	1 vegetable
Spinach, Raw	1 cup	12	0	0	0	0	0	44	2	3	2	1 vegetable
Squash, Summer, Fresh, Cooked	1/2 cup	18	0	0	0	0	0	1	4	1	<1	1 vegetable
Squash, Summer, Raw	1 cup	18	0	0	0	0	0	2	4	3	1	1 vegetable
Squash, Winter, Cooked	1 cup	39	<1	0	0	0	0	1	9	3	<1	1/2 starch

Succotash, Frozen, Cooked	1/2 cup	79	<1	0	0	0	38	17	4	4	1 starch
Tomato Juice	1/2 cup	21	0	0	0	0	440	5	<1	<1	1 vegetable
Tomato Paste, Canned	1/2 cup	110	1	9	<1	0	1034	25	6	5	1 starch, 1 vegetable
Tomato Sauce	1/2 cup	37	0	0	0	0	738	9	2	2	1 vegetable
Tomatoes, Canned	1/2 cup	24	0	0	0	0	250	6	1	1	1 vegetable
Tomatoes, Raw	1 cup	32	0	0	0	0	9	7	2	2	1 vegetable
Tossed Green Salad	3/4 cup	19	0	0	<1	0	11	4	1	<1	1 vegetable
Turnip Greens, Fresh, Cooked	1/2 cup	14	0	0	0	0	21	3	3	<1	1 vegetable
Turnips, Fresh, Cooked	1/2 cup	17	0	0	0	0	12	4	2	<1	1 vegetable
Vegetable Juice	1/2 cup	25	0	0	0	0	310	6	<1	<1	1 vegetable
Vegetable Juice Cocktail	1/2 cup	23	0	0	<1	0	442	6	1	<1	1 vegetable
Water Chestnuts, Canned	1/2 cup	40	0	0	0	0	18	9	3	<1	1 vegetable
Watercress, Raw	1 cup	4	0	0	0	0	14	<1	<1	<1	1 vegetable

VEGETABLES, VEGETABLE JUICES

	Serving	Calories	Fat (g)	Cal. from Fat	Sat. Fat (g)	Trans Fat (g)	Chol. (mg)	Sod. (mg)	Carb. (g)	Fiber (g)	Prot. (g)	Servings/Exchanges
Yams, Cooked	1/2 cup	79	0	0	0	0	0	5	19	3	1	1 starch
Yard-Long Beans, Fresh, Cooked	1/2 cup	24	0	0	0	0	0	2	5	2	1	1 vegetable
Zucchini, Fresh, Cooked	1/2 cup	14	0	0	0	0	0	3	4	1	<1	1 vegetable
Zucchini, Raw	1 cup	18	0	0	0	0	0	11	4	1	1	1 vegetable
Brands												
Betty Crocker												
Mashed Potatoes, Four Cheese	1/2 cup	170	7	30	2	0	5	490	22	1	4	1 1/2 starch, 1 fat
Mashed Potatoes, Roasted Garlic	1/2 cup	120	3.5	30	1	0.5	0	520	21	1	2	1 1/2 starch, 1 fat
Potatoes, Au Gratin	1/2 cup	150	5	50	1.5	1	<5	660	24	1	3	1 1/2 starch, 1 fat
Potatoes, Cheddar & Bacon	2/3 cup	140	5	45	1	1	0	690	23	1	3	1 1/2 starch, 1 fat

Potatoes, Cheesy Scalloped	1/2 cup	140	5	45	1	1	0	22	2	2	1 1/2 starch, 1 fat
Potatoes, Deluxe Loaded Au Gratin	2/3 cup	140	4	35	1	0	0	24	1	3	1 1/2 starch, 1 fat
Potatoes, Julienne	2/3 cup	140	5	45	1.5	1	<5	21	1	1	1 1/2 starch, 1 fat
Potatoes, Loaded Au Gratin	2/3 cup	140	4	35	2	0	5	24	1	3	1 1/2 starch, 1 fat
Potatoes, Scalloped	1/2 cup	130	3	30	1	0	<5	23	1	2	1 1/2 starch, 1 fat
Potatoes, Skillet Hash Browns	1/2 cup	120	4	35	1	0.5	0	18	2	2	1 starch, 1 fat
Potatoes, Sour Cream 'n Chive	2/3 cup	120	3	30	1	0	<5	22	1	2	1 1/2 starch, 1 fat
Potatoes, Three Cheese	2/3 cup	120	3	25	1	0	0	23	1	2	1 1/2 starch, 1 fat
Birds Eye											
Asian Vegetable in Sesame Ginger Sauce	1 cup	60	1	10	0	0	0	12	2	2	2 vegetable

VEGETABLES, VEGETABLE JUICES

	Serving	Calories	Fat (g)	Cal. from Fat	Sat. Fat (g)	Trans Fat (g)	Chol. (mg)	Sod. (mg)	Carb. (g)	Fiber (g)	Prot. (g)	Servings/Exchanges
Asparagus Stir-Fry	1 cup	90	0	0	0	0	0	30	16	2	4	2 vegetable
Baby Corn & Vegetable Blend	2/3 cup	50	1	10	0	0	0	10	9	3	2	1 vegetable
Baby Sweet Peas & Pearl Onions	2/3 cup	60	0	0	0	0	0	0	12	3	4	1 starch
Broccoli & Cauliflower Mixture	1 cup	25	0	0	0	0	0	25	4	2	1	1 vegetable
Broccoli & Cheese Sauce	1/2 cup	90	5	45	3	0	5	490	8	1	3	1 vegetable, 1 fat
California Blend & Cheddar Cheese	1/2 cup	80	4	35	2	0	5	390	8	1	2	1 vegetable, 1 fat
Creamed Spinach	1/2 cup	90	4	35	2.5	0	10	500	9	4	3	1 vegetable, 1 fat
Green Beans & Lightly Toasted Almonds	3/4 cup	80	3.5	30	0	0	0	410	8	3	3	1 vegetable, 1 fat

Food	Serving	Cal	Fat (g)	% Fat Cal	Sat Fat (g)	Chol (mg)	Sodium (mg)	Carb (g)	Fiber (g)	Protein (g)	Exchanges/Choices
Peas & Pearl Onions in Lightly Seasoned Sauce	2/3 cup	90	0	0	0	0	0	17	4	5	1 starch
Roasted Potatoes & Broccoli	2/3 cup	100	3.5	35	2	0	470	15	1	2	1 starch, 1 fat
Sweet Corn & Butter Sauce	1/2 cup	110	1.5	15	0.5	0	190	21	1	2	1 1/2 starch
Szechuan Vegetable in Sesame Sauce	1 cup	60	1.5	15	0	0	460	9	2	1	1 vegetable
Campbell's											
Tomato Juice	8 oz	50	0	0	0	0	680	10	2	2	2 vegetable
Tomato Juice, Low Sodium	8 oz	50	0	0	0	0	140	10	2	2	2 vegetable
V8 Calcium Enriched	8 oz	50	0	0	0	0	480	11	2	2	2 vegetable
V8 Diet Splash Berry Blend Juice Drink	8 oz	10	0	0	0	0	35	3	0	0	free

VEGETABLES, VEGETABLE JUICES

	Serving	Calories	Fat (g)	Cal. from Fat	Sat. Fat (g)	Trans Fat (g)	Chol. (mg)	Sod. (mg)	Carb. (g)	Fiber (g)	Prot. (g)	Servings/Exchanges
V8 Diet Splash Tropical Blend Juice Drink	8 oz	10	0	0	0	0	0	35	3	0	0	free
V8 High Fiber	8 oz	70	0	0	0	0	0	480	13	5	2	1 carb
V8 Low Sodium	8 oz	50	0	0	0	0	0	140	10	2	2	2 vegetable
V8 Spicy Hot	8 oz	50	0	0	0	0	0	480	10	2	2	2 vegetable
V8 Splash Strawberry Kiwi Juice Drink	8 oz	70	0	0	0	0	0	50	18	0	0	1 carb
V8 Vegetable Juice	8 oz	50	0	0	0	0	0	420	10	2	2	2 vegetable
Contadina												
Tomato Paste	2 Tbsp	30	0	0	0	0	0	20	6	1	2	1 vegetable
Tomato Paste, Italian	2 Tbsp	35	<1	0	0	0	0	290	7	1	1	1 vegetable
Tomato Sauce	1/4 cup	15	0	0	0	0	0	280	3	<1	<1	1 vegetable
Tomato Sauce with Italian Herbs	1/4 cup	15	0	0	0	0	0	320	4	1	<1	1 vegetable

Tomato Sauce, Extra Thick & Zesty	1/4 cup	20	0	0	0	0	340	3	1	1	1 vegetable
Tomatoes, Crushed	1/4 cup	20	0	0	0	0	150	3	<1	<1	1 vegetable
Tomatoes, Italian (Pear)	1/2 cup	25	0	0	0	0	220	4	1	1	1 vegetable
Tomatoes, Recipe Ready	1/2 cup	25	<1	0	0	0	570	5	1	1	1 vegetable
Tomatoes, Stewed	1/2 cup	35	0	0	0	0	220	9	1	1	2 vegetable
Tomatoes, Stewed with Italian Herbs	1/2 cup	35	0	0	0	0	260	8	1	1	1 vegetable
Tomatoes, Whole Peeled	1/2 cup	25	0	0	0	0	218	4	1	1	1 vegetable
Green Giant											
Alfredo Vegetables	1/2 cup	60	1.5	0	0	0	340	10	2	3	2 vegetable
Asparagus Cuts, No Sauce	1/2 cup	20	0	0	0	0	90	3	<1	2	1 vegetable
Baby Brussels Sprouts & Butter Sauce	1/2 cup	60	1	0.5	0	<5	320	9	3	3	2 vegetable

VEGETABLES, VEGETABLE JUICES

	Serving	Calories	Fat (g)	Cal. from Fat	Sat. Fat (g)	Trans Fat (g)	Chol. (mg)	Sod. (mg)	Carb. (g)	Fiber (g)	Prot. (g)	Servings/Exchanges
Baby Sweet Peas & Butter Sauce	3/4 cup	80	1.5	15	1	0	<5	340	14	4	5	1 starch
Baby Sweet Peas, No Sauce	1/2 cup	60	0.5	5	0	0	0	190	13	4	4	1 starch
Baby Vegetable Medley	3/4 cup	40	1	10	0	0	<5	250	9	2	1	2 vegetable
Broccoli & Carrots	3/4 cup	60	3	25	0	0	0	260	8	3	2	2 vegetable
Broccoli & Three Cheese Sauce	1/2 cup	45	1.5	15	0.5	0	0	420	7	2	3	1 vegetable
Broccoli Spears & Butter Sauce	3 spears	40	1.5	15	1	0	<5	330	6	2	2	1 vegetable
Broccoli Spears, No Sauce	3 spears	25	0	0	0	0	0	120	4	2	2	1 vegetable
Cream Style Corn	1/2 cup	110	1	10	0	0	0	320	24	2	2	1 1/2 starch
Creamed Spinach	1/2 cup	70	2.5	25	1.5	0	0	510	9	1	3	1 vegetable, 1 fat
Cut Green Beans	1/2 cup	20	0	0	0	0	0	400	4	1	1	1 vegetable

Cut Green Beans, 50% Less Sodium	1/2 cup	20	0	0	0	0	0	200	4	1	1	1 vegetable
Green Bean Casserole	2/3 cup	110	8	70	3	1	0	450	9	4	5	1 vegetable, 2 fat
Niblets Corn & Butter Sauce	2/3 cup	90	2	20	1	0	<5	320	15	3	3	1 starch
Sugar Snap Peas, No Sauce	1/2 cup	45	0	0	0	0	0	95	10	2	2	1/2 starch
Sweet Niblets Corn, No Added Salt	1/2 cup	90	1	10	0	0	0	0	18	1	2	1 starch
Sweet Peas	1/2 cup	60	0	0	0	0	0	400	12	3	4	1 starch
Sweet Peas, 50% Less Sodium	1/2 cup	60	0	0	0	0	0	200	11	3	4	1 starch
Teriyaki Vegetables	1 1/4 cup	40	4	40	0	0	0	400	9	2	2	2 vegetable
Libby's												
Bavarian Style Sauerkraut	2 Tbsp	10	0	0	0	0	0	200	3	<1	0	free

VEGETABLES, VEGETABLE JUICES

	Serving	Calories	Fat (g)	Cal. from Fat	Sat. Fat (g)	Trans Fat (g)	Chol. (mg)	Sod. (mg)	Carb. (g)	Fiber (g)	Prot. (g)	Servings/Exchanges
Pumpkin, Solid Pack, Canned	1/2 cup	40	0.5	5	0	0	0	5	9	5	2	2 vegetable
Ore-Ida												
Country Style Fries	3 oz	130	4.5	40	1	0	0	300	20	2	2	1 starch, 1 fat
Country Style Hash Browns	1 1/4 cup	70	0	0	0	0	0	20	16	1	2	1 starch
Crispers	3 oz	220	13	120	3	0	0	390	23	2	2	1 1/2 starch, 3 fat
Crispy Crowns	11 pieces	170	10	90	2.5	0	0	490	21	2	2	1 1/2 starch, 2 fat
Extra Crispy Easy Fries	3 oz	180	8	70	1.5	0	0	400	25	2	2	1 1/2 starch, 2 fat
Extra Crispy Fast Food Fries	3 oz	160	6	60	1	0	0	440	23	2	2	1 1/2 starch, 1 fat
Extra Crispy Golden Crinkles	3 oz	170	7	60	1.5	0	0	410	24	2	2	1 1/2 starch, 1 fat
Extra Crispy Seasoned Crinkles	3 oz	150	6	60	1	0	0	450	22	2	2	1 1/2 starch, 1 fat

Golden Crinkles	3 oz	120	3.5	35	2	0	0	310	20	2	2	1 starch, 1 fat
Golden Fries	3 oz	130	3.5	20	2	0	0	310	21	2	2	1 1/2 starch, 1 fat
Potatoes O'Brien	3/4 cup	60	0	0	0	0	0	40	13	2	1	1 starch
Shoestrings	3 oz	140	5	45	2.5	0	0	320	22	2	2	1 1/2 starch, 1 fat
Southern Style Hash Browns	2/3 cup	70	0	0	0	0	0	30	16	2	2	1 starch
Steak Fries	3 oz	110	3	25	1.5	0	0	300	19	2	2	1 starch, 1 fat
Steam n' Mash Cut Red Potatoes	3/4 cup	70	0	0	0	0	0	270	15	1	2	1 starch
Steam n' Mash Cut Russet Potatoes	3/4 cup	80	0	0	0	0	0	260	17	2	2	1 starch
Steam n' Mash Cut Sweet Potatoes	1 cup	90	0	0	0	0	0	30	20	3	1	1 starch
Tater Tots	9 pieces	170	8	70	1.5	0	0	420	20	2	2	1 starch, 2 fat
Zesties	3 oz	150	5	45	1	0	0	320	22	2	2	1 1/2 starch, 1 fat

VEGETARIAN FOODS

	Serving	Calories	Fat (g)	Cal. from Fat	Sat. Fat (g)	Trans Fat (g)	Chol. (mg)	Sod. (mg)	Carb. (g)	Fiber (g)	Prot. (g)	Servings/Exchanges
Bacon Strips, Soy Based	3 strips	68	3	25	0	0	0	428	2	<1	9	1 lean meat
Breakfast Links, Soy Based	1 link	64	5	45	<1	0	0	222	3	<1	5	1 med-fat meat
Breakfast Patty, Meatless, Soy Based	1 patty	79	3	25	0.5	0	0	270	3	2	10	1 lean meat
Chicken Slices, Soy Based	2 slices	132	8	72	1	0	0	474	4	3	10	1 med-fat meat, 1 fat
Edamame	1/2 cup	95	4	35	0.5	0	0	5	8	4	8	1/2 carb, 1 med-fat meat
Falafel	3 patties	170	9	80	1	0	0	150	16	2	7	1 carb, 1 med-fat meat, 1 fat
Frankfurter/Hot Dog, Meatless, Soy Based	1	70	2	20	0	0	0	280	6	1	8	1/2 carb, 1 lean meat

Food	Serving											Exchanges/Choices
Luncheon Meat, Soy Based	1 slice	188	11	100	2	0	0	576	6	3	17	1/2 carb, 2 med-fat meat
Meat Patties, Soy Based	1 patty	117	5	45	0.5	0	0	468	10	4	12	1/2 carb, 2 lean meat
Meatless Beef Crumbles, Soy Based	2 oz	60	0.5	5	0	0	0	270	6	3	13	1/2 carb, 2 lean meat
Meatless Sausage Crumbles, Soy Based	2 oz	60	0	0	0	0	0	490	8	2	7	1/2 carb, 1 lean meat
Meatless Burger, Vegetable & Starch Based	1 patty	130	3	25	1	0	15	290	12	4	13	1 carb, 1 lean meat
Miso	1/2 cup	274	8	70	1.5	0	0	5126	36	7	16	2 1/2 carb, 1 med-fat meat, 1 fat
Miso Sauce	1/2 cup	191	3	25	<1	0	0	2008	36	3	7	2 1/2 carb, 1 fat
Nuggets, Breaded, Soy Based	2	90	3.5	30	0.5	0	0	250	9	2	7	1/2 carb, 1 lean meat
Tempeh (Bean Cake)	1/4 cup	84	3	25	0	0	0	3	7	0	8	1/2 carb, 1 lean meat
Tofu Yogurt	1 cup	246	5	45	<1	0	0	92	42	<1	9	3 carb, 1 fat

VEGETARIAN FOODS

	Serving	Calories	Fat (g)	Cal. from Fat	Sat. Fat (g)	Trans Fat (g)	Chol. (mg)	Sod. (mg)	Carb. (g)	Fiber (g)	Prot. (g)	Servings/Exchanges
Tofu, Firm, Raw	1/2 cup	80	5	45	1	0	0	14	2	1	9	1 med-fat meat
Tofu, Lite, Firm, Silken	1/2 cup	45	2	20	0	0	0	82	2	0	8	1 lean meat
Brands												
Health Valley Organic												
No Salt Added Spicy Vegetarian Chili	1 cup	150	1	10	0	0	0	75	31	10	9	2 starch, 1 lean meat
Vegetarian Black Bean Chili	1 cup	150	1	10	0	0	0	480	32	8	10	2 starch, 1 lean meat
Vegetarian Chili with Three Beans	1 cup	150	1	10	0	0	0	480	32	10	10	2 starch, 1 lean meat
Lightlife												
Gimme Lean Beef	2 oz	70	0	0	0	0	0	350	10	2	7	1/2 carb, 1 lean meat
Gimme Lean Sausage	2 oz	60	0	0	0	0	0	310	7	3	7	1/2 carb, 1 lean meat
Honey BBQ Wings	4 wings	120	3	25	0	0	0	430	16	4	13	1 carb, 1 lean meat

Food	Serving	Cal	Fat (g)	Fat (%)	Sat Fat	Trans	Chol	Sodium	Carb	Fiber	Protein	Exchanges
Light Burgers, Original	1/3 cup	120	1.5	15	0	0	0	500	12	3	16	1 carb, 2 lean meat
Light Burgers, Veggie	1	140	4	35	0.5	0	0	370	16	4	10	1 carb, 1 med-fat meat
Organic Soy Tempeh	4 oz	230	8	70	1	0	0	10	16	12	22	1 carb, 3 lean meat
Smart Bacon	2 slices	20	1	10	0	0	0	140	0	0	2	free
Smart BBQ	1/4 cup	70	0	0	0	0	0	380	13	1	6	1 carb, 1 lean meat
Smart Chili	1 cup	260	0.5	5	0	0	0	820	44	12	19	3 carb, 1 lean meat
Smart Deli Bologna	4 slices	70	0	0	0	0	0	490	4	1	14	2 lean meat
Smart Deli Turkey	4 slices	100	3.5	30	0.5	0	0	300	5	2	13	2 lean meat
Smart Dogs	1	45	0	0	0	0	0	310	2	<1	8	1 lean meat
Smart Dogs Jumbo	1	80	1	5	0	0	0	560	3	2	15	2 lean meat
Smart Ground Original	1/3 cup	70	0	0	0	0	0	310	6	3	12	1/2 carb, 2 lean meat
Smart Links, Breakfast	2 links	100	3.5	30	0.5	0	0	580	8	4	10	1/2 carb, 1 lean meat
Smart Sausage, Chorizo Style	1 link	140	8	70	1	0	0	590	5	<1	12	2 lean meat
Smart Sausage, Italian Style	1	140	7	70	1	0	0	500	7	1	13	1/2 carb, 2 lean meat

VEGETARIAN FOODS

	Serving	Calories	Fat (g)	Cal. from Fat	Sat. Fat (g)	Trans Fat (g)	Chol. (mg)	Sod. (mg)	Carb. (g)	Fiber (g)	Prot. (g)	Servings/Exchanges
Smart Sausage, Smoked Style	1 patty	150	7	70	1	0	0	580	9	2	13	1/2 carb, 2 lean meat
Smart Strips, Chick'n	3 oz	80	0	0	0	0	0	520	6	4	14	1/2 carb, 2 lean meat
Tempehtations, Ginger Teriyaki	3 oz	160	5	45	1	0	0	560	18	5	11	1 carb, 1 med-fat meat
Tofu Pups	1	60	2.5	20	0.5	0	0	300	2	1	8	1 lean meat
Morningstar Farms												
Asian Veggie Patties	1 patty	100	4	35	0.5	0	0	490	10	2	7	1/2 carb, 1 lean meat
Breakfast Pattie, Organic Soy	1	80	3	25	0.5	0	0	240	4	1	8	1 lean meat
Buffalo Wing Veggie Wings	5	200	8	70	1	0	0	640	20	3	12	1 carb, 1 med-fat meat, 1 fat
Chik Patties Original	1	140	5	45	0.5	0	0	590	16	2	8	1 carb, 1 med-fat meat
Chik'n Nuggets	4	190	9	80	1.5	0	0	600	19	4	12	1 carb, 1 med-fat meat, 1 fat

Food	Serving											Exchanges
Classic Veggie Burgers, Organic Soy	1	150	6	50	0.5	0	0	280	10	3	14	1/2 carb, 2 lean meat
Garden Veggie Patties Veggie Burgers	1	110	3.5	30	0.5	0	0	350	9	3	10	1/2 carb, 1 lean meat
Grillers Chik'n Veggie Patties	1	80	3	30	0	0	0	350	7	5	9	1/2 carb, 1 lean meat
Grillers Original	1 burger	130	6	50	1	0	0	260	5	2	15	2 lean meat
Grillers Prime Veggie Burgers	1	170	9	80	1	0	0	360	4	2	17	2 lean meat
Hickory BBQ Riblets	1	220	3.5	30	0	0	0	810	35	5	18	2 carb, 2 lean meat
Italian Herb Chik Patties	1	170	5	45	0.5	0	0	480	22	2	10	1 1/2 carb, 1 med-fat meat
Maple Flavored Veggie Sausage Patties	1 patty	80	3	25	0.5	0	0	250	5	<1	10	1 lean meat
Meal Starters Chik'n Strips	12	140	3.5	30	0.5	0	0	510	6	1	23	1/2 carb, 3 lean meat

VEGETARIAN FOODS

	Serving	Calories	Fat (g)	Cal. from Fat	Sat. Fat (g)	Trans Fat (g)	Chol. (mg)	Sod. (mg)	Carb. (g)	Fiber (g)	Prot. (g)	Servings/Exchanges
Meal Starters Grillers Recipe Crumbles	2/3 cup	80	2.5	20	0	0	0	230	5	3	10	1 lean meat
Meal Starters Sausage Style Recipe Crumbles	2/3 cup	90	2.5	25	0	0	0	420	5	3	11	2 lean meat
Original Chik'n Tenders	2	190	7	60	1	0	0	580	20	3	12	1 carb, 1 med-fat meat
Spicy Black Bean Burger	1	210	7	65	1	1	0	700	24	7	17	1 1/2 carb, 2 lean meat
Veggie Bacon Strips	2 strips	60	4.5	40	0.5	0	0	230	2	1	2	1 fat
Veggie Bites, Broccoli Cheddar Snacks	3 pieces	180	10	90	2.5	0	5	550	15	2	8	1 carb, 1 med-fat meat, 1 fat
Veggie Bites, Spinach Artichoke Snacks	3 pieces	190	10	90	2.5	0	0	570	16	2	9	1 carb, 1 med-fat meat, 1 fat
Veggie Cakes, Ginger Teriyaki	1 patty	110	1.5	15	0.5	0	0	320	19	2	5	1 carb, 1 lean meat

Veggie Cakes, Southwestern Style	1 patty	130	3	30	1	0	5	340	21	2	6	1 1/2 carb, 1 lean meat
Veggie Italian Style Sausage	1 link	120	6	50	0.5	0	0	350	7	1	10	1/2 carb, 1 med-fat meat
Veggie Sausage Links	2 links	80	3	25	0.5	0	0	300	3	2	9	1 lean meat
Worthington/Loma Linda												
Chic-ketts	1 slice	110	5	45	1	0	0	390	3	2	14	2 lean meat
Dinner Roast	1 slice	180	11	100	1.5	0	0	580	6	3	14	1/2 carb, 2 med-fat meat
Fried Chik'n with Gravy	2 pieces	130	6	50	1	0	0	430	9	3	9	1/2 carb, 1 med-fat meat
FriPats	1 patty	130	6	50	1	0	0	320	5	3	15	2 lean meat
Leanies Links	1 link	100	7	60	1	0	0	430	2	1	8	1 med-fat meat
Meatless Chicken Roll	1 slice	90	4.5	40	0.5	0	0	240	2	1	9	1 med-fat meat
Prosage Link	2 links	80	3	30	0.5	0	0	320	3	2	9	1 lean meat
Stakelets	1 piece	150	7	70	1	0	0	480	7	2	14	1/2 carb, 2 lean meat

VEGETARIAN FOODS

	Serving	Calories	Fat (g)	Cal. from Fat	Sat. Fat (g)	Trans Fat (g)	Chol. (mg)	Sod. (mg)	Carb. (g)	Fiber (g)	Prot. (g)	Servings/Exchanges
Stripples	2 strips	60	4.5	40	0.5	0	0	220	2	1	2	1 fat
Yves Veggie Cuisine												
Chicken Skewers	1	100	1	10	0	0	0	450	7	4	15	1/2 carb, 2 lean meat
Classic Mac 'n' Soy Cheese	1 bowl	340	9	80	1.5	0	0	880	52	3	13	3 1/2 carb, 1 med-fat meat, 1 fat
Good Dog	1	70	3.5	30	0	0	0	430	1	0	8	1 lean meat
Hot Dog	1	50	0.5	5	0	0	0	400	2	0	10	1 lean meat
Meatless Breakfast Patties	2	80	2	15	0	0	0	350	4	2	11	2 lean meat
Meatless Canadian Bacon	3 slices	80	0.5	5	0	0	0	400	2	0	17	2 lean meat
Meatless Chicken Burger	1	100	3	25	0	0	0	420	5	2	15	2 lean meat
Meatless Chili	1 bowl	240	1	10	0	0	0	850	37	14	21	2 1/2 carb, 2 lean meat

Food	Serving										
Meatless Deli Bologna Slices	4 slices	80	2.5	20	0	0	480	2	0	14	2 lean meat
Meatless Deli Turkey Slices	4 slices	100	1.5	15	0	0	340	5	0	15	2 lean meat
Meatless Ground Round Original	1/3 cup	60	0.5	5	0	0	270	5	2	10	1 lean meat
Meatless Ground Turkey	1/3 cup	60	1	10	0	0	330	4	2	14	2 lean meat
Meatless Ham Slices	4 slices	100	2	20	0	0	480	5	0	15	2 lean meat
Meatless Lasagna	1 bowl	300	3	25	0.5	0	650	51	4	17	3 1/2 carb, 2 lean meat
Tofu Dogs	1	45	1	5	0	0	300	2	0	8	1 lean meat
Veggie Brat Classic	1	160	5	50	0	0	840	1	1	19	3 lean meat

Index